ESSENTIAL OILS
POCKET REFERENCE

SPECIAL THIRD EDITION
Printed by Life Science Publishing

All rights reserved. No part of this book may be reproduced or transmitted in any form or by any means, electronic or mechanical, including photocopying, recording, or by any information storage and retrieval system, without permission in writing from the publisher.

Third Edition
First Printing March 2004

Copyright ©2004 Life Science Publishing
1-800-336-6308
www.DiscoverLSP.com

ISBN 1-7337015-1-8

Printed in the United States of America

Disclaimer: The information contained in this book is for educational purposes only. It is not provided to diagnose, prescribe, or treat any condition of the body.
The information in this book should not be used as a substitute for medical counseling with a health professional. Neither the author nor publisher accepts responsibility for such use.

Acknowledgments

We wish to acknowledge D. Gary Young for his tremendous contribution to the rebirth of essential oils in North America. One of the pioneers in researching, cultivating, and distilling essential oils in North America, he has spent decades conducting clinical research on the ability of essential oils to combat disease and improve health. He has also developed new methods of application from which thousands of people have benefitted, especially his integration of therapeutic-grade essential oils with dietary supplements and personal care products. He is certainly one of the first, if not the first, to create these types of quality products.

Growing up as a farmer and rancher in Idaho, Gary developed a passion for the land, that has driven him to become one of the leading organic growers and distillers of essential oils in North America. With over 2,000 acres of land under cultivation in the US and Europe, he has set new standards for excellence that are redefining how therapeutic-grade essential oils are produced.

Gary's long experience as a grower, distiller, researcher, and alternative care practitioner not only gives him an unsurpassed insight into essential oils but also makes him an ideal spokespersona and educator on therapeutic properties of essential oils. Gary regularly travels throughout the world lecturing on the powerful potential of essential oils and how to produce therapeutic-grade essential oils that can consistently deliver results.

Much of the material contained in this book is derived from his research, lectures, and workshops, as well as the work of other practitioners and physicians who are at the forefront of understanding the clinical potential of essential oils to treat disease. To these researchers, the publisher is deeply indebted.

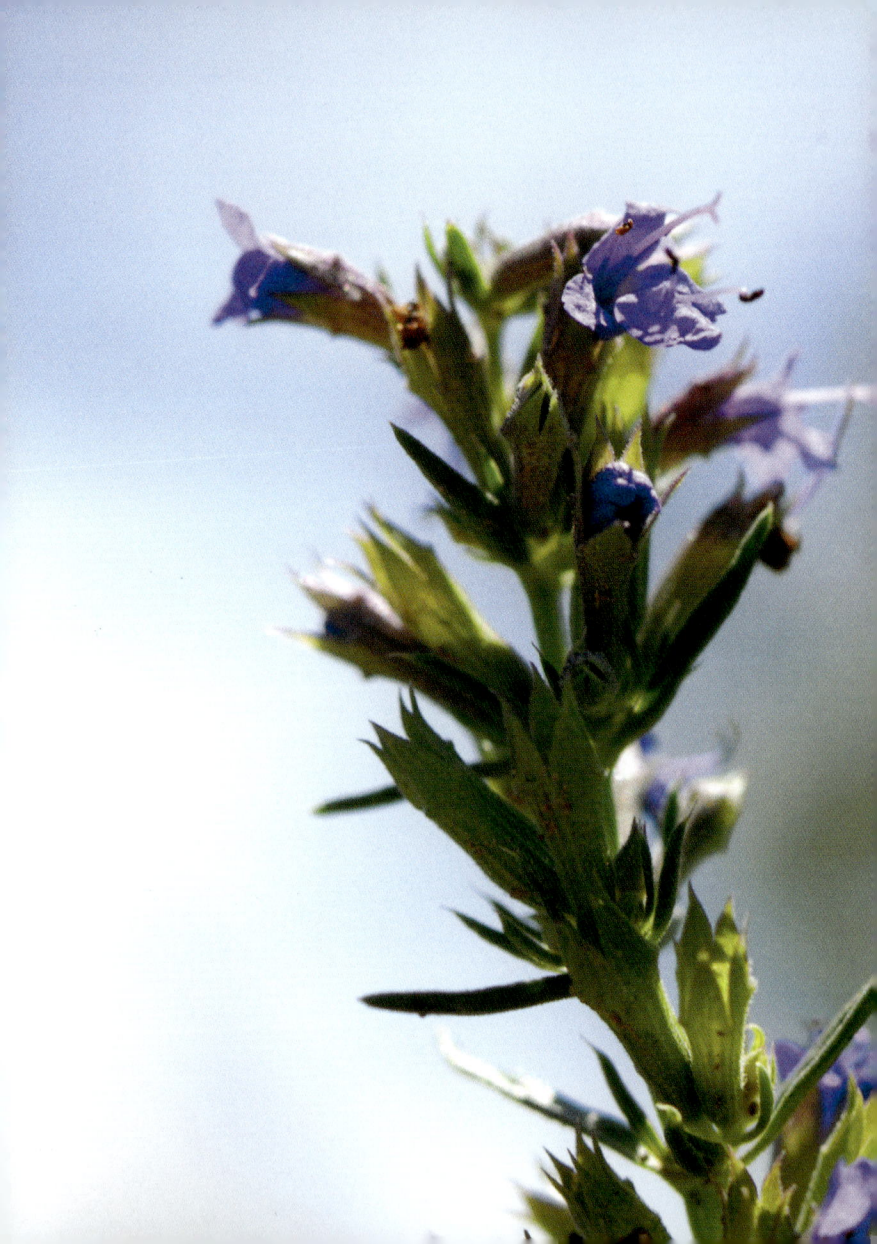

Contents

CHAPTER 1 – Essential Oils: The Missing Link in Modern Medicine
Yesterday's Wisdom, Tomorrow's Destiny 1
What Is an Essential Oil? 1
Different Schools of Application. 3
Mankind's First Medicine. 4
Early History of Essential Oil Extraction 5
Biblical and Ancient References to Essential Oils 6
Other Historical References 7
The Rediscovery 8

CHAPTER 2 – How Do Essential Oils Work?
Therapeutic-Grade Essential Oils 9
Science and Application 10
Using European AFNOR/ISO Standards to Identify Therapeutic-Grade Oils 11
Adulterated Oils and Their Dangers 13
Fact or Fiction: Myths and Misinformation 15
The Powerful Influence of Aromas on Both Mind and Body 15
Chemical Sensitivities and Allergies 17

CHAPTER 3 – How to Safely Use Essential Oils
Guidelines for Safe Use 19
Before You Start 20
Topical Application 21
Diffusing 24
Other Uses. 25

CHAPTER 4 – Vita Flex Technique 31

CHAPTER 5 – Raindrop Technique 35

CHAPTER 6 – Lymphatic Pump 55

CHAPTER 7 – Auricular Technique 57

CHAPTER 8 – Emotional Response with Essential Oils 61

CHAPTER 9 – The Personal Usage Reference 65

Appendix A – Essential Oil Application Codes 229

Appendix B – Body System Chart 233

Appendix C – Single Oil Data 245

Appendix D – Oil Blends Data 257

Index 265

Essential Oils: The Missing Link in Modern Medicine 1

Yesterday's Wisdom Tomorrow's Destiny

Plants not only play a vital role in the ecological balance of our planet, but they have also been intimately linked to the physical, emotional, and spiritual well-being of people since the beginning of time.

The plant kingdom continues to be the subject of an enormous amount of research and discovery. At least 30 percent of prescription drugs in the United States are based on naturally occurring compounds from plants. Each year, millions of dollars are allocated to universities searching for new therapeutic agents that lie undiscovered in the bark, roots, flowers, seeds, and foliage of jungle canopies, river bottoms, forests, hillsides, and vast wilderness regions throughout the world.

As the most powerful part of the plant, essential oils and plant extracts have been woven into history since time immemorial. Essential oils have been used medicinally to kill bacteria, fungi, and viruses. They provide exquisite fragrances to balance mood, lift spirits, dispel negative emotions, and create a romantic atmosphere. They can stimulate the regeneration of tissue or stimulate nerves. They can even carry nutrients to, and oxygenate the cells.

What Is an Essential Oil?

Essential oils are aromatic volatile liquids distilled from shrubs, flowers, trees, roots, bushes, and seeds.

The chemistry of essential oils is very complex: each one may consist of hundreds of different and unique chemical compounds. Moreover, essential oils are highly concentrated and far more potent than dried herbs. The distillation process is what makes essential oils so concentrated. It often requires an entire plant or more to produce a single drop of distilled essential oil.

Essential oils are also different from vegetable oils such as corn oil, peanut oil, and olive oil. They are not greasy and do not clog the pores like many vegetable oils can.

Vegetable oils can become oxidized and rancid over time and are not antibacterial. Most essential oils, on the other hand, cannot go rancid and are powerful antimicrobials. Pressed oils and essential oils high in plant waxes such as patchouli, if not distilled properly, could go rancid after time, particularly if exposed to heat for extended periods of time.

Essential oils are substances that definitely deserve the respect of proper education. Users need to be fully versed in the chemistry and safety of the oils. However, this knowledge is not being taught at universities in the United States. There is a disturbing lack of institutional information, knowledge, and training on essential oils and the scientific approach to aromatherapy. Only in the Middle East, the Orient, and Europe, with their far longer history of using natural products and botanical extracts, can one obtain adequate instruction on the chemistry and therapy of essential oils.

The European communities have a tight framework of controls and standards concerning botanical extracts and who may administer them. Only practitioners with proper training and certification can practice aromatherapy. However, in the United States, the regulatory agencies have not recognized these disciplines or mandated the type and degree of training required to distribute and apply essential oils. This means that in the U.S. individuals can bill themselves as "aromatherapists" after a brief class in essential oils, and apply oils to people—even though they may not have the experience or training to properly understand and administer them. This may not only undermine and damage the credibility of the entire discipline of aromatherapy, but it can be dangerous to patients.

Essential oils are not simple substances. They are mosaics of hundreds—or even thousands—of different chemicals. Any given essential oil may contain anywhere from 80 to 300 or more different chemical constituents. An essential oil like lavender is very complex with many of its constituents occurring in minute quantities—but all contributing to the oil's therapeutic effects to some degree. To understand these constituents and their functions requires years of study.

Even though an essential oil may be labeled as "basil" and have the botanical name Ocimum basilicum, it can have widely different therapeutic actions, depending on its chemistry. For example, basil high in linalool or fenchol is primarily used for its antiseptic properties. However, basil high in methyl chavicol is more anti-inflammatory than antiseptic. A third type, basil high in eugenol, has both anti-inflammatory and antiseptic effects.

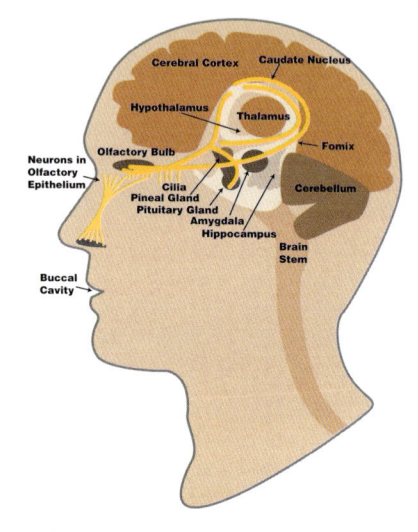

Limbic System: The procesing center of reason, motion, and smell

Additionally, essential oils can be distilled or extracted in different ways that have dramatic effects on their chemistry and medicinal action. Oils derived from a second or third distillation of the same plant material are obviously not going to be as potent as oils extracted during the first distillation. Also, oils that are subjected to high heat and pressure have a distinctly simpler (and inferior) profile of chemical constituents, since excessive heat and temperature fractures and breaks down many of the delicate aromatic compounds within the oil—some of which are responsible for its therapeutic action. In addition, oils that are steam distilled are far different from those that are solvent extracted.

Of greatest concern is the fact that some oils are adulterated, engineered, or "extended" with the use of synthetic chemicals. For example, pure frankincense is often extended with colorless, odorless solvents such as diethylphthalate or dipropylene glycol. The only way to distinguish the "authentic" from the "adulterated" is to subject the essential oil to rigorous analytical testing using state-of-the-art gas chromatography, mass spectroscopy, and NMR (nuclear magnetic resonance).

However, even gas chromatography doesn't identify a natural chemical from a synthetic one. That is why it is very easy to engineer oils or extend poor quality oils to make them smell and look good.

Unfortunately, a large percentage of essential oils marketed in the United States fall in this adulterated category. When you understand the world of synthetic oils as well as low-grade oils cut with synthetic chemicals, you realize why unsuspecting people with their untrained noses don't know the difference.

Different Schools of Application

Therapeutic treatment using essential oils follows three different models or frameworks: French, German, and English.

The English model advocates diluting a small amount of essential oil in a vegetable oil and massaging the body for the purpose of relaxation and relieving stress.

The French model prescribes the ingestion and neat (undiluted) topical application of therapeutic-grade essential oils. A common form of internal use is to add a few drops of an essential oil to agave nectar or honey, a piece of bread, or a small amount of vegetable oil. Many French practitioners have found that taking the oils internally yields excellent benefits.

The German model focuses on inhalation of essential oils. Research has shown that the effect of fragrance and aromatic compounds on the sense of smell can exert strong effects on the brain—especially on the hypothalamus (the hormone command center of the body) and limbic system (the seat of emotions). Some essential oils high in sesquiterpenes, such as myrrh, sandalwood, cedarwood, vetiver, melissa, and frankincense, can dramatically increase oxygenation and activity in the brain. This may directly improve the function of many systems of the body.

Together, these three models show how versatile and powerful essential oils can be. By integrating all three models with Vita Flex, auricular technique, touch therapy, spinal touch, lymphatic massage, and Raindrop Technique, the best possible results may be obtained.

In some cases, inhalation of essential oils might be preferred over topical application, if the goal is to increase growth hormone secretion, induce weight loss, or balance mood and emotions. Sandalwood, peppermint, vetiver, lavender, and white fir oils are effective for inhalation.

In other cases, however, topical application of essential oils would produce better results, particularly in the case of spinal or muscle injuries or defects. Topically applied, marjoram is excellent for muscles, lemongrass for ligaments, and wintergreen or birch for bones. For indigestion, a drop or two of peppermint oil taken orally may be very effective. However, this does not mean that peppermint cannot produce the same results when massaged on the stomach. In some cases, all three methods of application (topical, inhalation, and ingestion) are interchangeable and may produce similar benefits.

The ability of essential oils to act on both the mind and the body is what makes them truly unique among natural therapeutic agents. The fragrance of some essential oils can be very stimulating—both psychologically and physically. The fragrance of other essential oils may be calming and sedating, helping to overcome anxiety or hyperactivity. On a physiological level, essential oils may stimulate immune function and regenerate damaged tissue. Essential oils may also combat infectious disease by killing viruses, bacteria, and other pathogens.

Probably the two most common methods of essential oil application are cold-air diffusing and neat (undiluted) topical application. Other modes of application include incorporating essential oils into the disciplines of reflexology, Vita Flex, and acupressure. Combining these disciplines with essential oils enhances the healing response and often produces amazing results that can not be achieved by acupuncture or reflexology alone. Just 1–3 drops of an essential oil applied to an acupuncture meridian or Vita Flex point on the hand or foot can produce results within a minute or two.

Several years ago at a university in Europe, a professor well known in the field of aromatherapy commented that anyone who claims to cure diseases using essential oils is a quack. However, there are many people who are living proof that essential oils can be used to engineer recoveries from serious illness. Essential oils have been pivotal in helping many people live pain-free after years of intense pain. Patients have also witnessed firsthand how essential oils have corrected scoliosis and even restored hearing in those who were born deaf.

For example, a woman from Palisades Park, California, developed scoliosis after surviving polio as a teenager, which was further complicated by a serious fall and a dislocated shoulder. Suffering pain and immobility for 22 years, she had traveled extensively in a fruitless search to locate a practitioner who could permanently reset her shoulder. Upon learning about essential oils, she topically applied the oils of helichrysum and birch, among others, to the shoulder. Within a short time she became pain free as the shoulder relocated. She was able to raise her arm over her head for the first time in 22 years.

When one sees such dramatic recoveries, it is difficult to discredit the value and the power of essential oils and the potential they hold.

Mankind's First Medicine

For many centuries essential oils and other aromatics were used for religious rituals, the treatment of illness, and other physical and spiritual needs.

Records dating back to 4500 BC describe the use of balsamic substances with aromatic properties for religious rituals and medical applications. Ancient writings tell of scented barks, resins, spices, and aromatic vinegars, wines, and beers that were used in rituals, temples, astrology, embalming, and medicine. The evidence suggests that the people of ancient times had a greater understanding of essential oils than we have today.

The Egyptians were masters in using essential oils and other aromatics in the embalming process. Historical records describe how one of the founders of "pharaonic" medicine was the architect Imhotep, who was the Grand Vizier of King Djoser (2780 - 2720 BC). Imhotep is often given credit for ushering in the use of oils, herbs, and aromatic plants for medicinal purposes.

Many hieroglyphics on the walls of Egyptian temples depict the blending of oils and describe hundreds of oil recipes.

An ancient papyrus found in the Temple of Edfu contained medicinal formulae and perfume recipes used by alchemists and high priests in blending aromatic substances for rituals.

The Egyptians may have been the first to discover the potential of fragrance. They created various aromatic blends for both personal use and for ceremonies performed in the temples and pyramids.

Well before the time of Christ, the ancient Egyptians collected essential oils and placed them in alabaster vessels. These vessels were specially carved and shaped for housing scented oils. In 1922, when King Tut's tomb was opened, some 50 alabaster jars designed to hold 350 liters of oils were discovered. Tomb robbers had stolen nearly all of the precious oils leaving the heavy jars behind. Some of them still contained oil traces. The robbers chose oils over a literal king's ransom in gold, showing how valuable the fragrant essential oils were to this ancient civilization.

In 1817 the Ebers Papyrus, a medical scroll over 870 feet long, was discovered. Dating back to 1500 BC, the scroll included over 800 different herbal prescriptions and remedies. Other scrolls described a high success rate in treating 81 different diseases. Many of the remedies contained myrrh and honey. Myrrh is still recognized for its ability to help with infections of the skin and throat and to regenerate skin tissue. Because of its effectiveness in preventing bacterial growth, myrrh was used for embalming.

The physicians of Ionia, Attia, and Crete (ancient civilizations based in the Mediterranean Sea) came to the cities of the Nile to increase their knowledge. At this time, the school of Cos was founded and was attended by Hippocrates (460-377 BC), whom the Greeks, with perhaps some exaggeration, named the "Father of Medicine."

The Romans purified their temples and political buildings by diffusing essential oils. They also used aromatics in their steam baths to both invigorate the flesh and ward off disease.

Early History of Essential Oil Extraction

Ancient cultures found that aromatic essences or oils could be extracted from the plant by a variety of methods. One of the oldest and crudest forms of extraction was known as enfleurage. Raw plant material (usually stems, foliage, bark, or roots) was crushed and mixed with olive oil or animal fat. Other vegetable oils were also used. In the case of cedar, for example, the bark was stripped from the trunk and branches, ground into a powder, soaked with olive oil, and placed in a wool cloth. The cloth was then heated. The heat pulled the essential oil out of the bark particles into the olive oil, and the wool was pressed to extract the essential oil. Sandalwood oil was also extracted in this fashion.

Enfleurage was also used to extract essential oils from flower petals. In fact, the French word enfleurage means literally "to saturate with the perfume of flowers." For example, petals from roses or jasmine were placed in goose or goat fat. The essential oil molecules were pulled from the petals into the fat, which was then processed to separate the essential oils from the fat. This ancient technique was among the most primitive forms of essential oil extraction.

Other extraction techniques were also used. Some of these included:
- Soaking plant parts in boiling water
- Cold-pressing
- Soaking in alcohol
- Steam distillation by passing steam through the plant material and condensing the steam to separate the oil from the plant.

Many ancient cosmetic formulas were created from a base of goat fat. Ancient Egyptians formulated eyeliners, eyeshadows, and other cosmetics this way. They also stained their hair and nails with a variety of ointments and perfumes.

They probably used the same aromatic oils that were used in the temples. Such temple oils were commonly poured into evaporation dishes for fragrancing the chambers associated with sacred rituals and religious rites.

Fragrance "cones" made of wax and fragrant essential oils were worn by aristocratic Egyptian women who enjoyed the oils' rich scents as the cones melted with the heat of the day.

Ancient Arabians were another early culture that developed and refined a process of distillation. They perfected the extraction of rose oils and rose water, which were popular in the Middle East during the Byzantine Empire (330 AD - 1400 AD).

Biblical and Ancient References to Essential Oils

There are over 200 references to aromatics, incense, and ointments throughout the Old and New Testaments of the Bible. Aromatics such as frankincense, myrrh, galbanum, cinnamon, cassia, rosemary, hyssop, and spikenard were used for anointing and healing the sick. In Exodus, the Lord gave the following recipe to Moses for a holy anointing oil:

Myrrh	"five hundred shekels" (about 1 gallon)
Cinnamon	"two hundred and fifty shekels"
Calamus	"two hundred and fifty shekels"
Cassia	"five hundred shekels"
Olive Oil	"an hin" (about 1 1/3 gallons)

Psalms 133:2 speaks of the sweetness of brethren dwelling together in unity: "It is like the precious ointment upon the head, that ran down the beard, even Aaron's beard: that went down to the skirts of his garments." Another scripture that refers to anointing and the overflowing abundance of precious oils is Ecclesiastes 9:8: "Let thy garments be always white; and let thy head lack no ointment."

The Bible also lists an incident where an incense offering by Aaron stopped a plague. Numbers 16:46-50 records that Moses instructed Aaron to take a censer, add burning coals and incense, and to "go quickly into the congregation to make an atonement for them: for there is a wrath gone out from the Lord; the plague is begun." The Bible records that Aaron stood between the dead and the living and the plague was stayed. It is significant that according to the biblical and Talmudic recipes for incense, three varieties of cinnamon were involved. Cinnamon is known to be highly antimicrobial, anti-infectious, and antibacterial. The incense ingredient listed as "stacte" is believed to be a sweet, myrrh-related spice, which would make it anti-infectious and antiviral as well.

The New Testament records that wise men presented the Christ child with frankincense and myrrh. There is another precious aromatic, spikenard, described in the anointing of Jesus:

> And being in Bethany in the house of Simon the leper, as he sat at meat, there came a woman having an alabaster box of ointment of spikenard very precious; and she brake the box, and poured it on his head. Mark 14:3.

The anointing of Jesus is also referred to in John 12:3:

> Then took Mary a pound of ointment of spikenard, very costly, and anointed the feet of Jesus, and wiped his feet with her hair: and the house was filled with the odour of the ointment.

Other Historical References

Throughout world history, fragrant oils and spices have played a prominent role in everyday life.

Napoleon is reported to have enjoyed a cologne water made of neroli and other ingredients so much that he ordered 162 bottles of it. After conquering Jerusalem, one of the things the Crusaders brought back to Europe was solidified essence of roses.

The 12th century mystic, Hildegard of Bingen, used herbs and oils extensively in healing. This Benedictine nun founded her own convent and was the author of numerous works. Her book, Physica, has more than 200 chapters on plants and their uses for healing.

The Rediscovery

The reintroduction of essential oils into modern medicine first began during the late 19th and early 20th centuries.

During World War I, the use of aromatic essences in civilian and military hospitals became widespread. One physician in France, Dr. Moncière, used essential oils extensively for their antibacterial and wound-healing properties, and developed several kinds of aromatic ointments.

René-Maurice Gattefossé, PhD, a French cosmetic chemist, is widely regarded as the father of aromatherapy. He and a group of scientists began studying essential oils in 1907.

In his 1937 book, Aromatherapy, Dr. Gattefossé told the real story of his now-famous use of lavender essential oil to heal a serious burn. The tale has assumed mythic proportions in essential oil literature. His own words about this accident are even more powerful than what has been told over the years.

Dr. Gattefossé was literally aflame—covered in burning substances—following a laboratory explosion in July, 1910. After he extinguished the flames by rolling on a grassy lawn, he wrote that "both my hands were covered with rapidly developing gas gangrene." He further reported that, "just one rinse with lavender essence stopped the gasification of the tissue. This treatment was followed by profuse sweating and healing which began the next day."

Robert B. Tisserand, editor of The International Journal of Aromatherapy, searched for Dr. Gattefossé's book for 20 years. A copy was located and Tisserand edited the 1995 reprint. Tisserand noted that Dr. Gattefossé's burns "must have been severe to lead to gas gangrene, a very serious infection."

Dr. Gattefossé shared his studies with his colleague and friend, Jean Valnet, a medical doctor practicing in Paris. Exhausting his supply of antibiotics as a physician in Tonkin, China, during World War II, Dr. Valnet began using therapeutic-grade essential oils on patients suffering battlefield injuries. To his surprise, they exerted a powerful effect in combating and counteracting infection. He was able to save the lives of many soldiers who might otherwise have died.

Two of Dr. Valnet's students, Dr. Paul Belaiche and Dr. Jean-Claude Lapraz, expanded his work. They clinically investigated the antiviral, antibacterial, antifungal, and antiseptic properties in essential oils.

Because of the work of these doctors and scientists, the healing power of essential oils is again gaining prominence.

Today, it has become evident that we have not yet found permanent solutions for dreaded diseases such as the Ebola virus, hanta virus, AIDS, HIV, and new strains of tuberculosis and influenza. Essential oils may assume an increasingly important role in combating new mutations of bacteria, viruses, and fungi. More and more researchers are undertaking serious clinical studies on the use of essential oils to combat these types of diseases.

Research conducted at Weber State University in cooperation with D. Gary Young as well as other documented research, indicates that most viruses, fungi, and bacteria cannot live in the presence of many essential oils, especially those high in phenols, carvacrol, thymol, and terpenes. This, perhaps, offers a modern explanation why the Old Testament prophet Moses used aromatic substances to protect the Israelites from the plagues that decimated ancient Egypt. It may also help us understand why a notorious group of thieves, reputed to be spice traders and perfumers, was protected from the Black Plague as they robbed the bodies of the dead during the 15th century.

A vast body of anecdotal evidence (testimonials) suggests that those who use essential oils are less likely to contract infectious diseases. Moreover, oil users who do contract an infectious illness tend to recover faster than those using antibiotics.

How Do Essential Oils Work

Therapeutic-Grade Essential Oils

One of the factors that determines the purity of an oil is its chemical constituents. These constituents can be affected by a vast number of variables, including: the part(s) of the plant from which the oil was produced, soil condition, fertilizer (organic or chemical), geographical region, climate, altitude, harvesting methods, and distillation processes. For example, common thyme (Thymus vulgaris) produces several different chemotypes (biochemically unique variants within one species) depending on the conditions of its growth, climate, and altitude. One chemotype of thyme will yield an essential oil with high levels of thymol, depending on the time of year it is distilled. The later it is distilled in the growing season (ie., mid-summer or fall), the more thymol the oil will contain.

Proper cultivation assures that more specific chemotypes like Thymus vulgaris will maintain a good strain of thymol, where as with wildcrafting, you may produce linalol and eugenol thyme on the same mountainside.

An example of this was shown in studies at the University of Ege botany department in Izmir, Turkey where it was found that among Oreganum compactum plants within a 100 square foot radius, one plant would be very high in carvacrol and another would be high in another compound. Wildcrafting plants cannot guarantee the same chemotype even on the same hillside.

The key to producing a therapeutic-grade essential oil is to preserve as many of the delicate aromatic compounds within the essential oil as possible. Fragile aromatic chemicals are easily destroyed by high temperature and pressure, as well as contact with chemically reactive metals such as copper or aluminum. This is why all therapeutic-grade essential oils should be distilled in stainless steel cooking chambers at low pressure and low temperature.

The plant material should also be free of herbicides and other agrichemicals. These can react with the essential oil during distillation to produce toxic compounds. Because many pesticides are oil-soluble, they can also mix into the essential oil.

As we begin to understand the power of essential oils in the realm of personal, holistic healthcare, we will appreciate the necessity for obtaining the purest essential oils possible. No matter how costly pure essential oils may be, there can be no substitutes.

Although chemists have successfully recreated the main constituents and fragrances of some essential oils in the laboratory, these synthetic oils lack therapeutic benefits and may even carry risks. Why? Because essential oils contain hundreds of different chemical compounds, which, in combination, lend important therapeutic properties to the oil. Also, many essential oils contain molecules and isomers that are impossible to manufacture in the laboratory.

Anyone venturing into the world of therapy using essential oils must use the purest quality oils available. Inferior quality or adulterated oils most likely will not produce therapeutic results and could possibly be toxic. In Europe, a set of standards has been established that outlines the chemical profile and principal constituents that a quality essential oil should have. Known as AF-NOR (Association French Normalization Organization Regulation) and ISO (International Standards Organization) standards, these guidelines help buyers differentiate between a therapeutic-grade essential oil and a lower grade oil with a similar chemical makeup and fragrance. **All of the therapeutic effects of the essential oils in this book are based on oils that have been graded according to AFNOR standards.**

Science and Application

Essential oils and human blood share several common properties: They fight infection, contain hormone-like compounds, and initiate regeneration. Working as the chemical defense mechanism of the plant, essential oils possess potent antibacterial, antifungal, and antiviral properties. They also ward off attacks by insects and animals. The ability of some essential oils to work as hormones helps them bring balance to many physiological systems of the human body. Oils like clary sage and sage that contain sclerol, for example, have an estrogenic action. Essential oils also play a role in initiating the regeneration process for the plant, the same way the blood does in the human body.

This similarity goes even deeper. Essential oils have a chemical structure that is similar to that found in human cells and tissues. This makes essential oils compatible with human protein and enables them to be readily identified and accepted by the body.

Essential oils have a unique ability to penetrate cell membranes and diffuse throughout the blood and tissues. The unique, lipid-soluble structure of essential oils is very similar to the makeup of our cell membranes. The molecules of essential oils are also relatively small, which enhances their ability to penetrate into the cells. When topically applied to the feet or elsewhere, essential oils can travel throughout the body in a matter of minutes.

The ability of some essential oils, like clove, to decrease the viscosity or thickness of the blood can also enhance circulation and immune function. Adequate circulation is vital to good health, since it affects the function of every cell and organ, including the brain.

Research indicates that when essential oils are diffused, they can increase atmospheric oxygen and provide negative ions, which in turn inhibits bacterial growth. This suggests that essential oils could play an important role in air purification and neutralizing odors. Because of their ionizing action, essential oils have the ability to break down potentially harmful chemicals and render them nontoxic.

In the human body, essential oils stimulate the secretion of antibodies, neurotransmitters, endorphins, hormones, and enzymes. Oils containing limonene have been shown to prevent and slow the progression of cancer. Other oils, like lavender, have been shown to promote the growth of hair and increase the rate of wound healing. They increase the uptake of oxygen and ATP (adenosine triphosphate), the fuel for individual cells.

European scientists have studied the ability of essential oils to work as natural chelators, binding with heavy metals and petrochemicals and ferrying them out of the body.

Today approximately 300 essential oils are distilled or extracted, with several thousand chemical constituents and aromatic molecules identified and registered. The quantity, quality, and type of these aromatic compounds will vary depending on climate, temperature, and distillation factors. Ninety-eight percent of essential oils produced today are used in the perfume and cosmetic industry. Only about 2 percent are produced for therapeutic and medicinal applications.

Because essential oils are composites of hundreds of different chemicals, they can exert many different effects on the body. For example, clove oil can be simultaneously antiseptic and anaesthetic when applied topically. It can also be antitumoral. Lavender oil has been used for burns, insect bites, headaches, PMS, insomnia, stress, and hair growth.

Importantly, because of their complexity, essential oils do not disturb the body's natural balance or homeostasis: if one constituent exerts too strong an effect, another constituent may block or counteract it. Synthetic chemicals, in contrast, usually have only one action and often disrupt the body's homeostasis.

Using European AFNOR/ISO Standards to Identify Therapeutic-Grade Oils

As previously mentioned, one of the most reliable indicators of essential oil quality is the AFNOR (Association French Normalization Organization Regulation) or ISO certification (ISO is the International Standards Organization which has set standards for therapeutic-grade essential oils adopted from AFNOR). This standard is more stringent and differentiates true therapeutic-grade essential oils from similar oils with inferior chemistry.

The AFNOR standard was written by a team headed up by the government-certified botanical chemist Hervé Casabianca, PhD, while working with several analytical laboratories throughout France.

Dr. Casabianca recognized that the primary constituents within an essential oil had to occur in certain percentages in order for the oil to be considered therapeutic. He combined his studies with research conducted by other scientists and doctors, including the Central Service Analysis Laboratory certified by the French government for essential oil analysis.

As a result, many oils that are listed as therapeutic-grade such as frankincense or lavender, can be checked to see if they do indeed meet AFNOR standards. If some constituents are too high or too low, the oils cannot be certified.

For example, the AFNOR standard for Lavandula angustifolia (true lavender) dictates that the level of linalool should range from 25 to 38 percent and the level of linalyl acetate should range between 25 and 34 percent. As long as the oil's marker compounds are within the specified ranges, it can be recognized as a therapeutic-grade essential oil.

As a general rule, if two or more marker compounds in an essential oil fall outside the prescribed percentages, the oil does not meet the AFNOR standard. It cannot be recognized as therapeutic-grade essential oil, even though it is still of relatively high quality.

What distinguishes a therapeutic-grade essential oil from an essential oil that is not therapeutic-grade or AFNOR-certified? A lavender oil produced in one region of France might have a slightly different chemistry than that grown in another region and as a result may not meet the standard. It may have excessive camphor levels (1.0 instead of 0.5), a condition that might be caused by distilling lavender that was too green. Or the levels of lavandulol may be too low due to certain weather conditions at the time of harvest.

By comparing the gas chromatograph chemistry profile of a lavender essential oil with the AFNOR standard, you may also distinguish true lavender from various species of lavandin (hybrid lavender). Usually lavandin has high camphor levels, almost no lavandulol, and is easily identified. However, Tasmania produces a lavandin that yields an essential oil with naturally low camphor levels that mimics the chemistry of true lavender. Only by analyzing the chemical fingerprint of this Tasmanian lavandin using high resolution gas chromatography and comparing it with the AFNOR standard for genuine lavender can this hybrid lavender be identified.

Currently, there is no agency responsible for certifying that an essential oil is therapeutic grade. The only indication for a therapeutic-grade oil is if it meets AFNOR or ISO standards. **The therapeutic effects discussed in this book can only be achieved using essential oils which meet the AFNOR standards.**

In the United States, few companies use the proper analytical equipment and methods to properly analyze essential oils. Most labs use equipment best-suited for synthetic chemicals—not for natural essential oil analysis. Young Living Essential Oils uses the proper machinery and has made serious efforts to adopt the European testing standards, widely regarded as the "gold standard" for testing essential oils. In addition to operating its analytical equipment on the same standard as the European-certified laboratories, Young Living is continually expanding its analytical chemical library in order to perform more thorough chemical analysis.

Properly analyzing an essential oil by gas chromatography is a complex undertaking. The injection mixture, column diameter and length, and oven temperature must fall within certain parameters. Unless someone has gone to France and Turkey as Gary Young has and been trained in the analytical procedures of a gas chromatograph, they will not understand how to accurately test essential oils.

The column length should be at least 50 or 60 meters. However, almost all labs in the United States use a 30-meter column that is not long enough to achieve proper separation of all the essential oil constituents. While 30-meter columns are adequate for analyzing synthetic chemicals and marker compounds in vitamins, minerals, and herbal extracts, they are far too short to properly analyze the complex mosaic of natural chemicals found in an essential oil.

A longer column also enables double-phased ramping, which makes it possible to identify constituents that occur in very small percentages by increasing the separation of compounds. Without a longer column, it would be extremely difficult to identify these molecules, especially if they are chemically similar to each other or a marker compound.

While gas chromatography (GC) is an excellent tool for dissecting the anatomy of an essential oil, it does have limitations. Dr. Brian Lawrence, one of the foremost experts on essential oil chemistry, has commented that sometimes it can be difficult to distinguish between natural and synthetic compounds using GC analysis. If synthetic linalyl acetate is added to pure lavender, a GC analysis cannot really tell whether that compound is synthetic or natural, only that it is linalyl acetate. Adding a chiral column can help, however, in distinguishing between synthetic and natural oils. This addition allows the chemist to identify structural varieties of the same compound.

This is why oils must be analyzed by a chemist specially trained on the interpretation of a gas chromatograph chart. The chemist examines the entire chemical fingerprint of the oil to determine its purity and potency, measuring how various compounds in the oil occur in relation to each other. If some chemicals occur in higher quantities than others, these provide important clues to determine if the oil is adulterated or pure.

Adulteration is such a major concern that every batch of essential oil that comes into Young Living must be tested at either Central Service Laboratory or the Albert Vieille Laboratory, both AFNOR-certified laboratories, by chemists licensed to test therapeutic-grade essential oils. Batches that do not meet the standards are rejected and returned.

Adulteration of essential oils will become more and more common as the supply of top-quality essential oils dwindles and demand continues to increase. These adulterated essential oils will jeopardize the integrity of aromatherapy in the United States and may put many people at risk.

Adulterated Oils and Their Dangers

Today much of the lavender oil sold in America is the hybrid called lavandin, grown and distilled in China, Russia, France, and Tasmania. It is brought into France and cut with synthetic linalyl acetate to improve the fragrance. Then propylene glycol, DEP, or DOP (solvents that have no smell and increase the volume) are added and it is sold in the United States as lavender oil.

Often lavandin is heated to evaporate the camphor and then is adulterated with synthetic linalyl acetate. Most consumers don't know the difference, and are happy to buy it for $7 to $10 per half ounce in health food stores, beauty salons, grocery and department stores, and through mail order. This is one of the reasons why it is important to know about the integrity of the company or vendor from which you purchase your essential oils.

Frankincense is another example of a commonly adulterated oil. The frankincense resin that is sold in Somalia costs between $30,000 and $35,000 per ton. A great deal of time--12 hours or more--is required to properly steam-distill this essential oil from the resin, making the oil very expensive. Frankincense oil that sells for $25 per ounce or less is cheaply distilled with gum resins, alcohol, or other solvents, leaving the essential oil laden with harmful chemicals. Sadly, when these cut, synthetic, and adulterated oils cause rashes, burns, or other irritations, people wonder why they do not get the benefit they expected and conclude that essential oils do not have much value.

Some commercial statistics show that one large, U.S. corporation uses twice as much of a particular essential oil as is naturally grown and produced in the entire world! Where are these "phantom" essential oils coming from?

In France, production of true lavender oil (Lavandula angustifolia) dropped from 87 tons in 1967 to only 12 tons in 1998. During this same period the worldwide demand for lavender oil grew over 100 percent. So where did essential oil marketers obtain enough lavender to meet the demand? They probably used a combination of synthetic and adulterated oils. There are huge chemical companies on the east coast of the U.S. that specialize in creating synthetic chemicals that mimic every common essential oil. For every kilogram of pure essential oil that is produced, it is estimated there are between 10 and 100 kilograms of synthetic oil created.

Adulterated and mislabeled essential oils present dangers for consumers. One woman who had heard of the ability of lavender oil to heal burns used "lavender oil" purchased from a local health food store when she spilled boiling water on her arm. But the pain intensified and the burn worsened, so she later complained that lavender oil was worthless for healing burns. When her "lavender" oil was analyzed, it was found to be lavandin, the hybrid lavender that is chemically very different from pure Lavandula angustifolia. Lavandin contains high levels of camphor (12-18 percent) and can itself burn the skin. In contrast, true lavender contains virtually no camphor and has burn-healing agents not found in lavandin.

Adulterated oils that are cut with synthetic extenders can be very detrimental, causing rashes, burning, and skin irritations. Petrochemical solvents, such dipropylene glycol and diethyl-phthalate, can all cause allergic reactions, besides being devoid of any therapeutic effects.

Some people assume that because an essential oil is "100 percent pure," it will not burn their skin. This is not true. Some pure essential oils may cause skin irritation if applied undiluted. If you apply straight oregano oil to the skin of some people, it may cause severe reddening. Citrus and spice oils, like orange and cinnamon, may also produce rashes. Even the terpenes in conifer oils, like pine, may cause skin irritation on sensitive people.

Some writers have claimed that a few compounds, when isolated from the essential oil and tested in the lab, can exert toxic effects. Even so-called "nature-identical" essential oils (structured essential oils that have been chemically duplicated using 5 to 15 of the essential oil's primary chemical compounds in synthetic form) can produce unwanted side effects or toxicities. Isolated compounds may be toxic; however pure essential oils, in most cases, are not. This is because natural essential oils contain hundreds of different compounds, some of which balance and counteract each other's effects.

Many tourists in Egypt are eager to buy local essential oils, especially lotus oil. Vendors convince the tourists that the oils are 100 percent pure, going so far as to touch a lighted match to the neck of the oil container to show that the oil is not diluted with alcohol or other petrochemical solvents. However, this test provides no reliable indicator of purity. Many synthetic compounds can be added to an essential oil that are not flammable, including propylene glycol. Or, flammable solvents can be added to a vegetable oil base that will cause it to catch fire. Some natural essential oils high in terpenes can be flammable.

Fact or Fiction: Myths and Misinformation

Much of the published information available on essential oils should be regarded with caution. Many aromatherapy books are merely compilations of two or three other books. The content is similar, only phrased and worded differently. Because the information has been copied from sources that have never been documented, the same misinformation repeatedly surfaces.

Many aromatherapy books claim that essential oils, such as clary sage, fennel, sage, and bergamot, can trigger an abortion. Several years ago, a rumor circulated about a laboratory research project in which the uterus of a rat was turned inside out and a cold drop of clary sage oil was applied to the exposed uterine wall. When this caused a contraction of the muscle, clary sage was labeled as abortion-causing. One must ask, what would have happened if cold water had been dropped on the exposed uterus? The uterine wall would likely have contracted in response. Following this reasoning, water could be labeled as abortion-causing as well.

The truth is that to our knowledge, there has never been a single documented case that clary sage, lemon, sage, or bergamot essential oils have caused an abortion. Sclareol, a compound in clary sage, is not an estrogen, although it can mimic estrogen if there is an estrogen deficiency. If there is not an estrogen deficiency, sclareol will not create more estrogen in the body. As a rule, essential oils bring balance to the human body.

The belief that pure essential oils will not leave a stain when poured on a tissue is also unfounded. Any essential oil high in waxes will leave stains. Oils like frankincense, cedarwood, clove, ylang ylang, blue cypress, or German chamomile may also leave a noticeable residue. However, an essential oil spiked with synthetic diluents or solvent may or may not leave a stain.

The Powerful Influence of Aromas on Both Mind and Body

The fragrance of an essential oil can directly affect everything from your emotional state to your lifespan.

When a fragrance is inhaled, the odor molecules travel up the nose where they are trapped by olfactory membranes that are well protected by the lining inside the nose. Each odor molecule fits like a little puzzle piece into specific receptor cell sites that line a membrane known as the olfactory epithelium. Each one of these hundreds of millions of nerve cells is replaced every 28 days. When stimulated by odor molecules, this lining of nerve cells triggers electrical impulses to the olfactory bulb in the brain. The olfactory bulb then transmits the impulses to the gustatory center (where the sensation of taste is perceived), the amygdala (where emotional memories are stored), and other parts of the limbic system of the brain. Because the limbic system is directly connected to those parts of the brain that control heart rate, blood pressure, breathing, memory, stress levels, and hormone balance, essential oils can have profound physiological and psychological effects.

The sense of smell is the only one of the five senses directly linked to the limbic lobe of the brain, the emotional control center. Anxiety, depression, fear, anger, and joy all emanate from this region. The scent of a special fragrance can evoke memories and emotions before we are even consciously aware of it. When smells are concerned, we react first and think later. All other senses (touch, taste, hearing, and sight) are routed through the thalamus, which acts as the switchboard for the brain, passing stimuli onto the cerebral cortex (the conscious thought center) and other parts of the brain.

The limbic lobe (a group of brain structures that includes the hippocampus and amygdala located below the cerebral cortex) can also directly activate the hypothalamus. The hypothalamus is one of the most important parts of the brain, acting as our hormonal control center. It releases chemical messengers that can affect everything from sex drive to energy levels. The production of growth hormones, sex hormones, thyroid hormones, and neurotransmitters such as serotonin, are all governed by the hypothalamus. Thus, the hypothalamus is referred to as the "master gland."

Essential oils—through their fragrance and unique molecular structure—can directly stimulate the limbic lobe and the hypothalamus. Not only can the inhalation of essential oils be used to combat stress and emotional trauma, but it can also stimulate the production of hormones from the hypothalamus. This results in increased thyroid hormones (our energy hormone) and growth hormones (our youth and longevity hormone).

Essential oils may also be used to reduce appetite and produce significant reductions in weight because of their ability to stimulate the ventromedial nucleus of the hypothalamus, a section of the brain that governs our feeling of satiety or fullness following meals. In a large clinical study,[1] Alan Hirsch, MD, used fragrances, including peppermint, to trigger significant weight losses in a large group of patients who had previously been unsuccessful in any type of weight-management program. During the course of the six-month study involving over 3,000 people, the average weight loss exceeded

30 pounds. According to Dr. Hirsch, some patients actually had to be dropped from the study to avoid becoming underweight.

Another double-blind, randomized study by Hirsch[2] documents the ability of aroma to enhance libido and sexual arousal. When 31 male volunteers were subjected to the aromas of 30 different essential oils, each one exhibited a marked increase in arousal, based on measurements of brachial penile index and the measurement of both penile and brachial blood pressures. Among the scents that produced the most sexual excitement, was a combination of lavender and pumpkin fragrances. This study shows that fragrances enhance sexual desire by stimulating the amygdala, the emotional center of the brain.

In 1989, Dr. Joseph Ledoux at New York Medical University discovered that the amygdala plays a major role in storing and releasing emotional trauma.[3] From the studies of Dr. Hirsch and Dr. Ledoux the conclusion can be drawn that aromas may exert a profound effect in triggering a response from this almond-shaped neuro-structure.

In studies conducted at Vienna and Berlin Universities, researchers found that sesquiterpenes, found in essential oils such as vetiver, patchouli, cedarwood, sandalwood and frankincense, can increase levels of oxygen in the brain by up to 28 percent (Nasel, 1992). Such an increase in brain oxygen may lead to a heightened level of activity in the hypothalamus and limbic systems of the brain, which can have dramatic effects on not only emotions, learning, and attitude, but also many physical processes of the body, such as immune function, hormone balance, and energy levels. High levels of sesquiterpenes also occur in melissa, myrrh, cedarwood, and clove oil.

People who have undergone nose surgery or suffer olfactory impairment may find it difficult or impossible to detect a complete odor. The same is true of people who use makeup, perfume, cologne, hair sprays, hair coloring, perms, or other products containing synthetic odors. These people may not derive the full physiological and emotional benefits of essential oils and their fragrances.

Proper stimulation of the olfactory nerves may offer a powerful and entirely new form of therapy that could be used as an adjunct against many forms of illness. Essential oils, through inhalation, may occupy a key position in this relatively unexplored frontier in medicine.

Chemical Sensitivities and Allergies

Occasionally, individuals beginning to use quality essential oils will suffer rashes or allergic reactions. This may be due to using an undiluted spice, conifer, or citrus oil, or it may be caused by an interaction of the oil with residues of synthetic, petroleum-based personal care products that have leached into the skin.

When using essential oils on a daily basis, it is imperative to avoid personal care products containing ammonium or hydrocarbon-based chemicals. These include quaternary compounds such as quaternariums and polyquaternariums. These compounds are commonly found in a variety of hand creams, mouthwashes, shampoos, antiperspirants, after-shave lotions, and hair-care products. In small concentrations they can be toxic and present the possibility of reacting with essential oils and producing chemical by-products of unknown toxicity. These chemicals can be fatal if ingested, especially benzalkonium chloride, which unfortunately is used in many personal care products on the market.

Other compounds that present concerns are sodium lauryl sulfate, propylene glycol—extremely common in everything from toothpaste to shampoo—and aluminum salts found in many deodorants.

Of particular concern are the potentially hazardous preservatives and synthetic fragrances that abound in virtually all modern personal-care products. Some of these include methylene chloride, methyl isobutyl ketone, and methyl ethyl ketone. These are not only toxic, but they can also react with some compounds in natural essential oils. The result can be a severe case of dermatitis or even septicemia (blood poisoning).

A classic case of a synthetic fragrance causing widespread damage occurred in the 1970s. AETT (acetylethyltetramethyltetralin) appeared in numerous brands of personal care products throughout the United States. Even after a series of animal studies revealed that it caused significant brain and spinal cord damage, the FDA refused to ban the chemical. Finally, the cosmetic industry voluntarily withdrew AFTT after allowing it to be distributed for years. How many other toxins masquerading as preservatives or fragrances are currently being used in personal care products?

Many chemicals are easily absorbed through the skin due to its permeability. One study found that 13 percent of BHT (butylated hydroxytoluene) and 49 percent of DDT (a carcinogenic pesticide) can be absorbed into the skin upon topical contact (Steinman, 1997). Once absorbed, they can become trapped in the fatty subdermal layers of skin where they can leach into the blood stream. These chemicals can remain trapped in fatty tissues underneath the skin for several months or years, where they harbor the potential of reacting with essential oils that may be topically applied later. The user may mistakenly assume that the threat of an interaction between oils and synthetic cosmetics used months before is small. However, a case of dermatitis is a possibility.

Endnotes
1. Hirsch, AR, Inhalation of Odorants for Weight Reduction, Int J Obes, 1994, page 306
2. Alan R. Hirsch, MD, FACP, Dr. Hirsch's Guide to Scentsational Sex, Harper Collins, 1998 1993 Dec. 20;58(1-2):69-79
3. LeDoux, JE, Rationalizing Thoughtless Emotions, Insight, Sept. 1989

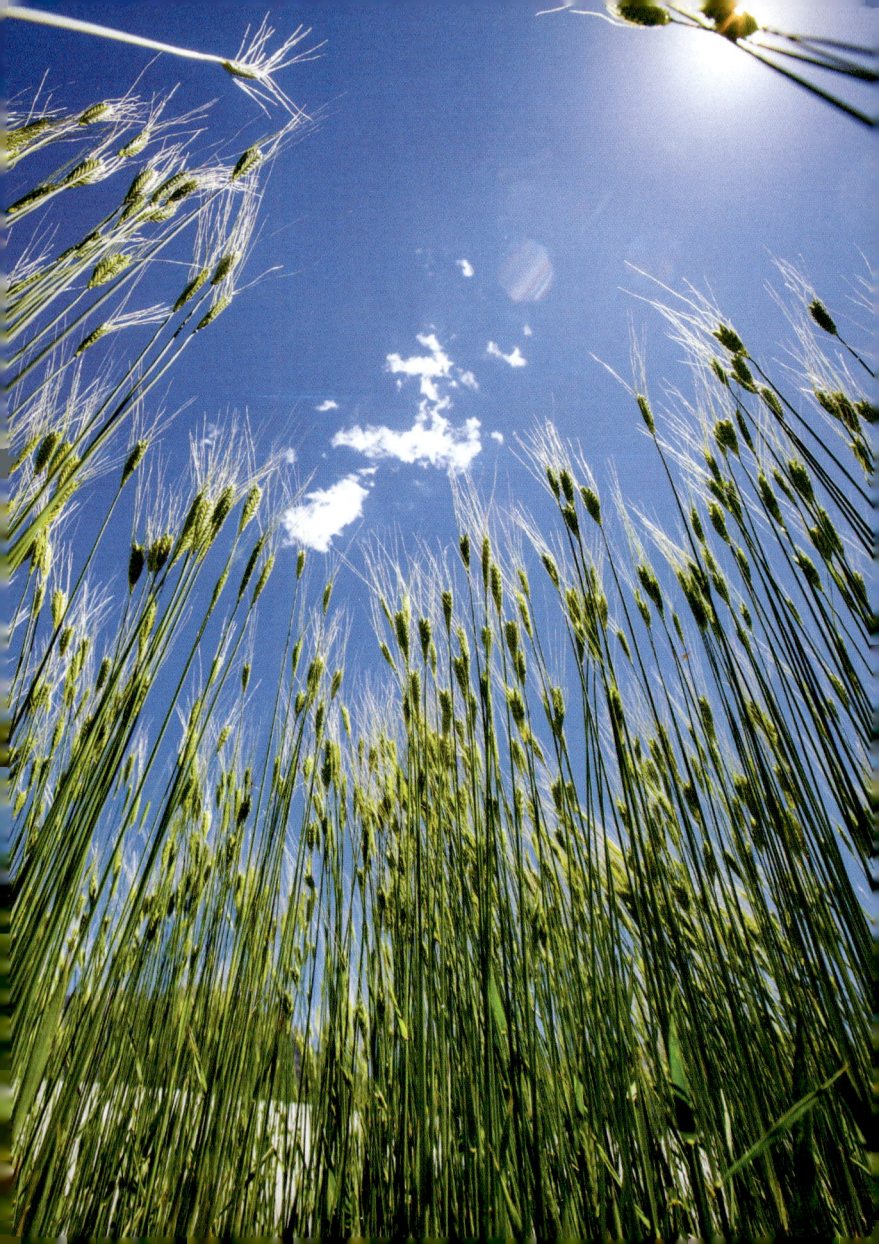

How To Safely Use Essential Oils 3

There are important guidelines to follow when using essential oils, especially if you are unfamiliar with the oils and their benefits. Many guidelines are listed below and are elaborated further throughout the chapter. However, no list of do's and don'ts can ever replace common sense. It is foolish to dive headlong into a pond when you don't know the depth of the water. The same is true when using essential oils. Start gradually, and patiently find what works best for you and your family members.

Basic Guidelines for Safe Use

1. Always keep a bottle of a pure vegetable oil handy when using essential oils. Vegetable oils dilute essential oils if they cause discomfort or skin irritation.

2. Keep bottles of essential oils tightly closed and store them in a cool location away from light. If stored properly, essential oils will maintain their potency for many years.

3. Keep essential oils out of reach of children. Treat them as you would any product for therapeutic use.

4. Essential oils rich in menthol (such as peppermint) should not be used on the throat or neck area of children under 30 months of age.

5. Angelica, bergamot, grapefruit, lemon, orange, tangerine, and other citrus oils are photosensitive and may cause a rash or dark pigmentation on skin exposed to direct sunlight or UV rays within 3-4 days after application.

6. Keep essential oils well away from the eye area and never put them directly into ears. Do not handle contact lenses or rub eyes with essential oils on your fingers. Even in minute amounts, oils with high phenol content, such as oregano, cinnamon, thyme, clove, lemongrass, and bergamot, may damage contacts and will irritate eyes.

7. Pregnant women should always consult a health care professional when starting any type of health program.

8. Epileptics and those with high blood pressure should consult their health care professional before using essential oils. Use caution with hyssop, fennel, basil, wintergreen/birch, nutmeg, rosemary, peppermint, sage, tarragon, and tansy oils.

9. People with high blood pressure should avoid using sage and rosemary.

10. People with allergies should test a small amount of oil on an area of sensitive skin, such as the inside of the upper arm, for 30 minutes, before applying the oil on other areas.

The bottom of the feet is one of the safest, most effective places to use essential oils.

11. Before taking GRAS essential oils internally, test your reactions by diluting one drop of essential oil in one teaspoon of an oil-soluble liquid like agave, olive oil, or rice milk. Never consume more than a few drops of diluted essential oil per day without the advice of a physician.

12. Do not add undiluted essential oils directly to bath water. Using Epsom salts or a bath gel base for all oils applied to your bath is an excellent way to disperse the oils into the bath water.

    When essential oils are put directly into bath water without a dispersing agent, they can cause serious discomfort on sensitive skin because the essential oils float, undiluted, on top of the water.

13. Keep essential oils away from open flames, sparks, or electricity. Some essential oils, including orange, fir, pine, and peppermint are potentially flammable.

Before You Start

Always skin test an essential oil before using it. Each person's body is different, so apply oils to a small area first. Apply one oil or blend at a time. When layering oils that are new to you, allow enough time (3-5 minutes) for the body to respond before applying a second oil.

Exercise caution when applying essential oils to skin that has been exposed to cosmetics, personal care products, soaps, and cleansers containing synthetic chemicals. Some of them—especially petroleum-based chemicals— can penetrate and remain in the skin and fatty tissues for days or even weeks after use. Essential oils may react with

> **CAUTION:** Essential oils will sting if applied in or around the eyes. Some oils may be painful on mucous membranes unless diluted properly. Immediate dilution is strongly recommended if skin becomes painfully irritated or if oil accidentally gets into eyes. Flushing the area with a vegetable oil should minimize discomfort almost immediately. DO NOT flush with water! Essential oils are oil-soluble, not water-soluble. Water will only spread the oils over a larger surface, possibly worsening the problem.

such chemicals and cause skin irritation, nausea, headaches, or other uncomfortable effects.

Essential oils can also react with toxins built up in the body from chemicals in food, water, and work environment. If you experience a reaction to essential oils, it may be wise to temporarily discontinue their use and start an internal cleansing program before resuming regular use of essential oils. In addition, double your water intake while using essential oils.

You may also want to try the following alternatives to a detoxification program to determine the cause of the problem:

- Dilute 1-3 drops of essential oil to 1/2 tsp. of massage oil, vegetable mixing oil, or any pure vegetable oil, such as almond or olive. More dilution may be needed, as necessary.

- Reduce the number of oils used at any time.

- Use single oils or oil blends, one at a time.

- Reduce the amount of oil used.

- Reduce the frequency of application.

- Drink more purified or distilled water.

- Ask your health care professional to monitor detoxification.

- Skin-test the diluted essential oil on a small patch of skin for 30 minutes. If any redness or irritation results, dilute the area immediately with a pure vegetable or massage oil. Then cleanse with soap and water.

- If skin irritation or other uncomfortable side effects persist, discontinue using the oil on that location and apply the oils on the bottoms of the feet.

You may also want to avoid using products that contain the following ingredients to eliminate potential problems:

- Cosmetics, deodorants, and skin care products containing aluminum, petrochemicals, or other synthetic ingredients.

- Perms, hair colors or dyes, and hair sprays or gels containing synthetic chemicals. Avoid shampoos, toothpaste, mouthwash, and soaps containing synthetic chemicals such as sodium laurel sulfate, propylene glycol, or lead acetate.

- Garden sprays, paints, detergents, and cleansers containing toxic chemicals and solvents.

You can use many essential oils anywhere on the body except on the eyes and in the ears. Other oils may irritate certain sensitive tissues. See recommended dilution rates in Appendix A

Keep all essential oils out of reach of children and only apply to children under skilled supervision. If a child or infant swallows an essential oil:

- Administer a mixture of milk, cream, yogurt, or another safe, oil-soluble liquid.

- Call a Poison Control Center or seek immediate emergency medical attention if necessary.

NOTE: If your body pH is low (meaning that your system is very acidic), you also could have a negative reaction to the oils.

Topical Application

Many oils are safe to apply directly to the skin. Lavender is safe to use on children without dilution. However, you must be sure what you are using is not lavandin labeled as lavender or genetically-altered lavender. When applying most other essential oils on children, dilute them with a carrier oil. For dilution, add 15–30 drops of essential oil to 1 oz. of a quality carrier oil as mentioned previously.

Carrier oils, such as a vegetable mixing oil, extend essential oils and provide more efficient use. When massaging, the vegetable oil helps lubricate the skin. Some excellent carrier oils include cold-pressed grapeseed, olive, wheat germ, and sweet almond oils, or a blend of any of these.

When starting an essential oil application, always apply the oil first to the bottom of the feet. This allows the body to become acclimated to the oil, minimizing the chance of a reaction. The Vita Flex foot charts (see Chapter 4) identify areas for best application. Start by applying 3–6 drops of a single or blended oil, spreading it over the bottom of each foot.

When applying essential oils to yourself, use 1–2 drops of oil on 2–3 locations twice a day. Increase to four times a day if needed. Apply the oil and allow it to absorb for 2–3 minutes before applying another oil or getting dressed (to avoid staining clothing).

As a general rule, when applying oils to yourself or another person for the first time, do not apply more than two single oils or blends at one time.

When mixing essential oil blends or diluting essential oils in a carrier oil, it is best to use containers made of glass or earthenware, rather than plastic. Plastic particles can leach into the oil and then into the skin once it is applied.

Before applying oils, wash hands thoroughly with soap and water.

Massage

Start by applying 2 drops of a single oil or blend on the skin and massaging it in. If you are working on a large area, such as the back, mix 1–3 drops of the selected essential oil into 1 tsp. of pure carrier oil (such as a vegetable mixing oil or a massage oil base).

Keep in mind that many massage oils such as olive, almond, or wheat germ oil may stain some fabrics.

Acupuncture

Licensed acupuncturists can dramatically increase the effectiveness of acupuncture by using essential oils. To start, place several drops of essential oil into the palm of your hand. Dip the acupuncture needle tip into the oil before inserting it. You can pre-mix several oils in your hand if you wish to use more than one oil.

Acupressure

When performing acupressure treatment, apply 1–3 drops of essential oil to the acupressure point with a finger. Using an auricular probe with a slender point to dispense oil can enhance the application. Start by pressing firmly and then releasing. Avoid applying pressure to any particular pressure point too long. You may continue along the acupressure points and meridians or use the reflexology or Vita Flex points as well. Once you have completed small point stimulation, massage the general area with the oil.

Warm Packs

For deeper penetration of an essential oil, use warm packs after applying oils. Dip a cloth in comfortably warm water. Wring the cloth out and place it on the location. Then cover the cloth loosely with a dry towel or blanket to seal in the heat. Allow the cloth to stand for 15–30 minutes. Remove the cloth immediately if there is any discomfort.

Cold Packs

Apply essential oils on the location, followed by cold water or ice packs when treating inflamed or swollen tissues. Frozen packages of peas or corn make excellent ice packs that will mold to the contours of the body part and will not leak. Keep the cold pack on until the swelling diminishes. For neurological problems, always use cold packs, never hot ones.

Layering

This technique consists of applying multiple oils one at a time. For example, place marjoram over a sore muscle, massage it into the tissue gently until the area is dry, and then apply a second oil, such as peppermint, until the oil is absorbed and the skin is dry. Then layer on the third oil, such as basil, and continue massaging.

Creating a Compress

- Rub 1–3 drops on the location, diluted or neat, depending on the oil used and the skin sensitivity at that location.

- Cover the location with a hot, damp towel.

- Cover the moist towel with a dry towel for 10–30 minutes, depending on individual need.

As the oil penetrates the skin, you may experience a warming or even a burning sensation, especially in areas where the greatest benefits occur. If burning becomes uncomfortable, apply a massage oil, vegetable mixing oil, or any pure vegetable oil such as olive or almond, to the location.

A second type of application is very mild and is suitable for children, or those with sensitive skin.

- Place 5–15 drops of essential oil into a basin filled with warm water.

- Water temperature should be approximately 100°F. (38°C.), unless the patient suffers neurological conditions; in this case, use cool water.

- Vigorously agitate the water and let it stand for 1 minute.

- Place a dry face cloth on top of the water to soak up oils that have floated to the surface.

- Wring out the water and apply the cloth on the location. To seal in the warmth, cover the location with a thick towel for 15–30 minutes.

Bath

Adding essential oils to bath water is challenging because oil does not mix with water. For even dispersion, mix 5–10 drops of essential oil in 1/4 cup of Epsom salts or bath gel base and then add this mixture under a running faucet. This method will help the oils disperse in the bath evenly and prevent stronger oils from stinging sensitive areas.

You can also use premixed bath gels and shampoos containing essential oils as a liquid soap in the shower or bath. Lather down with the bath gel, let it soak in, and then rinse. To maximize benefits, leave the soap or shampoo on the skin or scalp for several minutes to allow the essential oils to penetrate. You can create your own aromatic bath gels by placing 5–15 drops of essential oil in 1/2 oz. of an unscented bath gel base and then add to the bath water as described above.

Shower

Essential oils can be added to Epsom salts and used in the shower. There are special shower heads containing an attached receptacle that is filled with the essential oil/salts mixture. This allows essential oils to not only make contact with the skin, but also diffuses the fragrance of the oils into the air. The shower head receptacle can hold approximately 1/4 to 1/2 cup of bath salts.

Start by adding 5–10 drops of essential oil to 1/4 cup of bath salt. Fill the shower head receptacle with the oil/salt mixture. Make sure neither oils nor salts come in contact with the plastic seal on top of the receptacle. This should provide enough salt material for about 2–3 showers. Some shower heads have a bypass feature that allows the user to switch from aromatic salt water to regular tap water.

How to Enhance the Benefits of Topical Application

The longer essential oils stay in contact with the skin, the more likely they are to be absorbed. A high-quality lotion may be layered on top of the essential oils to reduce evaporation of the oils and enhance penetration. This may also help seal and protect cuts and wounds. Do not use ointments on burns until they are at least three days old.

Diffusing

Diffused oils alter the structure of molecules that create odors, rather than just masking them. They also increase oxygen availability, produce negative ions, and release natural ozone. Many essential oils such as lemongrass, orange, grapefruit, *Eucalyptus globulus*, tea tree, lavender, frankincense, and lemon, along with essential oil blends (Purification and Thieves), are extremely effective for eliminating and destroying airborne germs and bacteria.

A cold-air diffuser is designed to atomize a microfine mist of essential oils into the air, where they can remain suspended for several hours. Unlike aroma lamps or candles, a diffuser disperses essential oils without heating or burning, which can render the oil therapeutically less beneficial and even create toxic compounds. Burned oils may become carcinogenic. Research shows that cold air diffusing certain oils may:

- Reduce bacteria, fungus, mold, and unpleasant odors.
- Relax the body, relieve tension, and clear the mind.
- Help with weight management.
- Improve concentration, alertness, and mental clarity.
- Stimulate neurotransmitters.
- Stimulate secretion of endorphins.
- Stimulate growth hormone production and receptivity.
- Improve the secretion of IgA antibodies that fight candida.
- Improve digestive function.
- Improve hormonal balance.
- Relieve headaches.

Start by diffusing oils for 15–30 minutes a day. As you become accustomed to the oils and recognize their effects, you may increase the diffusing time to 1–2 hours per day.

Place the diffuser high in the room so that the oil mist falls through the air and removes the odor-causing substances.

By connecting your diffuser to a timer, you can gain better control over the length and duration of diffusing. For some respiratory conditions, you may diffuse the oils the entire night.

Do not use more than one blend at a time in a diffuser as this may alter the smell and the therapeutic benefit. However, a single oil may be added to a blend when diffusing.

Always wash the diffuser before using a different oil blend. Use natural soap and warm or hot water.

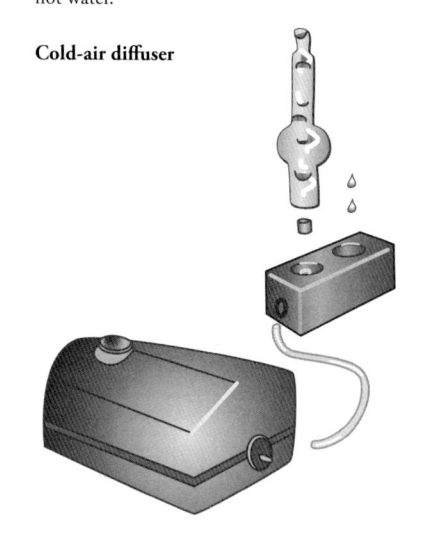

Cold-air diffuser

If you don't have a diffuser, you may add several drops of essential oil to a spray bottle, add 1 cup purified water, and shake. You can use this to mist your entire house, workplace, or car.

To freshen the air, use the following essential oil blend:
- 20 drops lavender
- 10 drops lemon
- 6 drops bergamot
- 5 drops lime
- 5 drops grapefruit

Diffuse neat, or mix with 1 cup of distilled water in a spray bottle; shake well before spraying.

Other Ways to Diffuse Oils
- Add essential oils to cedar chips to make your own potpourri.
- Put scented cedar chips in closets or drawers to deodorize them.
- Place any conifer essential oil such as spruce, fir (all varieties), cedar, or pine onto each log in the fireplace. As they burn, they will disperse an evergreen smell. This method has no therapeutic benefit, however.
- Put essential oil on cotton balls and place in your car or home air vents.
- Place a bowl of water with a few drops of oil on a wood stove.
- Dampen a cloth, apply essential oils to it, and place it near the intake duct of your heating and cooling system.

Humidifier and Vaporizer
Essential oils such as peppermint, lemon, Eucalyptus radiata, Melaleuca alternifolia, and frankincense make ideal additions to humidifiers or vaporizers.*

* NOTE: Test the oil in the vaporizer or humidifier first, some essential oils may damge the plastic parts of vaporizers.

Other Uses

Inhalation
Direct

- Place 2 or more drops into the palm of your left hand, and rub clockwise with the flat palm of your right hand. Cup your hands together over the nose and mouth and inhale deeply. (Do not touch your eyes!)

- Add several drops of an essential oil to a bowl of hot (not boiling) water. Inhale the steaming vapors that rise from the bowl. To increase the intensity of the oil vapors inhaled, drape a towel over your head and bowl before inhaling.

- Apply oils to a cotton ball, tissue, or handkerchief (do not use synthetic fibers or fabric) and place it in the air vent of your car.

- Inhale directly.

Indirect or Subtle Inhalation
(wearing as a perfume or cologne)

- Rub 2 or more drops of oil on your chest, neck, upper sternum, wrists, or under the nose and ears. Breathe in the fragrance throughout the day.

Vaginal Retention

For systemic health problems such as candida or vaginitis, vaginal retention is one of the best ways for the body to absorb essential oils.

- Mix 20–30 drops of essential oil in 2 tablespoons of carrier oil.
- Apply this mixture to a tampon (for internal infection) or sanitary pad (for external lesions). Insert and retain for 8 hours or overnight. Use tampons or sanitary pads made with organic cotton.

Rectal Retention

Retention enemas are the most efficient way to deliver essential oils to the urinary tract and reproductive organs. Always use a sterile syringe.

- Mix 15–20 drops of essential oil in a tablespoon of carrier oil.
- Place the mixture in a small syringe and inject into the rectum.
- Retain the mixture through the night (or longer for best results).
- Clean and disinfect the applicator after each use.

Water Distillers and Filters

You can apply oils like peppermint, lemon, clove, and cinnamon to the post-filter side of your water purifier. This will help purify the water.

Dishwashing Soap

To add fragrance or improve the antiseptic action of your liquid soap, add several drops of essential oils such as lavender, Melaleuca alternifolia, fir, spruce, pine, lemon, bergamot, and orange.

Cleaning and Disinfecting

A few drops of oil may be added to the dishwasher to help disinfect and purify. Some popular oils are pine, orange, tangerine, lemon, and peppermint, although any antibacterial oil would work well.

Painting

When painting, add 1 teaspoon of your favorite essential oil to one gallon of paint. Mix well. The oil will counteract the unpleasant smell of paint. Because essential oils are not fatty oils, they will not leave oil spots on the walls.

Laundry

Essential oils may be used to enhance the cleanliness and fragrance of your laundry. As unpleasant as it seems, dust mites live in your bedding, feeding from the dead skin cells you constantly shed. Recent research has shown that eucalyptus oil kills dust mites. To achieve effective dust mite control, add 25 drops of eucalyptus to each load, or approximately 1 tablespoon to a bottle of liquid laundry detergent.

You may also add several drops of essential oils to the rinse cycle, such as fir, spruce, juniper, lavender, cedarwood, wintergreen/birch, or rosewood.

Instead of using toxic and irritating softening agents in the dryer, place a washcloth dampened with 10 drops of lavender, lemon, melaleuca, bergamot, or other essential oils. While the oils will not reduce static cling, they will impart a distinctive fragrance to the clothes.

Surface Cleansers: Counters, Furniture, etc.

Instead of purchasing standard household cleaners for surfaces, you can create your own natural, safe version by filling a plastic spray bottle with water and a squirt of dishwashing soap.

Add 3 to 5 drops each of lavender, lemon, and pine essential oils. Shake the spray bottle well, and your homemade cleaner is ready to spray. This simple solution is extremely economical, yet it cleans and disinfects as well as any commercial cleaner.

Please keep in mind that some of the oils, if used directly, may stain some surfaces, such as linoleum.

Additional antibacterial and antiviral oils that are excellent for cleaning include cinnamon, clove, Eucalyptus globulus, thyme, juniper, Melaleuca alternifolia, spruce, lemongrass, and grapefruit.

Floors and Carpet

By combining essential oils with common household products, you can create your own nontoxic aromatic floor and carpet cleaners.

To clean non-carpeted floors, add 1/4 cup of white vinegar to a bucket of water. Then add 5–10 drops of lemon, pine, spruce, Melaleuca alternifolia, Antibacterial Blend, or another suitable oil. If the floor is especially dirty, add several drops of dishwashing soap. This will clean even the dirtiest floor.

To make a carpet freshener, add 16–20 drops of essential oils to a cup of baking soda or borax powder. Mix well and place in a covered container overnight so that the oil can be absorbed. Sprinkle over your carpet the next day and then vacuum the powder up.

You may also saturate a disposable cloth or tissue with several drops of essential oil and place it into the collecting bag of your vacuum. This will diffuse a pleasant odor as you clean. If your vacuum collects dirt into water, simply add a few drops into the water reservoir before cleaning. This refreshes both the carpet and the room.

Insecticide and Repellent: Dust Mites, Fleas, Ticks, Ants, Spiders, etc.

Many of us use synthetic chemicals to deal with insects. Single oils such as lavender, lemon, peppermint, lemongrass, cypress, Eucalyptus globulus, cinnamon, thyme, basil, citronella, and the Purification and Thieves blends, effectively repel many types of insects including mites, lice, and fleas. Peppermint placed on entryways prevents ants from entering.

If you need moth repellents for your linens and woolens, avoid toxic commercial mothballs made of naphthalene. Natural essential oils like citronella, lavender, lemongrass, Western red cedar, or rosemary can just as effectively repel moths and other insects. You can make a sachet by placing several drops of essential oil on a cotton ball. Wrap and tie this in a small handkerchief or square of cotton. Hang this cloth in storage areas or add it to your chest of linens. Refresh as often as necessary.

You can put this sachet in your bureau drawers to keep your clothes freshly scented. Lavender and rose are classic scents. For children's sleepwear, Roman chamomile is especially fragrant and relaxing. To scent stationery, stretch out an oil-scented cotton ball and place it in an envelope.

Hot Tubs and Saunas

Hot tubs, jacuzzis, and saunas act as reservoirs for germs, especially if used frequently. Lavender, cinnamon, clove, *Eucalyptus globulus*, thyme, lemon, or grapefruit can be used to disinfect and fragrance the water. Use 3 drops per person. For saunas, add several drops of rosemary, thyme, pine, or lavender to a spray bottle with water and then spray down the surfaces. Scented water can also be used to splash on hot sauna stones.

CAUTION: Some essential oils may damage plastic sauna/spa filters or hoses.

Deodorizing: Kitchens, Bathrooms, etc.

The kitchen and bathroom are often a source of odors and bacteria. Use the following mixtures to freshen, deodorize, and disinfect the air, work areas, cupboards, bathroom fixtures, sinks, tiles, woodwork, carpets, etc. These blends are safe for the family and the environment.

Since essential oils separate easily from water, always shake well and keep on shaking the bottle as you use these mixtures. They will deodorize and clean the air, instead of covering the odors.

Single oils:

Rosemary CT cineol with lemon, Eucalyptus globulus, and lavender

Blends:

Lavender with Purification

Recipe #1
Mix:
- 2 drops rosemary
- 4 drops lemon
- 3 drops *Eucalyptus globulus*
- 4 drops lavender with 1 quart water
- 1 cup water

Shake mixture well and use in a spray bottle.

Recipe #2
Mix:
- 3–4 drops lavender
- 5–6 drops Purification
- 1 cup water

Shake mixture well and use in a spray bottle.

Recipe #3
Mix:
- 7 drops pine with and equal amount of of chamomile, tea tree, lemongrass, or clove
- 1 cup water

Shake mixture well and use in a spray bottle

Cooking

Many essential oils make excellent food flavorings. They are so concentrated that only 1–2 drops of an essential oil is equivalent to a full bottle (1–2 oz. size) of dried herbs.

As a general rule, spice oils impart a far stronger flavor than citrus oils do. For strong spice oils (such as oregano, nutmeg, cinnamon, marjoram, tarragon, wintergreen, thyme, or basil), you can dip a toothpick into the oils and stir food (after cooking) with the toothpick. This controls the amount of essential oil that is put into the food.

Some oils that can be used as spices are: basil, cinnamon, clove, fennel, ginger, lemon, marjoram, nutmeg, oregano, peppermint, rosemary CT cineol, sage, spearmint, tarragon, coriander, grapefruit, mandarin, orange, wintergreen or birch, black pepper, and thyme.

For a recipe that serves 6–10 people, add 1–2 drops of an oil and stir in after cooking and just before serving, so the oil does not evaporate.

Internal and Oral Use as a Dietary Supplement

All essential oils that are Generally Regarded As Safe (GRAS) or certified as Food Additives (FA) by the FDA may be safely taken internally as dietary supplements. But ingesting essential oils should only be done under the direction of a knowledgeable health professional.

In fact, many oils are actually more effective when taken orally in very small amounts. Essential oils should always be diluted in vegetable oil, agave nectar or rice milk prior to ingestion. More or less dilution may be required, depending on how strong the oil is. More potent oils, such as cinnamon, oregano, lemongrass, and thyme, will require far more dilution than relatively mild oils, and very mild oils like lavender or lemon may not need any dilution at all.

As a general rule, dilute 1 drop of essential oil in 1 tsp. of agave nectar or in at least 4 ounces of a beverage.

Usually no more than 2 or 3 drops should be ingested at one time (during any 4–8 hour period). Because essential oils are so concentrated, 1–2 drops are often sufficient to achieve significant benefits.

<u>Essential oils should not be given as dietary supplements to children under six years of age. Parents should exercise caution before orally administering essential oils to any child, and again, oils should always be diluted prior to ingestion.</u>

Essential oils are extremely concentrated, so they should be kept out of reach of infants and children. If a large quantity of oil is ingested at one time (more than 5 drops), contact your health care physician and a Poison Control Center immediately.

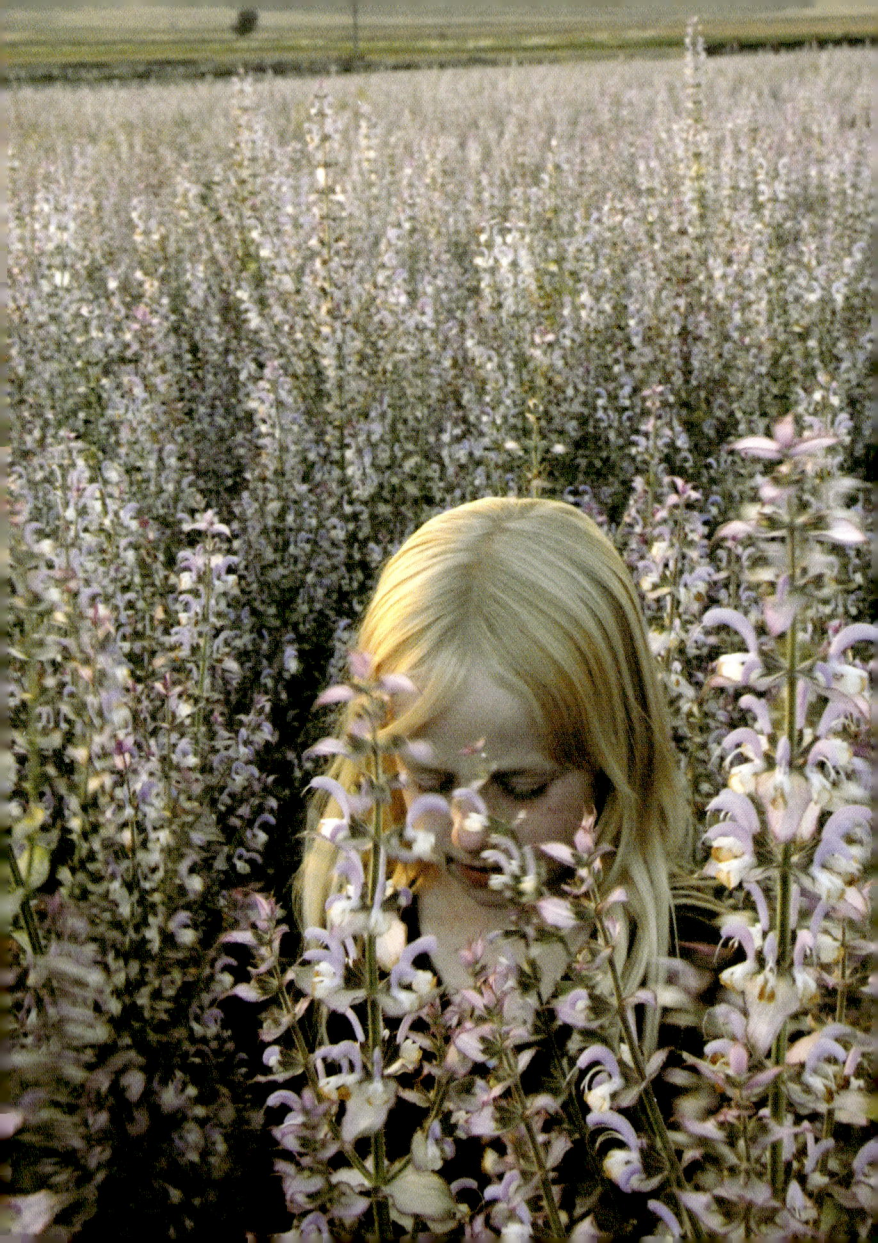

Vita Flex Technique 4

Vita Flex Technique means "vitality through the reflexes." It is a specialized form of hand and foot massage that is exceptionally effective in delivering the benefits of essential oils throughout the body. It is said to have originated in Tibet thousands of years ago, and was perfected in the 1960s by Stanley Burroughs long before acupuncture was popular in Western medicine.

It is based on a complete network of reflex points that stimulate all the internal body systems. Essential oils are applied to contact points, and energy is released through electrical impulses created by contact between the fingertips and reflex points. This electrical charge follows the nerve pathways to a break or clog in the electrical circuit usually caused by toxins, damaged tissues, or loss of oxygen. As with acupressure there are hundreds of Vita Flex reflex points throughout the human body, encompassing the entire realm of body and mind, that are capable of releasing many kinds of tension, congestion, and imbalances.

In contrast to the steady stimulation of Reflexology, Vita Flex uses a rolling and releasing motion that involves placing fingers flat on the skin, rolling onto the fingertips, and continuing over onto the fingernail using medium pressure. Then moving forward about half the width of the finger, this rolling and releasing technique is continually repeated until the Vita Flex point, or area, is covered. This movement is repeated over the area three times.

Combine this technique with 1-3 drops of essential oil applied to those areas of the feet that correspond to the system of the body you wish to support (see the diagrams on pages 32 and 33). Rapid and extraordinary results are experienced when combining essential oils with Vita Flex stimulation, as it increases the effect of both.

The diagram on page 34 shows the nervous system connection to the spine for the electrical points throughout the body.

Vita Flex Points - Right Foot

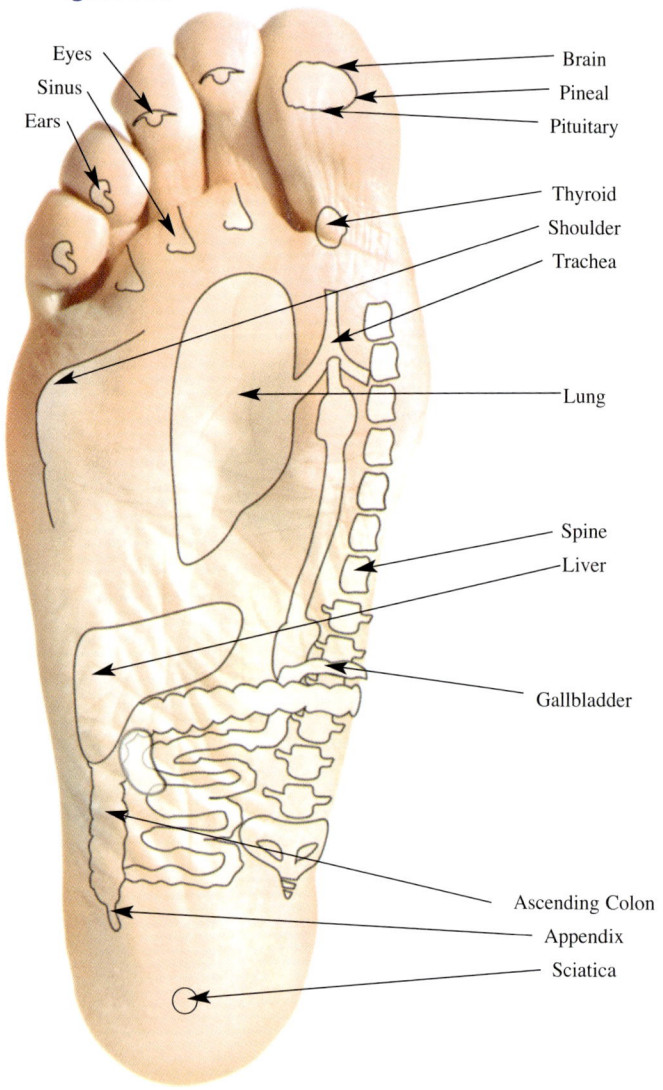

- Eyes
- Sinus
- Ears
- Brain
- Pineal
- Pituitary
- Thyroid
- Shoulder
- Trachea
- Lung
- Spine
- Liver
- Gallbladder
- Ascending Colon
- Appendix
- Sciatica

Vita Flex Points - Left Foot

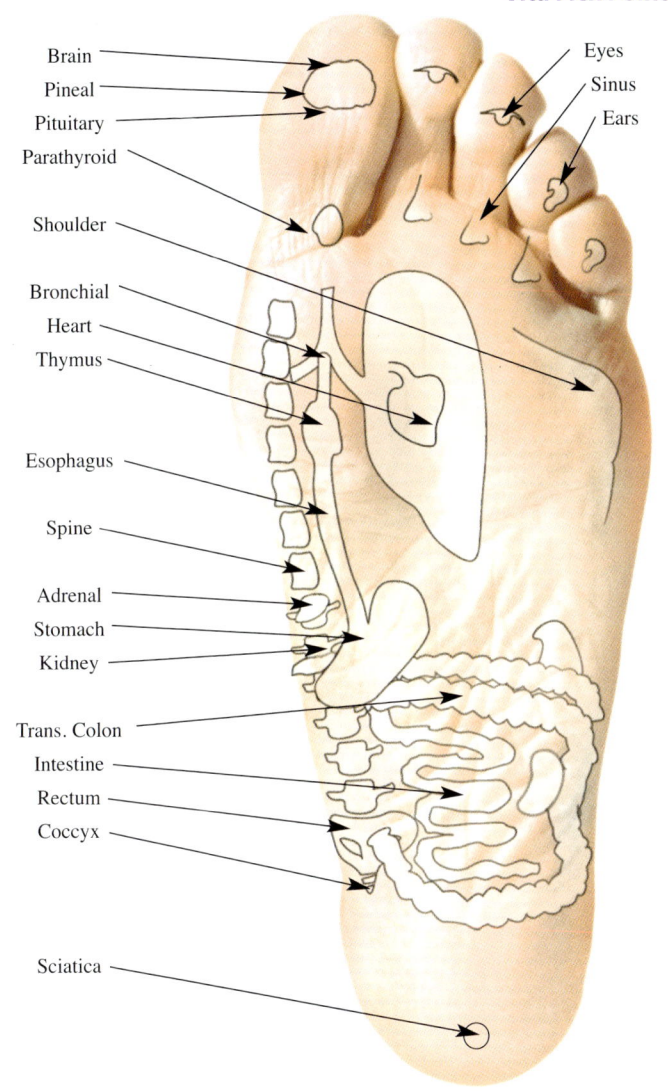

- Brain
- Pineal
- Pituitary
- Parathyroid
- Shoulder
- Bronchial
- Heart
- Thymus
- Esophagus
- Spine
- Adrenal
- Stomach
- Kidney
- Trans. Colon
- Intestine
- Rectum
- Coccyx
- Sciatica
- Eyes
- Sinus
- Ears

Nervous System Connection Points

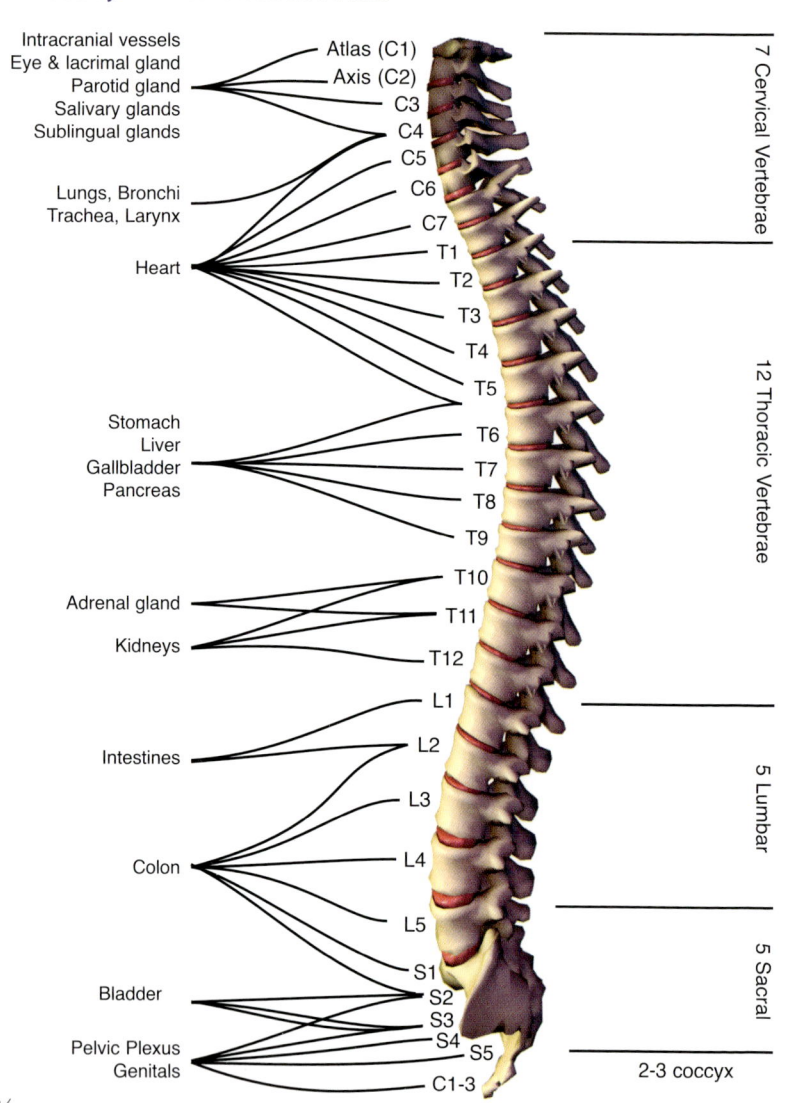

Organs/Areas	Vertebra	Section
Intracranial vessels	Atlas (C1)	7 Cervical Vertebrae
Eye & lacrimal gland	Axis (C2)	
Parotid gland	C3	
Salivary glands	C4	
Sublingual glands		
	C5	
Lungs, Bronchi	C6	
Trachea, Larynx	C7	
Heart	T1	12 Thoracic Vertebrae
	T2	
	T3	
	T4	
	T5	
Stomach	T6	
Liver	T7	
Gallbladder	T8	
Pancreas	T9	
	T10	
Adrenal gland	T11	
Kidneys	T12	
	L1	5 Lumbar
Intestines	L2	
	L3	
Colon	L4	
	L5	
	S1	5 Sacral
Bladder	S2	
	S3	
Pelvic Plexus	S4	
Genitals	S5	
	C1-3	2-3 coccyx

Raindrop Technique® 5

D. Gary Young developed the Raindrop Technique® (RT) during the 1980s based on his research with essential oils as antimicrobial agents, and prompted by some fascinating information he learned from an elder among the Lakota Indian Nation in South Dakota. This Lakota elder related that several generations ago, his ancestors regularly migrated north across the Canadian border into the northern regions of Saskatchewan and Manitoba, where they often witnessed the Aurora Borealis, or Northern Lights. When the Aurora Borealis was on display, those who were ill or had complicated health problems would stand facing the dancing lights and hold their hands out toward the lights and inhale deeply. Their belief was that the air was charged with healing energy from the Aurora Borealis. Mentally, they would "inhale" this energy into their spine and then out through nerve pathways to afflicted areas of the body.

This process stimulated an incredible healing effect for many of his ancestors. Effleurage (feathered finger stroking) became associated with this tradition after the borders were closed and the Lakota could no longer migrate north. Restricted to their reservations, they began practicing this energy process mentally, coupled with light stroking to facilitate the spreading of energy through the body.

It was this tradition that provided the promptings and began the process that gave birth to the development of Raindrop Technique (RT). Since 1989, RT has received an enormous amount of praise from users around the world for its ability to help ameliorate spinal abnormalities such as scoliosis and kyphosis, and facilitate tissue cleansing.

RT is based on the idea—now being explored in a number of scientific studies—that many types of scoliosis and spinal misalignments are caused by viruses or bacteria that lie dormant along the spine. These pathogens create inflammation, which, in turn, contorts and disfigures the spinal column.

RT is a powerful, non-invasive tool for assisting the body in correcting defects in the curvature of the spine by utilizing the antiviral, antibacterial, and anti-inflammatory action of several key essential oils. During the years that it has been practiced, it has resolved numerous cases of scoliosis, kyphosis, and chronic back pain. Further, it has eliminated the need for back surgery for hundreds of people. By integrating Vita Flex and massage, the power of essential oils brings the body into structural and electrical alignment.

Consistent with the French Model

The use of undiluted essential oils in RT is consistent with the French model for aromatherapy—which is the most extensively practiced and studied model in the world. With over 40 years of experience using essential oils clinically, the French have consistently recommended neat (undiluted) use of essential oils. An illustrious roster of 20th century French physicians provides convincing evidence that undiluted essential oils have a valuable place in the therapeutic arsenal of clinical professionals. René Gattefossé, PhD; Jean Valnet, MD; Jean-Claude Lapraz, MD; Daniel Pénoël, MD; and many others have long attested to the safe and effective use of undiluted essential oils and the dramatic and powerful benefits they can impart. According to Dr. Pénoël, "What happens when we use [essential oils] without diluting them? With many current essential oils, nothing dangerous or serious can happen."

In the case of Raindrop Technique®, the use of certain undiluted essential oils typically causes minor reddening and "heat" in the tissues. Normally, this is perfectly safe and not something to be overly concerned about. Blondes, redheads, and persons whose systems are toxic are more susceptible to this temporary reddening. Should the reddening or heat become excessive, it can be remedied within a minute or two by the immediate application of several drops of pure, quality vegetable oil to the affected area. This effectively dilutes the oils and the warming effect. Temporary mild warming is normal for RT. Typically it is even milder than that of many capsicum creams or sports ointments. Indeed, rather than being a cause of concern, this warming indicates that positive benefits are being imparted. In cases where the warmth or heat exceeds the comfort zone of the recipient, as mentioned before, the facilitator can apply any pure vegetable oil to the area until the comfort level is regained and reddening dissipates (usually within 2 minutes). NOTE: If a rash should appear, it is an indication of a chemical reaction between the oils and synthetic compounds in the skin cells and interstitial fluid of the body (usually from conventional personal care products). Some misconstrue this as an allergic reaction, when in fact the problem is not caused by an allergy but rather by foreign chemicals already imbedded in the tissues.

A number of medical professionals throughout the United States have adopted RT in their clinical practice and have found it to be an outstanding resource for aiding sciatica, scoliosis, kyphosis, and chronic back pain. Ken Krieger, DC, a chiropractor practicing in Scottsdale, Arizona, states, "As a chiropractor, I believe that the dramatic results of RT are enough for me to rewrite the books on scoliosis." Similarly, Terry Friedmann, MD, of Westminster, Colorado, states that "these essential oils truly represent a new frontier of medicine; they have resolved cases that many professionals had regarded as hopeless."

Do Infections Cause Scoliosis and Sciatica?

A growing amount of scientific research shows that certain microorganisms lodge near the spinal cord and contribute to deformities. Studies at Western General Hospital in Edinburgh, Scotland, linked virus-like particles to idiopathic scoliosis.[1,2] Researchers at the University of Bonn have also found the varicella zoster virus can lodge in the spinal ganglia throughout life.[3]

Research in 2001 further corroborated the existence of infectious microorganisms as a cause of spine pain and inflammation. Alistair Stirling and his colleagues at the Royal Orthopedic Hospital in Birmingham, England, found that 53 percent of patients with severe sciatica tested positive for chronic, low-grade infection by gram-negative bacteria (particularly Propionibacterium acnes) which triggered inflammation near the spine. Stirling suggested that the reason these bacteria had not been identified earlier was because of the extended time required to incubate disc material (7 days).[4]

The tuberculosis mycobacterium has also

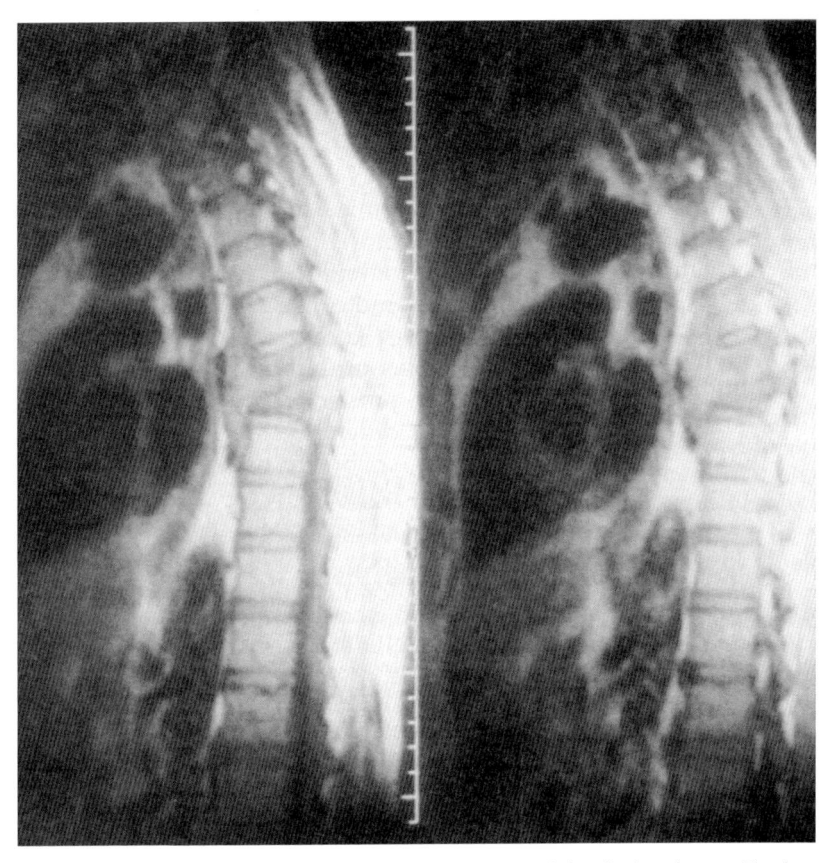

Example of kyphosis (hunchback) caused by an infectious microorganism (tuberculosis) in the spine. The above X-rays show two views of the spine of a 62 year-old man with a 3-month history of increasing back pain and inflammation due to kyphosis. The problem had become so severe that he could no longer walk unaided; however, there was no history of tuberculosis. The X-rays show the collapse of the seventh thoracic vertebra. He subsequently underwent back surgery to help correct the problem. Specimens taken during the surgery did not immediately show a bacterial infection, but after 12 weeks of incubation, the presence of Mycobacterium tuberculosis was detected, confirming the original diagnosis of spinal tuberculosis.

Source: Jenks, Peter J. and Stewart, Bruce. Images in Clinical Medicine. Vertebral Tuberculosis. New England Journal of Medicine, 1998 June 4, 338 (23);1677.

been shown to contribute to spinal disease and possibly deformations. Research at the Pasteur Institute in France, published in The New England Journal of Medicine, documented increasing numbers of patients showing evidence of spinal disease (Pott's disease) caused by tuberculosis.[5, 6, 7, 8]

In addition, vaccines made from live viruses have been linked to spinal problems. A 1982 study by Pincott and Taff found a connection between oral poliomyelitis vaccines and scoliosis.[9]

Powerful Infection-Fighters

Essential oils are some of the most powerful inhibitors of microbes known, and as such are an important new weapon in combating many types of tissue infections. A 1999 study by Marilena Marino and colleagues found that thyme oil exhibited strong action against stubborn gram-negative bacteria.[10] Similarly, basil essential oil also demonstrated strong bactericidal action against microorganisms Aeromonas hydrophila and Pseudomonas fluorescens.[11] A study at the Central Food Technological Institute in Mysore, India, found that a large number of essential oil components had tremendous germ-killing effects, inhibiting the growth of Staphylococcus, Micrococcus, Bacillus, and Enterobacter strains of bacteria. These compounds included menthol (found in peppermint), eucalyptol (found in rosemary, eucalyptus, and geranium), linalool (found in marjoram), and citral (found in lemongrass).[12] A 2001 study conducted by D. Gary Young, Diane Horne, Sue Chao, and colleagues at Weber State University in Ogden, Utah, found that oregano, thyme, peppermint, and basil exhibited very strong antimicrobial effects against pathogens such as Streptococcus pneumoniae, a major cause of illness in young children and death in elderly, and immune-weakened patients.[13] Many other studies confirm these findings.[14]

The ability of essential oils to penetrate the skin quickly and pass into bodily tissues to produce therapeutic effects has also been studied. Hoshi University researchers in Japan found that cyclic monoterpenes (including menthol, which is found in peppermint) are so effective in penetrating the skin that they can actually enhance the absorption of water-soluble drugs.[15] North Dakota State University researchers have similarly found that cyclic monoterpenes such as limonene and other terpenoids such as menthone and eugenol easily pass through the dermis, magnifying the penetration of pharmaceutical drugs such as tamoxifen.[16]

It is interesting to note that many essential oils used in RT—in addition to being highly antimicrobial—are also among those classified as GRAS (Generally Regarded As Safe) for internal use by the U.S. Food and Drug Administration. These include basil, marjoram, peppermint, oregano, and thyme. These and many other GRAS essential oils have a decades-long history of being consumed as foods or flavorings with virtually no adverse reactions.

In sum, RT is one of the safest, noninvasive techniques available for spinal health. It is also an invaluable tool to promote healing from within using topically applied essential oils.

Introduction to the Technique

Raindrop Technique® uses a sequence of highly antimicrobial essential oils synergistically combined to simultaneously kill the responsible viral agents and reduce inflammation. The principle single oils used include:

- oregano (*Origanum compactum*)
- thyme (*Thymus vulgaris*)
- basil or balsam fir (*Ocimum basilicum* or *Abies balsamea*)

- cypress (*Cupressus sempervirens*)
- wintergreen or birch (*Gaultheria procumbens* or *Betula alleghaniensis*)
- marjoram (*Origanum majorana*)
- peppermint (*Mentha piperita*).

The oils are dispensed like little drops of rain from a height of about six inches above the back and very lightly massaged along the vertebrae and back muscles. Although the entire process takes about 45 minutes to complete, the oils will continue to work in the body for up to one week following treatment, with continued re-alignment taking place during this time.

One caution: RT is not a cure-all or a magic bullet. A healthy balanced body is the result of a well-rounded program of exercise and proper diet. Health is everything we do, say, hear, see, and eat. RT is only one tool to help restore balance in the body. Healthy eating habits and a positive, open mind will also help prepare the body and skin to accept the oils better and more rapidly.

Although this technique is explained as simply as possible, you may want to contact Essential Science Publishing to purchase a demonstration video. Every step of the technique is carefully demonstrated in an actual hands-on presentation. You can order the video by visiting the ESP website at www.essentialscience.net or by calling toll-free 800-336-6308. Viewing this video and following the outline presented here will make this revolutionary technique easy to understand and easy to put into practice.

The Raindrop Technique®

It is recommended that RT be performed in a quiet, semi-darkened area free of distractions. Soft and relaxing music will make the recipient more comfortable. The temperature should be cool enough to prevent sweating, but warm enough to be comfortable as the recipient's back and legs will be exposed. In describing the technique, "facilitator" refers to the person giving the Raindrop Technique; "recipient" refers to the person receiving it.

For This Technique, You Will Need:

1. Massage table (ideally) or a comfortable, flat surface for the recipient to lie on. The surface should be high enough that the facilitator can perform the technique without back strain. It is best to cover the surface with sheets or towels that are expendable as several of the oils may stain certain fabrics. Also, some of the oils can react with the vinyls used to cover massage tables so be sure vinyl surfaces are covered well.
2. Two medium-sized towels and a twin-sized bed sheet. The towels will be used to make a warm compress; the sheet to protect the modesty of the recipient.
3. Easy access to hot water.
4. Timer, clock, or watch.
5. A stable tray on which to place oils (and instructions, if needed) near the receiver.
6. Each of the 10 oils listed throughout this chapter. (Seven single oils, two blends and a vegetable or massage oil.)

Preparation
- Both the facilitator and the recipient should remove all jewelry. This includes watches, pendants, chains, rings, bracelets, belts, earrings, etc.
- The facilitator should wear clothing that is loose and comfortable, and may wish to remove their shoes.
- The recipient should be draped in a bed sheet or towel, or dressed in hospital gown-attire so the facilitator can apply essential oils to the shoulders, neck, back, legs, and feet of the recipient.
- The facilitator should make sure their fingernails are clipped and filed down as short as possible to prevent unintentionally scratching the recipient's skin, particularly when doing the Vita Flex Technique.
- The facilitator should make sure fingernails are free of fingernail polish. Essential oils remove many polishes and lacquers.
- Only perform RT if you are feeling healthy, energized, and emotionally/ mentally clear and focused.
- For optimum results, the recipient should drink extra purified or distilled water for the first few days following RT. This will aid the body in flushing toxins from the tissues.

NOTE: Facilitators may choose to apply frankincense to themselves (on wrists, shoulders, neck, and top of the head) to help counter any negative energies coming from the recipient.

To begin:
- The recipient should lie on their back, face up on the massage table with the head resting in the face cradle.
- The recipient should lie as straight as possible with the hips flat on the table. The arms should rest alongside the body.
- The facilitator should keep constant physical contact with the recipient to prevent feelings of insecurity, anxiousness, or abandonment.
- Check for evenness of feet and in the length of the legs. Hold recipient's ankles just below the shin bone (with the right hand on the left ankle and the left hand on the right ankle) with the index finger of each hand touching the center of the outside ankle bone. While holding the ankles in this position, the thumbs of the facilitator should be even with one another. Unevenness could indicate a pelvic rotation or structural misalignment.

If you intend to offer the Raindrop Technique® as a service, please be advised that some states require that you be a licensed massage therapist, aesthetician or chiropractor prior to offering any service where physical touch is involved. Please check the regulations for your jurisdiction.

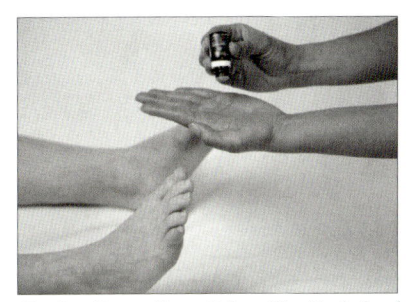

Fig. A — Putting Energy Balance Blend in the hand

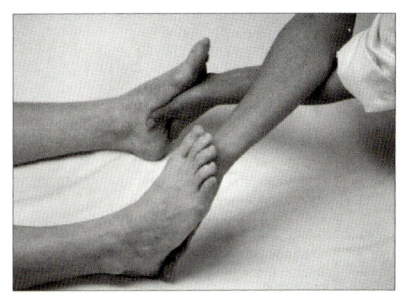

Fig. B — Placing hands on the recipient's feet

STEP 1 – Apply Valor blend to feet and shoulders

Oregano, thyme, and the Valor blend are the foundation oils for all Raindrop Technique work. The technique always begins with the application of Valor to the feet and shoulders. This is one of the most important steps for a successful RT because it works on the physical, electrical, spiritual, and emotional levels, supporting the physical and energy alignment of the body. The key to using this oil blend is patience. Once the frequencies begin to balance, a structural alignment will much more likely begin to occur.

This first step forms the foundation for everything that follows.

- According to energy medicine principles, female energy relates to the left side of the body, male energy to the right side. So this application begins differently for males and females.
- Put 6 drops of Valor into your left hand and apply to the left foot first if the recipient is a woman (See Fig. A); put the oil in the right hand and apply to the right foot first if the recipient is a man. Then apply the oil on the other foot.

STEP 2 – Place hands on recipient's feet and shoulders

Step 2 works best if there are two facilitators: one to hold the feet, the other to make contact at the shoulders. However, if you are working by yourself, the application works well just holding the feet, which is the most important. You may kneel or sit while holding the feet or shoulders of the recipient. You should be in a comfortable position to maintain contact for several minutes.

- Cross your hands and place your palms as flat as possible against the soles of the receiver's feet. This hand crossing enables the facilitator to place the right palm on the right foot and the left palm on the left foot. The facilitator should hold this position for at least 5 minutes. (See Fig. B)
- If two facilitators are available, the second should sit or stand at the recipient's head and apply three drops of Valor to each shoulder. The right palm is placed on the recipient's right shoulder and left palm is placed on the left shoulder at the same time (without crossing arms). There must be as much palm-to-shoulder contact as possible.
- Let your mind be free and peaceful. Encourage the recipient to take deep breaths, inhaling

and exhaling deeply and slowly, so they engage in their own healing. The recipient may feel a little heat or tingling on the feet, or an energy working up through the legs to the back, even moving as high as the head. Some facilitators may feel their hands become warm or tingly. Sometimes the facilitator may feel a pulsating effect. The facilitator should try to feel the energy coming through the recipient's feet. Look for:

- Temperature change
- A "pulsing" feeling
- Subtle vibration

Once you feel energy and it is equal in both feet, you can release.

The vertebrae can achieve some realignment with this initial application alone. However, if there are people present with hidden negative attitudes, the results may be less than optimal. Only perform the RT if you are feeling healthy, energized, and emotionally/mentally clear and focused.

CAUTION: If there is a fold in the skin on the back of the neck or elsewhere, please note that essential oils can accumulate there. Be aware of this as you proceed, and if the recipient notices a burning sensation in a skin fold, be prepared to add V6 Oil Complex or massage oil there.

STEP 3 – Apply seven essential oils to the feet

In this step we will apply the seven single oils in a specific order to the spinal Vita Flex area of the soles of the feet (see chart on pages 32-33) using the Vita Flex Technique. The seven oils in their application sequence are:

- Oregano has potent antimicrobial and anti-inflammatory properties.
- Thyme is highly antimicrobial, inhibiting the growth of infectious microorganisms. It easily penetrates the skin and travels throughout the body.
- Basil or Balsam Fir: Basil has antispasmodic properties that relax muscles. It is also anti-inflammatory and antimicrobial. Balsam fir is an excellent substitute for basil and is less irritating to sensitive skin.
- Cypress oil improves circulation, relieves spasms and swelling, and helps heal damaged tissue.
- Wintergreen and Birch are virtually identical chemically. They are anti-inflammatory and analgesic (pain-relieving) due to their high methyl salicylate content. They are excellent for bones and joints.

NOTE: Be careful of your sources in obtaining either of these oils. It is my experience in the market that there is very little natural birch essential oil available worldwide. Additionally, much of the wintergreen sold today has been chemically extended and adulterated with synthetic methyl salicylate.

- Marjoram oil is antispasmodic and muscle-relaxing.
- Peppermint enhances the effects of all the preceding essential oils. It also has pain-killing and antimicrobial properties, stimulating circulatio n and cooling inflamed tissue.

The procedure for this portion of RT involves a series of substeps as follows:

A. Place 2-3 drops of oregano (small feet require only 1-2 drops of essential oil) in the palm of the left hand. Dip the fingertips of the right hand in the oil, stir clockwise three times and apply along the spine Vita Flex points of the right foot (see chart on pages 32-33). This is the area along the bottom inside edge of the foot from the heel to the tip of the big toe. Massage with Vita Flex Technique the full length of this area three times. Remember

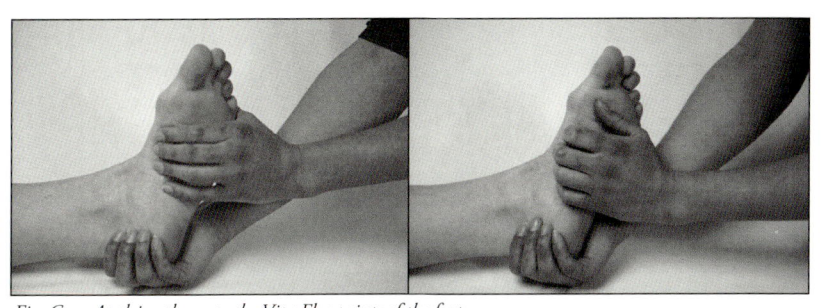

Fig. C — Applying thyme to the Vita Flex points of the foot

to use the right hand for both oil application and Vita Flex massage on the right foot. (See Fig. C)

B. Place 2-3 drops of thyme essential oil in the palm of the left hand. Dip two fingertips of the right hand in the oil, stir clockwise three times and apply—just as above with oregano oil—along the spinal Vita Flex area of the right foot. Massage along the full length of this spinal area using the Vita Flex Technique once to apply the oil, then two more times.

C. Apply 2-3 drops of basil or balsam fir in the same manner as above on the right foot.

D. Apply 2-3 drops of cypress in the same manner as above on the right foot.

E. Apply 2-3 drops of wintergreen or birch in the same manner as above on the right foot.

F. Apply 2-3 drops of marjoram in the same manner as above on the right foot.

G. Apply 2-3 drops of peppermint in the same manner as above on the right foot.

Repeat steps A-G, on the left foot, placing the oils in the palm of the right hand and applying them and doing Vita Flex on the left foot with the left hand.

STEP 4 – Apply oregano and thyme to spine

- Have the recipient turn over on their stomach to expose the back. Do this carefully to protect the recipient's modesty.
- Hold the bottle six inches above the skin and evenly space **2-4 drops** of oregano oil along the center of the spine from bottom to top (sacrum to atlas). (See Fig. D)
- Immediately after applying oregano, with 6-inch brush-like strokes, brush the backs of your fingertips along the spine as you "feather up" the back from the sacrum (base of spine) to the atlas (hair line on back of neck). Repeat this feathering process two more times. (See Fig. E)
- In the same way as above, evenly space 3-5 drops of thyme oil along the center of the spine from bottom to top. Feather in the thyme just as you did for oregano.

CAUTION: More is not better. If there is a slight warming or burning sensation along the spine or on the neck, apply a pure vegetable or massage oil. The high phenol content of oregano and thyme essential oils can produce excess warming or reddening to the skin, particularly with fair-skinned people. Following the application of thyme and oregano, if the recipient becomes

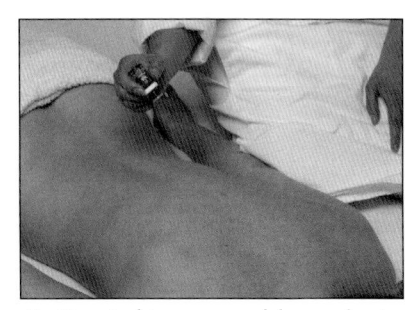

Fig. D — Applying oregano and thyme to the spine

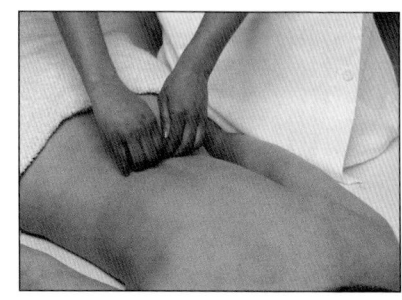

Fig. E — Brush strokes up the spine

uncomfortable with burning sensations, apply 5-10 drops of vegetable or massage oil over affected areas.

STEP 5 – Apply basil or balsam fir; massage spinal muscles using circular motions

- Evenly drop **6-10 drops** of basil or balsam fir evenly along the center of the spine.
- Spread the oil over the back by using the feathering technique described in step 4.
- In small circular clockwise motions (using the pads of the fingertips of both hands placed side by side) massage the muscles on each side of the spine. Start at the sacrum and work up to the atlas, using the fingertips to gently push or pull the tissue away from the spine. After finishing one side of the spine, start on the other side. Do not work directly on the spine, but on the muscles on either side of the spine. Do not apply direct pressure to the vertebrae. Repeat this step two more times. (See Fig. F)

STEP 6 – Apply cypress and do a finger straddle/hand "saw" massage

- Evenly drop **6-10 drops** of cypress along the center of the spine.

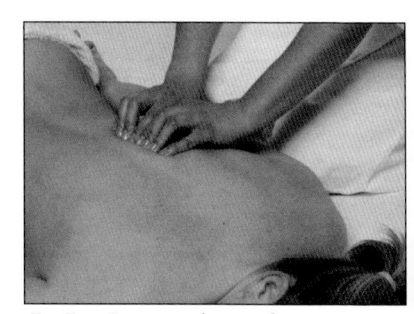

Fig. F — Easing muscles away from spine

- Spread the oil over the spine and spinal muscles using the feathering technique described in Step 4.
- Stand on the recipient's left side (right side if the facilitator is left handed) near the shoulder area, facing the recipient's feet. Straddle the spine at the sacrum (base) with the index and middle fingers of the non-dominant hand. Place the bottom edge of the dominant hand (ulnar or pinky side down) just below the middle joints of the two straddling fingers. (See Fig. G)

Simultaneously perform the following two motions:

1. Apply moderate downward pressure with the straddling fingers while pulling them slowly to the atlas (top) of the spine.
2. Using an equal downward pressure, "saw" the dominant hand back and forth, using short, rapid 1-inch strokes, moving the two straddling fingers back and forth as you slide them up the spine all the way to the hairline. Repeat this step two more times.

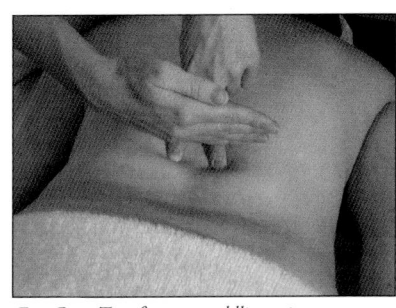

Fig. G — Two fingers straddling spine

STEP 7 – Apply wintergreen or birch and thumb-roll up the spine

- Evenly drop **6-10 drops** of wintergreen or birch along the center of the spine.
- Spread the oil over the spine and spinal muscles using the feathering technique described in Step 4.
- With your thumbs one inch apart on either side of the spine, use the Vita Flex method of thumb-rolling to work up the spine a thumbwidth at a time, from the sacrum to the atlas. Apply mild pressure. You may want to offset your thumbs by one inch to avoid bumping thumbs on the inward roll. Continue to roll your thumbs lightly over onto the nails and then release. Repeat this step two more times. (See Figs. H and I)

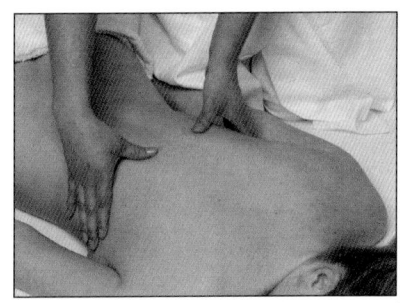

Fig. H — Thumb-rolling up spine (Down position)

STEP 8 – Apply marjoram and peppermint to spinal muscles using flared feather strokes

In this step we apply the last two single essential oils—in the sequence listed—to the muscles along either side of the spine and feather them to the rib and shoulders areas of the back. The two oils are marjoram and peppermint.

- Evenly drop (Raindrop-style) **6-10 drops** (depending on the length of the recipient's spine) of marjoram onto the muscles along

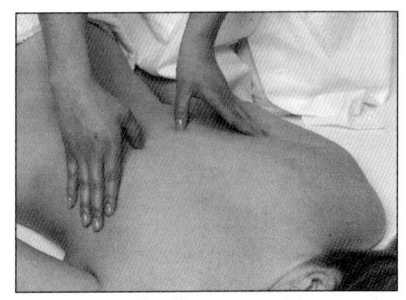

Fig. I — Thumb-rolling up spine (Up position)

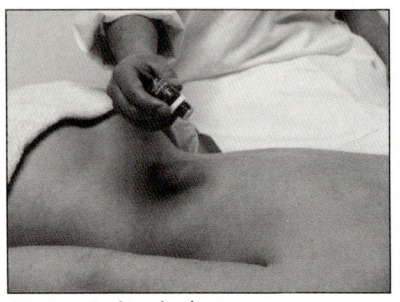

Fig. J — Applying basil, wintergreen, cypress, marjoram, and peppermint to muscles on each side of spine

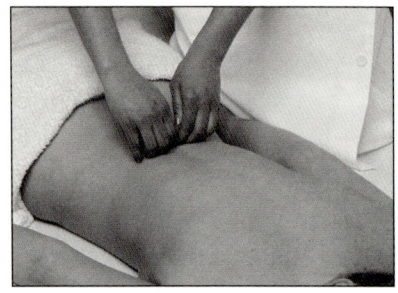

Fig. K — Brush strokes up the back muscles

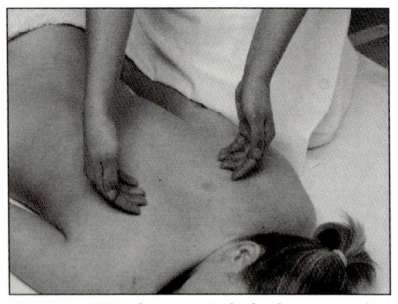

Fig. L — "Feathering up" the back over muscles next to the spine

each side of the spine (12-20 drops total). (See Fig. J)

- After applying marjoram, with the nail side of your fingertips, use 6-inch brush-like strokes to feather the oil up the spine from the sacrum to the atlas. Repeat this step two more times. (See Fig. K)
- Then, extending the feather strokes (about 8 inches), lightly flare the fingertips out towards the sides of the back as you feather up the spine. Flare right hand to the right side of the back, and the left hand to the left side of the back, moving all the way to the side of the rib cage. Repeat this step two more times. This light stroking, or feathering, is called "effleurage." (See Fig. L)
- Starting at the sacrum, do a second set of flared feather strokes moving up the full length of the spine to the atlas (the hairline on the back of the neck). Flare your fingertips out over the shoulders and neck when you reach the atlas. Repeat this two more times, for a total of three times.
- Apply and feather a total of **6-10 drops** of peppermint essential oil using the same process.

STEP 9 – Apply Aroma Siez to the back

The Aroma Siez blend contains several highly antispasmodic essential oils that help relax sore, tense, or inflamed muscles.

- Apply at least **6-8 drops** of Aroma Siez over the entire length of each side of the spine (**12-16 drops** total). Feather in the blend as in Step 8, then, using circular motions with the flat of the hands, gently massage into the back muscles. Include the areas along the outer edges of the rib cage and shoulders that have not been previously worked.

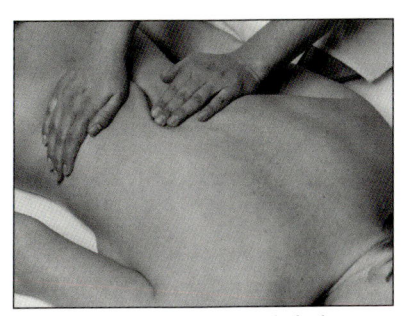

Fig. M — Palm rub massage on the back

STEP 10 – Massage entire back and neck with a quality vegetable or massage oil, finishing with palm rub

This application helps to seal in the essential oils, enhancing penetration.

- Put **12-20 drops** (depending on the size of the back) of V6 Oil Complex or massage oil, in your palm to warm the oil before spreading onto the muscles of the entire back and back of the neck. Use a gentle massage to evenly spread the massage oil.
- Place both hands on the receiver's back, palms down, near the base of the spine, one hand close to you, one hand on the far side of the back. Then slide the palms, with mild downward pressure, in opposite directions from the far side of the back to the near side, working slowly up the back toward the neck. Continue this alternating back and forth massage up to the nape of the neck. (See Fig. M) Do this massage up and down the back three times.

STEP 11 – Apply Valor to the spine

Apply **6-10 drops** of Valor, raindrop-style, along the center of the spine, from the sacrum to the atlas. Feather in the blend as in Step 8. Gently massage into the spine and spinal muscles using circular motions with the flats of your hands, moving from the sacrum to the atlas. Repeat two more times.

> CAUTION: Special care must be taken with this step because the back can become hot! The heat will usually build slowly and peak in about 3-8 minutes, before cooling down to the point where it feels quite pleasant. The greater the inflammation and viral infection along the spine, the hotter the area along the spine will become.
>
> If the heat becomes uncomfortable, place a dry, folded towel between the back and the damp towel (see first point below). If the warming sensation continues to be uncomfortable, remove all towels and massage the area with 10-15 drops of vegetable or massage oil.

STEP 12 – Apply moist warm towel; perform back press

- Soak one of the towels in warm water, wring it out, fold it in thirds, and lay it along the entire length of the spine.
- Place the other dry towel (folded in half) over the wet towel.
- Allow the heat from the wet towel to penetrate, usually about 8–10 minutes. If the heat fades before 8 minutes are up, it may be helpful to apply the warm moist towel a second time.
- Pay very close attention to the recipient's comfort. Ask questions.
- After the warmth of the oils has subsided (from 8–15 minutes), with the towels still in place, perform the back press by crossing the hands and placing them 1-2 inches apart at the base of the back. Gently press the hands

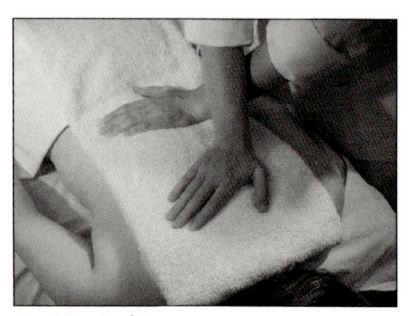

Fig. N — Back Press

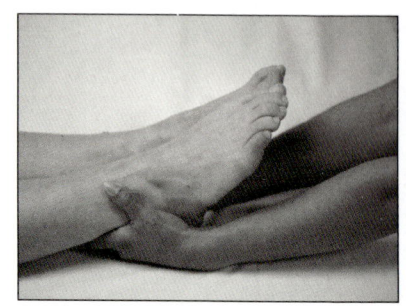

Fig. O — Stretching the spine

down and away from each other, vibrating the hands and spreading them slightly. Repeat this process of pressing, vibrating and spreading the hands 3-5 times, each time starting further up the spine, until reaching the top of the spine (See Fig. N). Repeat this step two more times.

STEP 13 – Remove towels and inspect spine

- Remove the towels. Make sure the person is lying with their head snug in the head cradle of the massage table and with their spine straight (hips aligned with shoulders).
- Check the spine. Corrections may or may not be visible. Results may take several days to take full effect. You may need to perform another technique at a later time.

STEP 14 – Gently stretch the back and neck

- Have the recipient turn over onto their back. Be careful to keep the receiver covered to protect modesty.
- If you are working alone, hold the ankles firmly and apply light pressure to stretch the back as shown (See Fig. O). If there is a second facilitator, they should hold the ankles while you cradle the individual's head in your hands (see cranial hold on next page), place your thumbs around the chin, and gently lift and ease back to create slight tension. Hold for 3 seconds, then release for 3 seconds. Repeat three times.

Best results are achieved when two people perform this stretching step: one gently tensioning the neck while the other holds the legs. If there is only one facilitator, this step can be done in two sequential steps—ankles first, then neck.

STEP 14A – Finger placement for cranial hold

- Place both hands under the recipient's neck, with the fingers touching each other and the thumbs just below the jaw. (See Fig. P)

STEP 14B – Basic cranial hold

- Gently pull the recipient's head back from the torso using the cranial hold. Pull back gently for 3 seconds, then release for 3 seconds. Repeat this cycle slowly and gently three times. Check with the recipient during this process to verify that they are not experiencing any pain. If there is pain, immediately discontinue the stretch. (See Fig. Q)

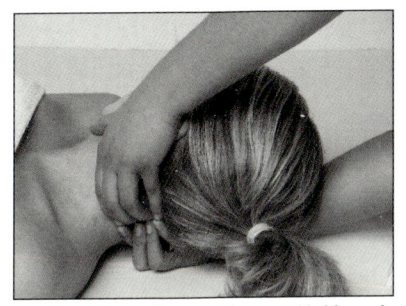

Fig. P — Finger placement for cranial hold stretch

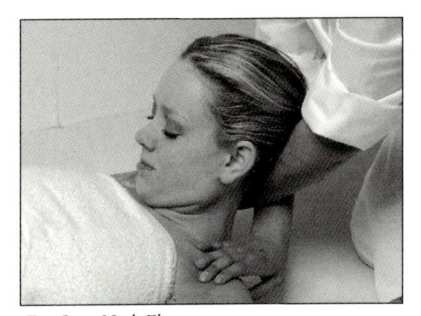

Fig. S — Neck Flex

STEP 14C – Modified cranial hold

This is an alternate version of the cranial hold, which differs in the hand placement on the receiver's head.

- Hold the recipient's head with one hand under the neck, palm up, and the other hand cradling the receiver's chin. Gently create tension in the neck by slowly pulling the head away from the torso. Hold for 5 seconds, then release for 5 seconds. Repeat two more times. (See Fig. R)
- Do not pull too hard. An assistant, if available, can anchor the feet while you gently tension the neck.

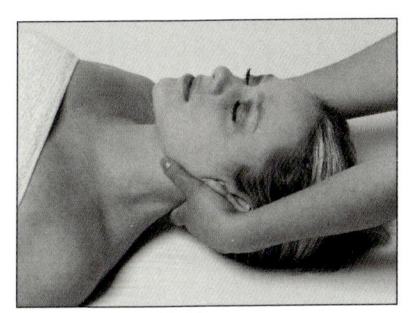

Fig. Q — Cranial hold

STEP 15 – Neck Flex

- Kneel or sit so that your shoulders are parallel to the recipient's shoulders.
- Cross your arms and place your hands (palm side down) on the recipient's shoulders (left hand on the right shoulder and visa versa).
- Make sure the recipient's tongue is not between their teeth.
- Raise your elbows in order to gently lift and stretch the recipient's neck until their chin touches the chest.
- Repeat this step two more times. (See Fig. S)

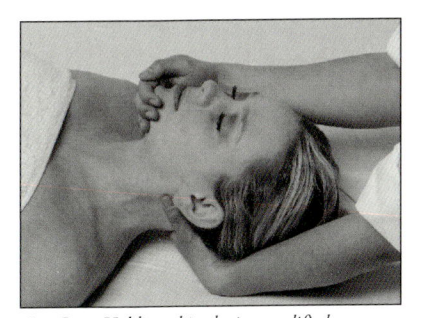

Fig. R — Holding chin during modified cranial hold

- For optimum results, the recipient should drink extra purified or distilled water for the first few days following RT. This will aid the body in flushing toxins from the tissues.

Customizing Raindrop Technique® to Address Specific Health Issues

Raindrop Technique can be customized to address different health issues that are not directly related to back problems. Lung infections, digestive complaints, hormonal problems, liver insufficiencies, and other problems can all be dealt with by substituting standard RT essential oils with other oils that are specifically targeted for that body system.

As a rule, when customizing RT, you will generally want to start with the Valor, oregano, and thyme. These three oils form the basis or "hub" of all Raindrop applications. (For extra antiviral effect, add mountain savory.) The other essential oils such as basil, wintergreen, marjoram, thyme, or cypress can be omitted or replaced by essential oils specific for the condition being treated.

For example, if a lung infection is present, basil and wintergreen should be replaced with ravensara, cypress replaced with Eucalyptus radiata, and marjoram replaced with mountain savory. (See diagram above)

There are several variations to the basic Raindrop Technique. These variations are not easy to explain and require class instruction and demonstration.

SUMMARY:

Raindrop Technique (RT) is a powerful tool that assists both professionals and lay people to achieve true balance in the body. Out of the thousands of RT sessions that have been performed, there have been hundreds of instances where the results were amazingly profound and immediate. Here are just a few examples:

A young man from Denver, Colorado who suffered from chronic scoliosis was able—for the first time in eight years—to fully bend over after the application of RT. With an overhead camera televising an image of his spine as he bent over, an audience of over 400 watched the vertebrae in his spine literally move into place. When he stood up, he was measured and had gained an inch in height.

Another case involved a professional model in her early 40s, who had developed early adult-onset scoliosis. She had to alter clothing so it would fit properly for modeling sessions. She wasn't able to sit still for any length of time. After receiving RT, her spine straightened to such a degree that she, too, gained an inch in height. She followed up with more RT in the next few months and reported that all discomfort was gone. She now dances and rides horses pain-free.

It is quite common that individuals with scoliosis who receive RT will gain 1/2 an inch or more in stature from a single application. Many others have reported pain relief, congestion relief, and cold and flu relief as a result of RT. This is why RT has captured so much interest among those involved in the healing arts.

Older children can benefit from RT, but it is critical to adjust the amount of oil used in proportion to their body size. Amounts should be adjusted to reflect the difference in body size relative to an adult.

Body System Oils Wheel

Center: Valor, oregano, thyme

- **BRAIN**: cardemom, peppermint, Clarity, M-Grain, Peace & Calming
- **JOINTS/BONES**: wintergreen, spruce, helichrysum, Pan Away
- **LONGEVITY**: thyme, frankincense, Longevity
- **COLON/DIGESTION**: tarragon, fennel, cumin, spearmint, Di-Tone
- **HORMONE BALANCE**: clary sage, fleabane, Endo Flex, Dragon Time, Mister
- **LUNG**: ravensara, eucalyptus radiata, myrtle, Raven, Melrose
- **LIVER**: ledum, carrot seed, German chamomille, Juva Flex
- **HEART/CIRCULATION**: clove, nutmeg, goldenrod, cypress, Aroma Life

---

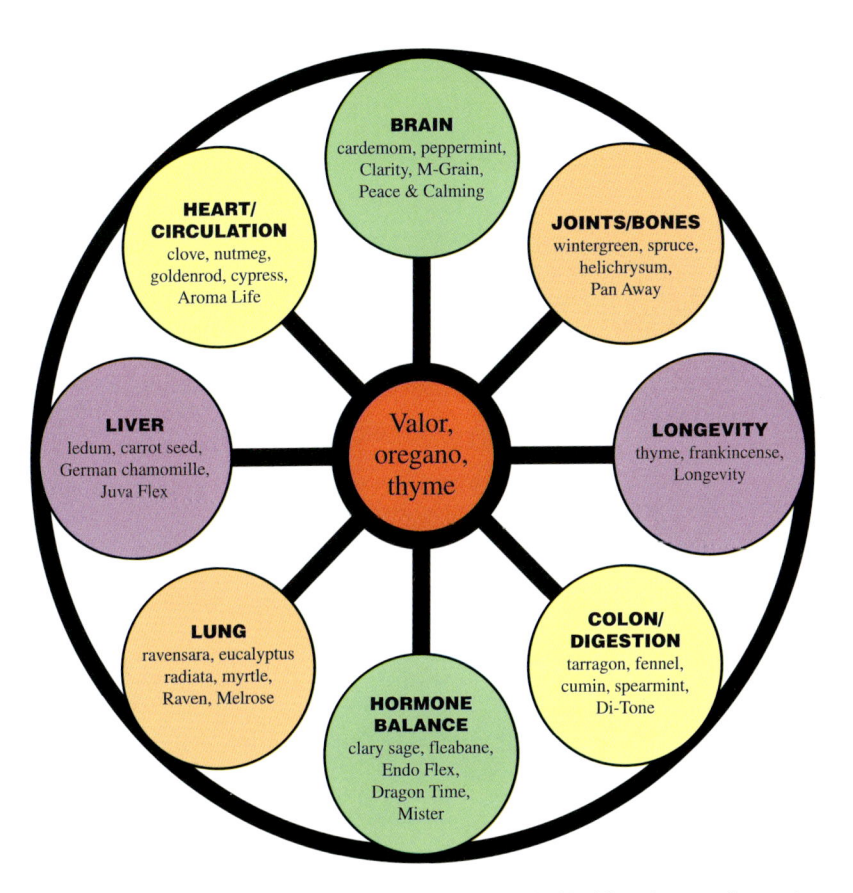

Every person is biochemically different, and what works for one may not work for another. Different body types respond to the applications in ways you may not expect. Learn to be sensitive to the person on whom you are working so that you can respond to their needs.

The question is often asked, "How long do the effects of this application last?" Again, each person responds differently. Generally speaking, a high level of health and proper diet are key factors, as are exercise and attitude. The effects of one application may last several months for one person, but for another it may be necessary to have repeated applications weekly until the body begins to respond. The goal is to retrain the tissues of the body. This may take a few weeks or even a full year.

Spinal alignment may have a completely

different look when the individual is lying down, rather than sitting. There is more torque on the spine in a sitting or standing position, so these are the positions in which X-rays are usually taken. The spine may appear to be totally corrected when the receiver is lying down, but then appear to be crooked when they are in a sitting position. This variance is normal and may be apparent until a total retraining of the muscles occurs. The object is to achieve proper alignment in all positions.

Endnotes

1. Green RJ, Webb JN, Maxwell MH. The nature of virus-like particles in the paraxial muscles of idiopathic scoliosis. J Pathol. 1979 Sep;129(1):9-12.
2. Webb JN, Gillespie WJ. Virus-like particles in paraspinal muscle in scoliosis. Br Med J. 1976 Oct 16;2(6041):912-3.
3. Wolff MH, Buchel F, Gullotta F, Helpap B, Schneweiss KE. Investigations to demonstrate latent viral infection of varicella-Zoster virus in human spine ganglia. Verh Dtsch Ges Pathol. 1981;65:203-7.
4. Stirling AL, et al., Association between sciatica and Propionibacterium acnes. Lancet 2001:V357.
5. Nagrath SP, Hazra DK, Pant PC, Seth HC. Tuberculosis spine—a diagnostic conundrum. Case report. J Assoc Physicians India. 1974 May;22(5):405-7.
6. Jenks PJ, Stewart B. Images in clinical medicine. Vertebral tuberculosis. N Engl J Med. 1998 June 4;338(23):1677.
7. Monaghan D, Gupta A, Barrington NA. Case report: Tuberculosis of the spine—an unusual presentation. Clin Radiol. 1991 May;43(5):360-2.
8. Petersen CK, Craw M, Radiological differentiation of tuberculosis and pyogenic osteomyelitis: a case report. J Manipulative Physiol Ther. 1986 Mar;9(1):39-42.
9. Pinott JR, Taffs LF. Experimental scoliosis in primates: a neurological cause. J Bone Joint Surg Br. 1982;64(4):503-7.
10. Marino M, Bersani C, Comi G. Antimicrobial activity of the essential oils of Thymus vulgaris L. measured using a bioimpedometric method. Journal of Food Protection, Vol. 62, No. 9, 1999 pp. 1017-1023.
11. Wan J, Wilcock A, Coventry MJ. The effect of essential oils of basil on the growth of Aeromonas fluorescens. Journal of Applied Microbiology, 1998, 84, 152-158.
12. Beuchat LR. Antimicrobial properties of spices and their essential oils. Center for Food Safety and Quality Enhancement, Department of Food Science and Technology, University of Georgia, Griffin, Georgia.
13. Horne D, et al., Antimicrobial effects of essential oils on Streptococcus pneumoniae. Journal of Essential Oil Research, (September/October 2001). 13, 387-392.
14. Moleyar V, Narasimham P. Antibacterial activity of essential oil components. International Journal of Food Microbiology, Vol. 16 (1992) 337-32.
15. Obata Y, et al. Effect of pretreatment of skin with cyclic monoterpenes on permeation of diclofenac in hairless rat. Biol Pharm Bull. 1993 Mar;16(3)312-4.
16. Zhao K, Singh J. Mechanisms of percutaneous absorption of tamoxifen by terpenes: eugenol, d-limonene and menthone. Control Release. 1998. Nov 13;55(2-3)253-60.

Lymphatic Pump 6

Maintaining lymph circulation is one of the keys to keeping the immune system adequately functioning. This technique is designed to promote lymph circulation. It is an excellent tool for those who are sedentary or bedridden.

1. With the recipient lying on their back, hold one leg with one hand just above ankles with your palm on the underside of the leg (covering the Achille's tendon).
2. Place the other hand on the bottom of the recipient's foot with your palm over the ball of their feet and your fingers curled around their toes.
3. Push the top of the recipient's foot away from you. (See Fig. A)
4. Then, pull the recipient's foot toward you by the toes until the ball of the foot is as close to the table as possible. (See Fig. B)
5. Check with the recipient during the pump to verify that the muscles in their feet are not being overextended. This should be an active process, but not a painful one.
6. Pull and push their foot using this "pumping motion" at least 10 times on each leg for maximum benefit. Note that their entire body should move during each step of the Lymphatic Pump.

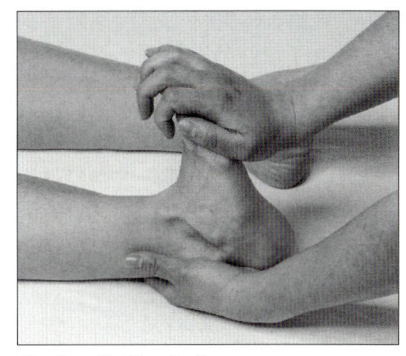

Fig. A — Pushing the foot

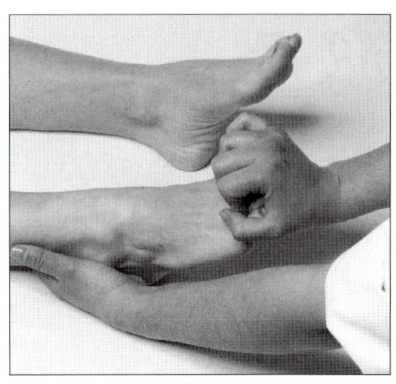

Fig. B — Pulling the foot

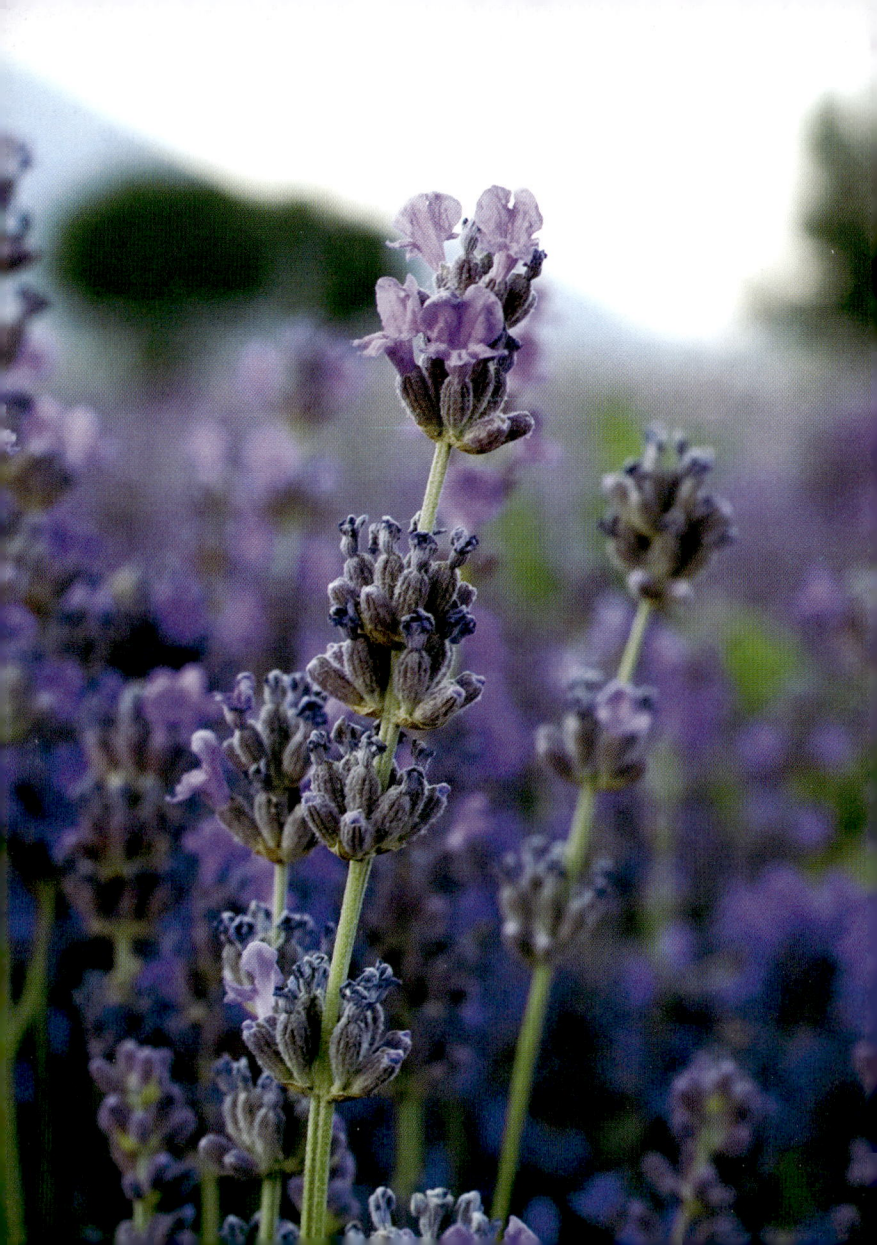

Auricular Technique 7

D. Gary Young developed auricular aroma technique, the integration of essential oils with standard auricular technique, after using essential oils in acupuncture applications in his clinic. He found that using essential oils in conjunction with acupuncture was extremely beneficial. He also found that acupuncture stimulation with essential oils was noticeably greater than either acupuncture or essential oil applications by themselves.

Acupuncture with essential oils seems to enhance benefits substantially. As Gary left his first clinical practice and began researching, farming, and teaching, he knew he could not continue the practice of acupuncture, so he started developing a simplified technique that everyone could use. That technique is called auricular probe technique, using a small, pen-shaped instrument with a rounded end to apply the oils to the acupuncture meridians or Vita Flex points on the ears. This concept can be used in both the emotional and physical realm.

For working the spine and dealing with neurological problems that exist because of spinal cord injury, auricular probe technique was found to be extremely beneficial to deliver the oils to the exact location of the neurological damage.

Auricular probe technique is a program that Gary continues to research and develop, and teach to doctors. It has shown tremendous potential and will grow to be a well-known modality in the future.

Emotional Ear Chart

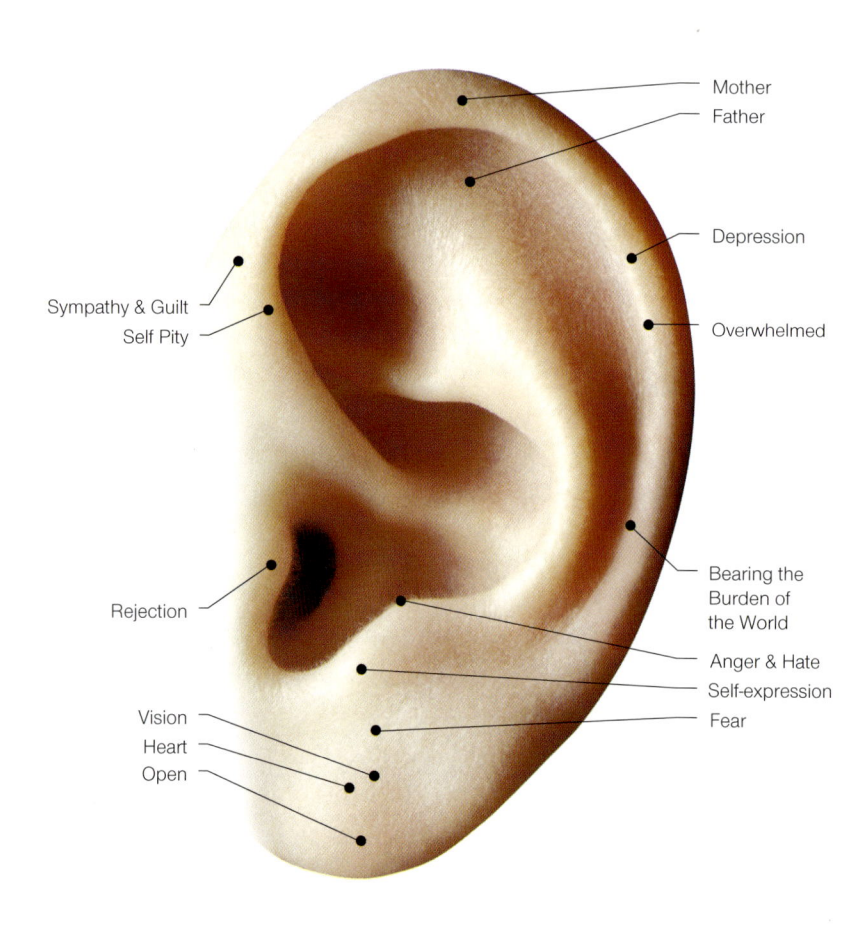

- Mother
- Father
- Depression
- Overwhelmed
- Sympathy & Guilt
- Self Pity
- Bearing the Burden of the World
- Anger & Hate
- Self-expression
- Fear
- Rejection
- Vision
- Heart
- Open

Physical Ear Chart

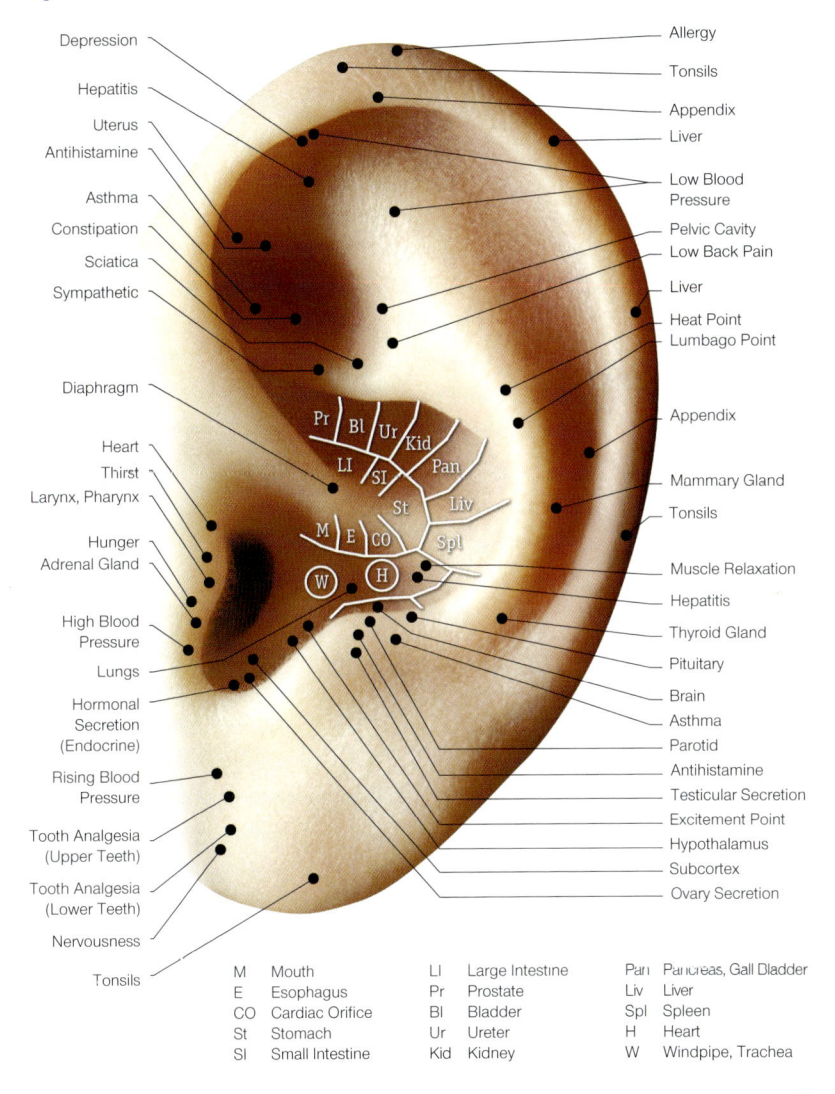

Labels (clockwise from top-left):
- Depression
- Hepatitis
- Uterus
- Antihistamine
- Asthma
- Constipation
- Sciatica
- Sympathetic
- Diaphragm
- Heart
- Thirst
- Larynx, Pharynx
- Hunger
- Adrenal Gland
- High Blood Pressure
- Lungs
- Hormonal Secretion (Endocrine)
- Rising Blood Pressure
- Tooth Analgesia (Upper Teeth)
- Tooth Analgesia (Lower Teeth)
- Nervousness
- Tonsils
- Ovary Secretion
- Subcortex
- Hypothalamus
- Excitement Point
- Testicular Secretion
- Antihistamine
- Parotid
- Asthma
- Brain
- Pituitary
- Thyroid Gland
- Hepatitis
- Muscle Relaxation
- Tonsils
- Mammary Gland
- Appendix
- Lumbago Point
- Heat Point
- Liver
- Low Back Pain
- Pelvic Cavity
- Low Blood Pressure
- Liver
- Appendix
- Tonsils
- Allergy

M	Mouth	LI	Large Intestine	Pan	Pancreas, Gall Bladder
E	Esophagus	Pr	Prostate	Liv	Liver
CO	Cardiac Orifice	Bl	Bladder	Spl	Spleen
St	Stomach	Ur	Ureter	H	Heart
SI	Small Intestine	Kid	Kidney	W	Windpipe, Trachea

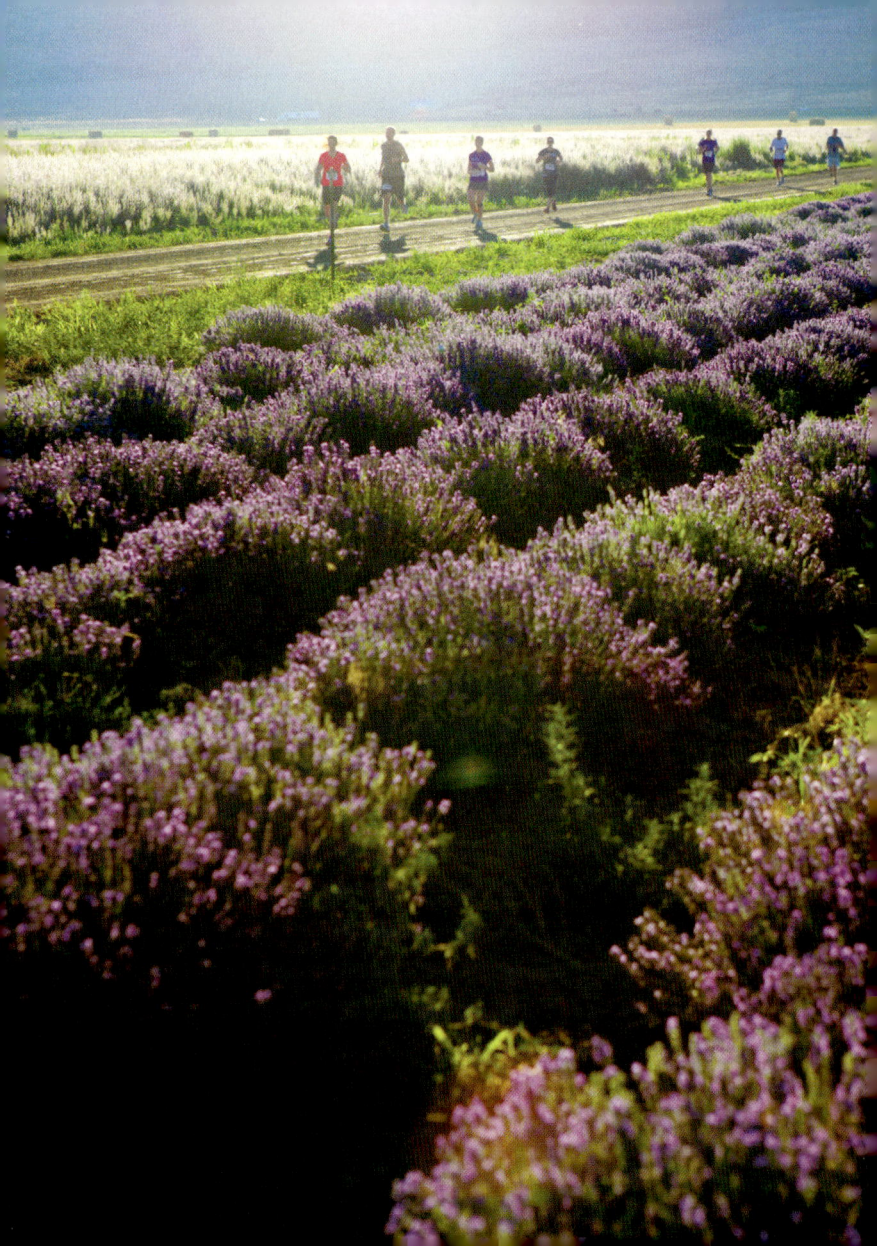

Emotional Response with Essential Oils 8

Today, we live in a society of emotional turmoil. There is more focus on emotional behavior and psychological conditions of the body now than at any time in our history. Many doctors are recognizing the possibility that a number of diseases are caused by emotional problems that link back to infancy and perhaps even to the womb. These emotional problems may have compromised our immune system or genetic structuring, causing children to become allergic to something that the mother ingested while pregnant.

Essential oils play an important role in assisting people to move beyond these emotional barriers. The aldehydes and esters of certain essential oils are very calming and sedating to the central nervous system (including both the sympathetic and parasympathetic systems). These substances allow us to relax instead of letting anxiety build up in our body. Anxiety creates an acidic condition that activates the transcript enzyme which then transcribes that anxiety on the RNA template and stores it in the DNA. That emotion then becomes a predominant factor in our lives from that moment on.

When we encounter an emotionally charged situation, instead of being overwhelmed by it, we can diffuse essential oils, put them in our bath, or wear them as cologne. The aromatic molecules will absorb into the bloodstream from the nasal cavity to the limbic system. They will activate the amygdala (the memory center for fear and trauma) and sedate and relax the sympathetic/parasympathetic system. The oils help support the body in minimizing the acid that is created so that it does not initiate a reaction with the transcript enzyme.

Because essential oils affect the amygdala and pineal gland in the brain, they can help the mind and body by releasing emotional trauma and sharpening focus.

People have many distractions in today's fast-paced world. Essential oils may assist people to stay centered in their goals. Those who are struggling to retain or remember information can breathe the essential oils of peppermint, cardamom, or rosemary to stimulate the brain and memory functions for better concentration. Those who find it difficult to stay focused can breathe the essential oils of galbanum, frankincense, sandalwood, and melissa. These oils are extremely beneficial for clarifying one's purpose. The blend Gathering will also bring focus to people's minds. For emotional clearing and release, the combination of essential oils called Trauma Life is especially helpful.

Oils For Emotional Applications

ABUSE
Single Oils: Geranium, ylang ylang, sandalwood.
Blends: SARA, Hope, Joy, Peace & Calming, Inner Child, Grounding, Trauma Life, Valor, Forgiveness, White Angelica

AGITATION
Single Oils: Bergamot, cedarwood, clary sage, frankincense, geranium, juniper, lavender, myrrh, marjoram, rosewood, rose, ylang ylang, sandalwood.
Blends: Peace & Calming, Joy, Valor, Harmony, Forgiveness, Chivalry

ANGER
Single Oils: Bergamot, cedarwood, Roman chamomile, frankincense, lavender, lemon, marjoram, myrrh, orange, rose, sandalwood, ylang ylang.
Blends: Release, Valor, Sacred Mountain, Joy, Harmony, Hope, Forgiveness, Present Time, Trauma Life, Surrender, Christmas Spirit, White Angelica

ANXIETY
Single Oils: Orange, Roman chamomile, ylang ylang, lavender.
Blends: Valor, Hope, Peace & Calming, Present Time, Joy, Citrus Fresh, Surrender, Believe

APATHY
Single Oils: Frankincense, geranium, marjoram, jasmine, orange, peppermint, rosewood, rose, sandalwood, thyme, ylang ylang
Blends: Joy, Harmony, Valor, 3 Wise Men, Hope, White Angelica, Motivation, Passion, Highest Potential

ARGUMENTATIVE
Single Oils: Cedarwood, Roman chamomile, eucalyptus, frankincense, jasmine, orange, thyme, ylang ylang.
Blends: Peace & Calming, Joy, Harmony, Hope, Valor, Acceptance, Humility, Surrender, Release, Chivalry

BOREDOM
Single Oils: Cedarwood, spruce, Roman chamomile, cypress, frankincense, juniper, lavender, rosemary, sandalwood, thyme, ylang ylang, black pepper.
Blends: Dream Catcher, Motivation, Valor, Awaken, Passion, Gathering, En-R-Gee

CONCENTRATION
Single Oils: Cedarwood, cypress, juniper, lavender, lemon, basil, helichrysum, myrrh, orange, peppermint, rosemary, sandalwood, ylang ylang.
Blends: Clarity, Awaken, Gathering, Dream Catcher, Magnify Your Purpose, Brain Power

CONFUSION
Single Oils: Cedarwood, spruce, cypress, peppermint, frankincense, geranium, ginger, juniper, marjoram, jasmine, rose, rosewood, rosemary, basil, sandalwood, thyme, ylang ylang.
Blends: Clarity, Harmony, Valor, Present Time, Awaken, Brain Power, Gathering, Grounding

DAY-DREAMING
Single Oils: Ginger, spruce, lavender, helichrysum, lemon, myrrh, peppermint, rosewood, rose, rosemary, sandalwood, thyme, ylang ylang.
Blends: Sacred Mountain, Gathering, Valor, Harmony, Present Time, Dream Catcher, 3 Wise Men, Magnify Your Purpose, Envision, Brain Power, Highest Potential

DEPRESSION
Single Oils: Frankincense, lemon, sandalwood, geranium, lavender, angelica, orange, grapefruit, ylang ylang.
Blends: Valor, Motivation, Passion, Hope, Joy, Brain Power, Present Time, Envision, Sacred Mountain, Harmony, Highest Potential

DESPAIR
Single Oils: Cedarwood, spruce, clary sage, frankincense, lavender, geranium, lemon, orange, lemongrass, peppermint, spearmint, rosemary, sandalwood, thyme, ylang ylang.
Blends: Joy, Valor, Harmony, Hope, Gathering, Grounding, Forgiveness, Motivation

DESPONDENCY
Single Oils: Bergamot, clary sage, cypress, geranium, ginger, orange, rose, rosewood, sandalwood, ylang ylang.
Blends: Peace & Calming, Inspiration, Harmony, Valor, Hope, Joy, Present Time, Gathering, Inner Child, Trauma Life, Envision, Chivalry

DISAPPOINTMENT
Single Oils: Clary sage, frankincense, geranium, ginger, juniper, lavender, spruce, orange, thyme, ylang ylang.
Blends: Hope, Joy, Valor, Present Time, Harmony, Dream Catcher, Gathering, Legacy, Magnify Your Purpose, Passion, Motivation

DISCOURAGEMENT
Single Oils: Bergamot, cedarwood, frankincense, geranium, juniper, lavender, lemon, orange, spruce, rosewood, sandalwood.
Blends: Valor, Sacred Mountain, Hope, Joy, Dream Catcher, Into the Future, Legacy, Magnify Your Purpose, Envision, Believe

FEAR
Single Oils: Bergamot, clary sage, Roman chamomile, cypress, geranium, juniper, marjoram, myrrh, spruce, orange, sandalwood, rose, ylang ylang.
Blends: Valor, Present Time, Hope, white Angelica, Trauma Life, Gratitude, Highest Potential

FORGETFULNESS
Single Oils: Cedarwood, Roman chamomile, frankincense, rosemary, basil, sandalwood, peppermint, thyme, ylang ylang.
Blends: Clarity, Valor, Present Time, Gathering, 3 Wise Men, Dream Catcher, Acceptance, Brain Power, Highest Potential

FRUSTRATION
Single Oils: Roman chamomile, clary sage, frankincense, ginger, juniper, lavender, lemon, orange, peppermint, thyme, ylang ylang, spruce.
Blends: Valor, Hope, Present Time, Sacred Mountain, 3 Wise Men, Humility, Peace & Calming, Surrender, Live With Passion, Gratitude

GRIEF/SORROW
Single Oils: Bergamot, Roman chamomile, clary sage, *Eucalyptus globulus*, juniper, lavender.
Blends: Valor, Release, Inspiration, Inner Child, Gathering, Harmony, Present Time, Magnify Your Purpose

GUILT
Single Oils: Roman chamomile, cypress, juniper, lemon, marjoram, geranium, rose, frankincense, sandalwood, spruce, thyme.
Blends: Valor, Release, Inspiration, Inner Child, Gathering, Harmony, Present Time, Magnify Your Purpose, Gratitude

IRRITABILITY
Single Oils: All oils except eucalyptus, peppermint, black pepper.
Blends: Valor, Hope, Peace & Calming, Surrender, Forgiveness, Present Time, Inspiration

JEALOUSY
Single Oils: Bergamot, *Eucalyptus globulus*, frankincense, lemon, marjoram, orange, rose, rosemary, thyme.
Blends: Valor, Sacred Mountain, White Angelica, Joy, Harmony, Humility, Forgiveness, Surrender, Release, Gratitude

MOOD SWINGS
Single Oils: Bergamot, clary sage, sage, geranium, juniper, fennel, lavender, peppermint, rose, jasmine, rosemary, lemon, sandalwood, spruce, yarrow, ylang ylang.
Blends: Peace & Calming, Gathering, Valor, Dragon Time, Mister, Harmony, Joy, Present Time, Envision, Magnify Your Purpose, Brain Power

OBSESSIVENESS
Single Oils: Clary sage, cypress, geranium, lavender, marjoram, rose, sandalwood, ylang ylang, helichrysum.
Blends: Sacred Mountain, Valor, Forgiveness, Acceptance, Humility, Inner Child, Present Time, Awaken, Motivation, Surrender, Live With Passion

PANIC
Single Oils: Bergamot, Roman chamomile, frankincense, lavender, marjoram, wintergreen or birch, myrrh, rosemary, sandalwood, thyme, ylang ylang, spruce.
Blends: Harmony, Valor, Gathering, White Angelica, Peace & Calming, Trauma Life, Awaken, Grounding, Believe

RESENTMENT
Single Oils: Jasmine, rose, tansy.
Blends: Forgiveness, Harmony, Humility, White Angelica, Surrender, Joy

RESTLESSNESS
Single Oils: Angelica, bergamot, cedarwood, basil, frankincense, geranium, lavender, orange, rose, rosewood, ylang ylang, spruce, valerian
Blends: Peace & Calming, Sacred Mountain, Gathering, Valor, Harmony, Inspiration, Acceptance, Surrender

SHOCK
Single Oils: Helichrysum, basil, Roman chamomile, myrrh, ylang ylang, rosemary CT cineol.
Blends: Clarity, Valor, Inspiration, Joy, Grounding, Trauma Life, Brain Power, Highest Potential, Australian Blue

Personal Usage Reference 8

How Essential Oils Work

Essential oils can work through inhalation, ingestion, topical application, or rectal/vaginal retention.

Although topical use is perhaps best known, dietary use of essential oils may be one of the most effective ways of unlocking their health benefits. Many essential oils have been used as food flavorings or as a part of patent medicines for centuries, endowing them with a long history of safe use. Recent research suggests that certain high ORAC essential oils act as potent antioxidants that can actually raise antioxidant levels in the body and prevent premature aging.

Many of the oils listed in this section are classified as "GRAS" by the U.S. Food and Drug Administration. This means they are "generally regarded as safe" for human consumption.

Topical application is probably the most common means of using essential oils. According to researcher Jean Valnet, M.D., an essential oil that is directly applied to the skin can pass into the bloodstream and diffuse throughout the tissues in 20 minutes or less. More recent studies have also documented the ability of essential oils to penetrate the stratum corneum (the upper layer of skin) to reach the subdermal tissues and blood vessels beneath.[1,2]

Some of the compounds in essential oils that work synergistically to enhance permeation include alpha-pinene (frankincense, valerian, basil, cistus), beta-pinene (galbanum, hyssop, fir, rosemary), alpha-terpineol (bay laurel, *Melaleuca ericifolia*, ravensara), 1,8-cineole (*Eucalyptus globulus, E. radiata, E. dives*, rosemary) and d-limonene (white fir, tangerine, orange, lemon, grapefruit).

Inhalation is an effective means of therapeutically using and delivering an essential oil. The fragrance of an essential oil can have a direct influence on both the body and mind due to its ability to stimulate the brain's limbic system (a group of subcortical structures including the hypothalamus, the hippocampus, and the amygdala). This can produce powerful effects that can effect everything from emotional balance and energy levels to appetite control, heart, and immune function.

Some researchers believe that the inhalation of an essential oil can also enhance the body's frequency, which can have a direct impact on disease. Disease and emotional trauma foster a negative frequency that may be disrupted or broken by essential oils. Oils with higher frequencies can elevate the entire frequency of the body whether topically or orally administered, thereby creating an internal environment that opposes the establishment of some disease conditions.

When to Mix Oils and Blends

The essential oils and blends that are listed for a specific condition can be used either separately or together. By combining a single oil with another recommended single oil or blend, a synergistic or additive effect is produced that results in stronger total effect than the sum of the actions produced by each oil or blend separately.

As a rule, when a list of oils or blends is recommended and does not list specific quantities, usually 1-3 drops of each oil should be used. For example, if the list reads, "Lavender, lemongrass, marjoram, ginger," this means that 1 drop of lavender should be mixed with one drop of any 2-4 of these oils for a synergistic blend. Normally it is best to avoid using more than 3 oils in any given blend at a time.

How to Choose an Essential Oil

The essential oils listed for a specific condition are not designed to be a comprehensive or complete list; they are merely a starting point. Other oils that are not listed can also be effective.

In addition, essential oils are not listed in any particular order. This is because one oil might be more compatible with one person's unique body chemistry than another's for aromatic purposes and skin sensitivity, not necessarily for physical response. If results are not felt within several minutes, try another oil, blend, or combination, on the next application.

How to Use Essential Oils

Essential oils should be used in moderation as they are highly concentrated. In most cases, one or two drops is sufficient to produce significant effects. It is strongly recommended that most essential oils be diluted in vegetable oil prior to either topical or internal application (particularly if you have not used essential oils previously).

When using essential oils topically, first do a skin test with 1 drop of essential oil on the inside of the upper arm. Use no more than 10 to 20 drops during one topical application.

Many essential oils can be used as dietary supplements. All essential oils should be diluted prior to oral use unless directed by a physician or one trained in the oral use of essential oils. No more than 2-4 drops should be consumed at one time (in a single serving) unless indicated otherwise. The simplest way to dilute essential oils for ingestion is to mix a drop in a teaspoon of honey (do not give honey to children age 1 or under) or a cup of almond or rice milk. If taste is a problem, oils can be diluted 50-50, placed in a gelatin capsule and swallowed.

When using essential oils always increase fluid intake because the oils can accelerate the detoxification process in the body. If you are not taking in adequate fluids, toxins could recirculate causing nausea, headaches, etc.

Avoid Petrochemicals

Exercise caution when applying essential oils to skin that has been exposed to cosmetics, personal care products, or soaps and cleansers containing synthetic or petroleum-based chemicals. Essential oils may react with such chemicals and cause skin irritation, nausea, or headaches. Essential oils can also react with toxins built up in the body from chemicals in food, water, and the work environment. If you experience a reaction to essential oils, temporarily discontinue their use and start an internal cleansing program (30 days using the Cleansing Trio) before resuming regular use of essential oils.

Tip on Safe Use:

Skin-test the diluted essential oil on a small patch of skin. If any redness or irritation results, cleanse skin thoroughly and reapply. If skin irritation persists, discontinue using that oil or oil blend.

How to Use This Reference Guide

This Guide has two parts, which must be used together in order to correctly and safely develop regimens for essential oil application.

The first part of the guide is a list of 18 standard application methods found on the next pages 69 and 70. For each of these applications, dilution rates, mixtures and procedures are listed in detail. These applications are listed in five basic groups: TOPICAL, RETENTION, ORAL, INGESTION and INHALATION. The details of each application method are listed here at the beginning of this chapter to avoid unnecessary repetition throughout the remainder of the chapter. It is recommended that you read through all these application methods to familiarize yourself with them before using this guide.

The second part of the guide, comprising the rest of the chapter, includes application suggestions for over 300 different illnesses and injuries with single essential oils, blends, dietary supplements and topical treatments, which are appropriate for those conditions. Each topic contains some or all of the following headings pointing to the products to use and how to use them:

Singles	Dietary Supplements
Blends	Topical Treatments
EO Applications	Other

Within each 'EO Applications' heading is a listing of keywords indicating which of the 18 application methods are appropriate and effective for that condition. It is important to note that abbreviated keywords are listed in the body of this guide. Readers must return to the application methods explanations on pages 69 and 70 to get the full detail of how to use the oils in each particular application method.

As explained in earlier sections of this book, essential oils are very concentrated natural substances—easily 100 times more concentrated than the natural herbs they come from. So dilution of an essential oil is a very important aspect of using it therapeutically. Some essential oils are so mild that dilution is simply not necessary, even for use on infants. Others are so strong that dilution is mandatory. (See Appendix A for a list of recommended safe dilutions for all the oils mentioned in this book).

A Sample Lookup

Here is an example of how to develop an application program using the two parts of the guide. Let's say that you are experiencing a sore throat and want to know what you can do to treat that condition with the products in this reference book.

Step 1: Locate the disease/injury topic alphabetically in the Personal Usage Guide

In this case, the heading you are looking for is a subhead located under the main heading of THROAT INFECTIONS. It is found on page 211.

Step 2: Note the recommended essential oils – both singles and blends – to be used.

In this case, the section on Sore Throat lists 10 single oils, 3 standard blends, and 2 custom blends that all may be helpful when used according to the methods listed in the EO Applications section.

Although this listing shows 15 possible oils, only 1-3 oils or blends should be used at any given time. You will need to select 1-3 oils or blends that you will use based on availability, budget and aroma (for example, some oils are strong enough that you may not want to be using or wearing them at work.)

Step 3: Make a list of the recommended essential oil (EO) applications listed for the illness/injury you are checking.

In this case, under the THROAT INFECTIONS heading, quite a variety of methods is listed. Altogether 10 different application methods are listed, ranging from Direct Inhalation to Raindrop Technique. (Not all conditions have this many application methods. Most recommend only one or two.) The 10 listed application methods for a sore throat are intended to show all possible application methods for using essential oils in treating that condition.

<u>Normally, only 1-3 different applications should be used at any given time.</u> This is a matter of both convenience and safety. If someone were to attempt all 10 applications for a sore throat at once, it would require an enormous investment of time, be extremely inconvenient and would put more essential oil in that person's body than is needed or helpful.

Again, cross check the keyword application method descriptions under each disease heading with the detailed application descriptions on the next two pages. This will provided important additional information, such as dilution rates and frequency of application.

Step 4: Note any additional dietary supplements and topical treatments listed for the condition.

Step 5: Make a written personal regimen that includes the 1-3 oils you have selected, the 1-3 EO application methods you will be using, the dietary supplements and the topical treatments, if any.

This will save you from having to look up everything again each time you do your applications.

Step 6: Make sure you understand the proper essential oil dilution levels.

If you do not properly link oils with their application method details, you could make a mistake here. For example, one of the applications for sore throat is Direct Inhalation, in which the oils are used in their 'neat,' or undiluted state. However, for Topical Application to the skin, the dilution rate is 50-50 or 1 part essential oil to 1 part vegetable oil. (V6 Oil Complex)

Step 7: Be faithful with your regimen.

Therapeutic-grade essential oils are wonderful, natural, healing substances, and they work extremely well with the body's own defenses to solve problems. However, they are not drugs, and they may not always work in seconds, or even minutes. Essential Oils will enhance and speed up the benefits of dietary supplements, but it is still a 'natural' process. Sometimes it can take hours or even days to see the improvement.

The 18 Basic Essential Oil Application Methods

NOTE: Please read this information carefully as all directions in the following personal guide section will refer to the 18 methods outlined here.

TOPICAL (On the skin surface)

- NEAT: Apply neat (undiluted) as directed to affected area. (See Appendix A)
- DILUTE 50-50: 1 part essential oil (s) to 1 part V6 Oil Complex. (See Appendix A)
- DILUTE 20-80: 1 part essential oil(s) to 4 parts V6 Oil Complex. (See Appendix A)
- VITA FLEX: Apply 1-3 drops neat to the Vita Flex points on the feet as directed. See Vita Flex chart found in Chapter 4 for point locations.
- COMPRESS: Dilute 1 part essential oil(s) with 4 parts V6 Oil Complex and apply 8-10 drops on affected area. Cover with a HOT, moist hand towel. Then cover the moist towel with a dry towel for 10-15 minutes. Can also use a cool, moist hand towel instead of a hot one, to create a COLD compress.
- BATH SALT: Mix thoroughly 10-15 drops of essential oil into 2 tablespoons of Epsom salts or baking soda. Dissolve in warm bathwater as tub is filling and soak for at least 20 minutes before using soap or shampoo; or place in special shower head designed to hold salt/essential oil mixture and shower for 10 minutes.
- BODY MASSAGE: Apply diluted in a 20:80 ratio (1 part essential oils to 4 parts V6 Oil Complex) in a full-body massage.
- RAINDROP Technique: (See Chapter 5)

RETENTION

- RECTAL: Dilute the recommended essential oil(s) in 40:60 ratio (4 parts essential oil to 6 parts V6 Oil Complex), insert 1-2 tablespoons in rectum with a bulb syringe and retain up to 8 hours or overnight.

    Caution: The outer skin surrounding the anus is usually more sensitive to the oil mixture than internal tissues. Be very careful when inserting the oils, to keep them from touching the outside skin. One way to do this is to insert the oils using 2-4 gelatin capsules lubricated with olive oil or V6 Oil Complex.

- TAMPON: Dilute the recommended essential oil(s) in 40:60 ratio (4 parts essential oil to 6 parts V6 Oil Complex). Apply 1-2 tablespoons to a tampon and insert into vagina (for internal infection) OR apply to a sanitary pad (for external lesions). Retain up to 8 hours or overnight. Use only tampons or sanitary pads made with non-perfumed, non-scented organic cotton.

ORAL

- GARGLE: Add 2-3 drops essential oil with 4 tablespoons purified water, shake or mix vigorously. Gargle for 30 seconds.
- TONGUE: Apply 1 drop of essential oil neat to the back of the tongue with cotton swab or fingertip. Retain, allowing oil to combine with saliva, for at least 1 minute, then swallow. Note: this should NOT be done with essential oils which have a **20-80** application code. (See Appendix A)

INHALATION

- **DIFFUSION:** Diffuse neat in a cold-air diffuser (cold air diffusers are not designed to handle vegetable oils because they are thicker and may clog the diffuser mechanism).

- **DIRECT:** Apply 2-3 drops of essential oil(s) to the palm of one hand; rub palms together; cup hands over nose and mouth (being careful not to touch the skin near your eyes) and inhale vapors deeply 6-8 times.

- **VAPOR:** Run hot, steaming water into a sink or large bowl. Water should be at least 2 inches deep to retain heat for a few minutes. Drape a towel over your head, covering the hot water also, enclosing your face over the steaming water. Add 3-6 drops of essential oils(s) into the hot water. Inhale vapors as deeply as possible several times, through the nose, as they rise with the steam. Recharge vapors with additional hot water.

INGESTION

- **CAPSULE:** Unless directed otherwise, use a clean medicine dropper to fill the larger half of an empty gelatin capsule (available at health food stores) half-way with essential oil(s); then fill the remainder with V6 Advanced Oil Complex or a high quality cold-pressed vegetable oil, seal with the other half of the gel cap and take as directed.

    There are two basic dosages used for capsules, indicated by capsule size. '00' size capsules (which contain a 400 mg dose when filled with a 50-50 dilution of essential oil) and '0' size capsules (which contain a 200 mg dose when filled with a 50-50 dilution of essential oil). If '0' size capsules are not readily available, you can half fill '00' size capsules.

- **RICE MILK:** Add the essential oil to rice milk and take as directed. Use 3-5 drops in 1/2 cup of rice milk. Goat milk may be substituted for rice milk.

- **SYRUP:** Add the essential oil to Agave nectar or Grade B Maple Syrup. Use 3 drops in 1 tsp. maple syrup. Hold in mouth for 30 seconds before swallowing. Agave nectar (a low-glycemic natural sweetener derived from the Agave plant) seems to work more effectively than maple syrup.

ABSCESS (Skin)
(See SKIN DISORDERS)

ABSENTMINDEDNESS

Clinical studies on Ningxia wolfberry *(Lycium barbarum)* have shown that it has an anti-senility effect. Clinical studies at University of Colorado Health Sciences Center found that high antioxidant foods such as spinach (found in JuvaPower) and blueberry (found in Berry Young Juice) dramatically improved learning and cognition.[3,4] (See BRAIN DISORDERS)

Single Oils:
Peppermint, cardamom, vetiver, frankincense, sandalwood, rosemary, basil

Blends:
Clarity, Brain Power, M-Grain

EO Applications:
INHALATION:
DIFFUSION, 15 min every 2 hours, as needed
DIRECT, 2-4 times daily, as needed
TOPICAL:
NEAT, 1-2 drops on temples and/or back of neck, as needed.

Dietary Supplementation:
Power Meal, Ultra Young, Sulfurzyme, VitaGreen, Essential Omegas, Mineral Essence, JuvaPower/Spice, Berry Young Juice.

ABUSE (mental and physical)

The trauma from mental and physical abuse can result in self-defeating behavior that can undermine success later in life. Through their powerful effect on the limbic system of the brain (the center or stored memories and emotions), essential oils can help release pent-up trauma, emotions, or memories.

Single Oils:
Geranium, sandalwood, or melissa.

Blends:
SARA, Trauma Life, Release, Acceptance, Forgiveness, Surrender, Humility, Joy, White Angelica, Inner Child, Harmony, Hope, Brain Power, Citrus Fresh, Christmas Spirit, Valor

EO Applications:
INHALATION:
DIFFUSION, 15 min. every 2 hours as needed
DIRECT, 2-3 times daily, as needed
TOPICAL:
NEAT, 1-2 drops on temples and/or back of neck as needed. Also apply 2-3 drops on the Vita Flex liver point of the right foot. Also apply a trace under the nose.

Dietary Supplementation:
Power Meal, Super C, Super C Chewable, Super B

Other:

Physical Abuse: Begin with application of 2-3 drops Forgiveness, unless suicidal. It is most effective around the navel. Follow with 1-2 drops Release over the Vita Flex points, especially the liver point of right foot, and under the nose.

Parental, Sexual or Ritual Abuse: 1-3 drops SARA over the area where abuse took place; then Forgiveness, Trauma Life, Release, Joy, or Present Time.

Spousal Abuse: Use Forgiveness, Trauma Life, Acceptance, Release, Valor, Joy, or Envision.

Feelings of Revenge: 1-2 drops of Surrender on the sternum over the heart, 2-3 drops of Present Time on the thymus, and 2-3 drops Forgiveness over navel.

Suicidal: 2 drops Hope on rim of ears. Melissa, Brain Power, or Present Time may be beneficial also.

Protection/Balance: 1-2 drops of White Angelica on each shoulder, 1-2 drops Harmony over thymus and on energy centers or chakras of the body.

ACID/ALKALINE BALANCE
(See FUNGAL INFECTIONS, ACIDOSIS, and ALKALOSIS)

ACIDOSIS
(See FUNGAL INFECTIONS)

Acidosis is a condition where the pH of the intestinal tract and the blood serum become excessively acidic. This can promote the growth of pathogenic fungi like candida and exacerbate yeast infections. Acidic blood can stress the liver and eventually lead to many forms of chronic and degenerative diseases.

To raise pH, avoid acid-ash foods, overuse of antibiotics, and monitor the pH of the saliva (6.4-6.5) and blood (7.3-7.6).

Single Oils:
Peppermint, lemon

Blends:
Di-Tone

EO Applications:
 INGESTION:
   CAPSULE, 00 Size, 2 daily between meals, if possible, otherwise with meals.

Dietary Supplementation:
Royaldophilus, AlkaLime, Coral Sea, Mega Cal, JuvaPower/Spice, Essentialzyme, Polyzyme, VitaGreen, Wolfberry Crisp, BerryGize Bar

Other Regimens:

Take Royaldophilus and Polyzyme with peppermint until acid level is balanced, then add Essentialzyme.

To reduce acid indigestion and prevent fermentation that can contribute to bad dreams and interrupted sleep: 1 tsp. AlkaLime in water before bedtime.

To raise pH, take 2-6 capsules of VitaGreen 3 times daily and take 1 tsp. AlkaLime in water one hour before or two hours after meals each day. For maintenance, take 1 tsp. AlkaLime once per week.

To stimulate enzymatic action in the digestive tract: Mix together or use individually, raw carrot juice, alfalfa, trace minerals, and papaya.

ACNE
(See SKIN DISORDERS)

A.D.D.
(See ATTENTION DEFICIT DISORDER)

ADDICTIONS

Many food and chemical dependencies, such as addictions to tobacco, caffeine, drugs, alcohol, and sugar may originate in the liver. Cleansing and detoxifying the liver is a crucial first step toward breaking free of these addictions. Increasing intake of alkaline calcium can help bind bile acids and prevent fatty liver. A colon and tissue cleanse is also important.

Using stevia, stevioside, or FOS can help reduce sugar cravings. Stevia is a supersweet noncaloric extract derived from an ancient South American herb, while FOS is a sweet-tasting indigestible sugar derived from chicory roots and Jerusalem artichokes with no calories and important health benefits.

Trace mineral and mineral deficiencies can also play a part in some addictions. Magnesium, potassium, calcium, and zinc should all be included in the diet.

Blends:
Harmony, Peace & Calming, JuvaCleanse, JuvaFlex

EO Applications:
 INHALATION:
   DIFFUSION, 15 min every 2 hours as needed
   DIRECT, 2-3 times daily, as needed
 TOPICAL:
   NEAT, 1-2 drops on temples and/or back of neck 4 times daily
   COMPRESS, warm, over liver

Dietary Supplementation:
JuvaTone, JuvaPower/Spice, Stevia, Wolfberry Crisp, Mineral Essence, Coral Sea, SuperCal, Mega Cal, Stevia Select, Comfort-Tone, Essentialzyme, ICP
(See LIVER and SMOKING CESSATION)

ADDISON'S DISEASE
(See ADRENAL GLAND IMBALANCE)

ADRENAL GLAND IMBALANCE

The adrenal glands consist of two sections: An inner part called the medulla produces stress hormones and an outer part called the cortex secretes critical hormones called glucocorticoids and aldosterone. Because of these hormones, the cortex has a far greater impact on overall health than the medulla does.

Why are aldosterone and glucocorticoids so important? Because they directly affect blood pressure and mineral content and help regulate the conversion of carbohydrates into energy.

Addison's Disease

In cases like Addison's disease, adrenal cortex hormones are no longer produced or severely limited. This can lead to life-threatening fluid and mineral loss unless these hormones are replaced.

Because Addison's disease is an autoimmune disease in which the body's own immune cells destroy the adrenal glands, it may be treated with MSM. MSM is an important source of organic sulfur that has been shown to have positive effects with many types of autoimmune diseases, including lupus, arthritis, and fibromyalgia.

If adrenal insufficiency is accompanied by a lack of thyroid hormone, the condition is known as Schmidt's syndrome.

Symptoms:
- Severe fatigue
- Lightheadedness when standing
- Nausea
- Depression/irritability
- Craving salty foods
- Loss of appetite
- Muscle spasms
- Dark, tan-colored skin

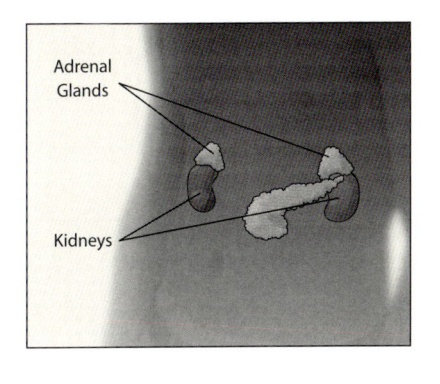

Essential oils can play a part in correcting deficiencies in adrenal cortex function. Nutmeg, for example, has adrenal-like activity that raises energy levels.

Single Oils:
Nutmeg, sage, clove, rosemary, basil

Blends:
EndoFlex, Joy, En-R-Gee

EO Applications:
  TOPICAL:
  COMPRESS, warm, over the adrenal gland area (on back, over the kidneys)
  INGESTION:
  CAPSULE, 00 size, 2 daily

Other:
The following essential oil blend recipe is designed to be used with a compress over the adrenal area:
- 3 drops clove
- 3 drops nutmeg
- 7 drops rosemary
- 20 drops massage oil or V-6 Mixing Oil.

Dietary Supplementation:
Thyromin, VitaGreen, Royal Essence, Super B, Master Formula, Mineral Essence

Other:
Supplementation regimen for adrenal support
- Thyromin: 1 immediately after awakening.
- Super B: 1 after meals. If you experience a niacin flush (skin becoming red and itchy for about 15 minutes), use only 1/2 of a tablet.
- Master Formula: 2-6 tablets, 3 times daily according to blood type and need.

Cushing's disease

Cushing's disease is the opposite of Addison's disease. It is characterized by the overproduction of adrenal cortex hormones. While these hormones are crucial to sound health in normal amounts, their unchecked overproduction can cause as much harm as their underproduction. This results in the following symptoms:
- Slow wound healing
- Low resistance to infection
- Obesity
- Acne
- Moon-shaped face
- Easily-bruised skin
- Weak or wasted muscles
- Osteoporosis

Supporting the Adrenal Glands

Add essential oils to 1/4 teaspoon of massage oil and apply as a warm compress over the adrenal glands (located on top of the kidneys).

- 3 drops clove
- 3 drops nutmeg
- 7 drops rosemary

Although Cushing's disease can be caused by a malfunction in the pituitary, it is usually triggered by excessive use of immune-suppressing corticosteroid medications—such as those used for asthma and arthritis. Once these are discontinued, the disease often abates.

Single Oils:
Lemon, peppermint, fleabane, nutmeg

Blends:
ImmuPower, Thieves, Endoflex

EO Applications:
TOPICAL:
   COMPRESS, warm, over adrenal area (on back, over kidneys)
INGESTION:
   CAPSULE, 00 size, 2 daily

Dietary Supplementation:
Exodus, ImmuPro, ImmuneTune

AGE-RELATED MACULAR DEGENERATION (AMD)

AMD is one of the most common causes of blindness among people over 60 years of age. In fact 30% of all people over 70 years of age suffer to some degree from this disease. The most common form of the disease is DRY in which macular cells degenerate irreversibly. The WET form of the disease is marked by abnormal blood vessel growth that results in macula-damaging blood leaks. The disease results in a steady loss of central vision until eyesight is totally impaired.

For dry AMD, the best prevention will be foods rich in antioxidants and carotenoids. The Ningxia wolfberry, the highest known antioxidant food, is also extremely high in lutein, which is vital for preserving eye health. Other foods rich in carotenoids that are also powerful antioxidants include blueberries and spinach. Clove oil, the highest known antioxidant nutrient, can also be a front line treatment.

Single Oils:
Clove

Blends:
Longevity
EO Applications:
Capsule, 00 size, 1 daily
Dietary Supplementation:
Longevity Capsules, ImmuPro, Berry Young Juice, Wolfberry Crisp, Super C Chewable

AGENT ORANGE EXPOSURE
Single Oils:
Ledum, German chamomile, carrot seed
Blends:
JuvaFlex, JuvaCleanse, EndoFlex
EO Applications:
TOPICAL:
NEAT, 4-6 drops JuvaFlex, JuvaCleanse over liver area and 2-4 drops of EndoFlex over adrenal gland area, 2 times daily
COMPRESS, warm, over liver area, 1-2 times daily
Dietary Supplementation:
ImmuPro, ImmuneTune, Cleansing Trio, JuvaTone, Thyromin
Other:
The following is a regimen for liver cleansing support to aid in relieving effects of toxic exposure:
- Essentialzyme: 3 servings daily
- ComforTone, ICP, and JuvaTone: 3 servings daily
- ImmuneTune: 4 servings daily
- Rub 3 drops EndoFlex on the thyroid (hollow at base-front of neck) and 3 drops over the kidneys 3 times daily. Also rub 3 drops on the thyroid and kidney Vita Flex points of the feet.
- After 90 days on the program, gradually reduce the above amounts but stay on the program for a full year.
- Add 1 cup Epsom salts and 4 ounces of 35 percent food-grade hydrogen peroxide to bath water once daily.
- Take a 30-minute bath with 6 cups of Epsom salts per tub of water. Drink 3 glasses of Master Cleanse lemonade and 1 ounce of Berry Young Juice while bathing.

AGITATION
Single Oils:
Lavender, orange, Roman chamomile
Blends:
Peace & Calming, Forgiveness, Surrender, Joy
EO Applications:
INHALATION:
DIFFUSION, 15 min. every 2 hours, as needed
DIRECT, 2-3 times per day, as needed
TOPICAL:
NEAT, 1-2 drops on temples and/or back of neck
VITA FLEX, 1-2 drops on brain and heart points
Dietary Supplementation:
Super B, Super C, Super C Chewable, Super Cal.

AIDS (Acquired Immune Deficiency Syndrome)
The AIDS virus attacks and infects immune cells that are essential for life.

Essential oils such as lemon, cistus, thyme, and lavender have immune building properties. Other oils like cumin *(Cuminum cyminum)* have an inhibitory effect on viral replication. In May 1994, Dr. Radwan Farag of Cairo University demonstrated that cumin seed oil had an 88 to 92 percent inhibition effect against HIV, the virus responsible for AIDS. Other antiviral essential oils include oregano, frankincense, sandalwood, grapefruit, and tsuga.

Single Oils:
Cistus, lemon, cumin, blue cypress, sandalwood, tsuga, grapefruit, myrrh, frankincense

Blends:
Brain Power, Exodus II, Valor, Thieves, ImmuPower

EO Applications:
Essential oil regimen:
1. Valor and Thieves: 4-6 drops on feet daily for 3 weeks
2. Exodus II: 6-8 drops along spine 3 times weekly
3. ImmuPower: 6 drops daily in a capsule
4. Raindrop Technique: 2 times weekly

Dietary Supplementation:
Cleansing Trio, JuvaTone, Rehemogen, Thyromin, ImmuPro, ImmuneTune, VitaGreen, Sulfurzyme, Exodus, Super B, Berry Young Juice, Ultra Young, Mighty Mist

Other:
Supplementation regimen:
1. ImmuPro: Chew 4-8 tablets before going to bed; also take 2 in morning and 2 in afternoon.
2. Cleansing Trio for 120 days with JuvaTone.
3. ImmuGel: 1/2 tsp., 3 times daily. Hold in mouth for better absorption, swallow slowly.
4. Thyromin: Start with 2 at night, 1 in morning.
5. ImmuneTune: 6-8 capsules daily.
6. VitaGreen: 6-10 capsules daily.
7. Sulfurzyme: 1 tablespoon.
8. Exodus: Up to 18 capsules daily.
9. Super B: 1 tablet daily with a meal.
10. Ultra Young: 3 sprays on inside of each cheek, 4-5 times daily.
11. Eat 5-6 mini-meals daily, primarily Power Meal (3 times daily) and fish for protein. Do not eat beef or chicken for first 3-4 weeks to allow more energy for immune building.

ALCOHOLISM
(See also ADDICTIONS)

Single Oils:
Lavender, Roman chamomile, orange, helichrysum, elemi, rosemary

Blends:
JuvaFlex, JuvaCleanse, Forgiveness, Acceptance, Surrender, Motivation, Joy

EO Applications:
INHALATION:
DIFFUSION, 15 min every 2 hours as needed
DIRECT, 2-3 times daily, as needed
TOPICAL:
NEAT, 1-2 drops on temples and/or back of neck 4 times daily
COMPRESS, warm, over liver

Dietary Supplementation:
JuvaTone, JuvaPower/Spice, Cleansing Trio, Thyromin, Power Meal, Detoxyme, Mega Cal, Mineral Essence

ALKALOSIS
(See also ACIDOSIS)

Alkalosis is a condition where the pH of the intestinal tract and the blood becomes excessively alkaline. While moderate alkalinity is essential for good health, excessive alkalinity can cause problems and result in fatigue, depression, irritability, and sickness.

The best solution is to lower, or acidify, the internal pH of the body using a high protein diet. Ultrafiltered whey is the best solution for excess alkalinity (it is contained in Wheyfit and Berrygize Bar). Rudolf Wiley, Ph.D., recommends courses of action to accomplish this in

BioBalance: The Acid/Alkaline Solution to the Food-Mood-Health Puzzle.

Single Oils:
   Ginger, tarragon, anise
Blends:
   Di-Tone
EO Applications:
   INGESTION:
   CAPSULE, 00 Size, 2 daily between meals, if possible, otherwise with meals
Dietary Supplementation:
   Essentialzyme, Sulfurzyme, WheyFit, Wolfberry Crisp, Berrygize Bar

ALLERGIES

Allergies can be triggered by food, pollen, environmental chemicals, dander, dust, and insect bites and can impact:

   Respiration—wheezing, labored breathing
   Mouth—swelling of the lips or tongue, itching lips
   Digestive tract—diarrhea, vomiting, cramps
   Skin—rashes, dermatitis
   Nose—sneezing, congestion

Food Allergies

Food *allergies* are different from food *intolerances*. The former involve an immune system reaction, whereas the latter involves a gastrointestinal reaction (and is far more common). For example, peanuts often produce a lifelong allergy in adults due to peanut proteins being targeted by immune system antibodies as foreign invaders. In contrast, intolerance of pasteurized cow's milk that causes cramping and diarrhea is due to the inability to digest lactose (milk sugar) because of a lack of the enzyme lactase.

Food allergies are often associated with the consumption of peanuts, shellfish, nuts, wheat, cow's milk, eggs, and soy. Infants and children are far more susceptible to food allergies than adults, due to the immaturity of their immune and digestive systems.

A thorough intestinal cleansing is one of the best ways to combat most allergies. Start with the Cleansing Trio and JuvaTone.

Hay fever (allergic rhinitis)

Hay fever is an allergic reaction triggered by airborne allergens (pollen, animal hair, feathers, dust mites) that cause the release of histamines and subsequent inflammation of nasal passages and sinus-related areas. Allergies resemble asthma, which manifests in the chest and lungs.

Symptoms: Inflammation of the nasal passages, sinuses, and eyelids that causes sneezing, runny nose, watery, red, itchy eyes, and wheezing.

Single Oils:
   Lavender, ledum, German chamomile, Roman chamomile
Blends:
   Harmony, Valor, Juva Cleanse
EO Applications:
   INHALATION:
   DIFFUSION, 15 min every 2 hours, as needed
   DIRECT, 2-4 times daily, as needed
   INGESTION:
   CAPSULE, 00 size, 2 times daily
Dietary Supplementation:
Sulfurzyme, Detoxzyme, Essentialzyme, Polyzyme, Royaldophilus, VitaGreen, Cleansing Trio, JuvaTone

ALOPECIA AREATA (Hair Loss)

Alopecia is an inflammatory hair-loss disease that is the second-leading cause of baldness in the U.S. A randomized, double-blind study at the Aberdeen Royal Infirmary in Scotland found that certain essential oils were extremely effective in combating this disease. [5, 6]

Single Oils:
Thyme, rosemary, lavender, cedarwood
EO Applications:
  TOPICAL:
    DILUTE 20-80, (5 drops essential oils in 20 drops olive, grapeseed or fractionated coconut oil). Massage into scalp before sleep nightly.

ALUMINUM TOXICITY
(See METAL TOXICITY, Aluminum)

ALZHEIMER'S
(See BRAIN DISORDERS)

ANALGESIC

An 'analgesic' is defined as a compound that binds with a number of closely related specific receptors in the central nervous system to block the perception of pain or affect the emotional response to pain. A number of essential oils have analgesic properties.

Single Oils:
Peppermint, elemi, wintergreen/birch, clove, lavender, lemongrass, Idaho tansy

Blends:
PanAway, Thieves
Additional simple blends for pain relief:
1. Equal parts helichrysum and clove
2. Equal parts tea tree and rosemary
3. Equal parts wintergreen/birch, spruce and black pepper
4. 3 parts tea tree with 5 parts rosemary

EO Applications:
  TOPICAL:
    DILUTE 50-50, apply 4-6 drops on location, as needed
  Topical Treatments:
  Peppermint Cedarwood Moisturizing Bar Soap can be a topical treatment for mild pain.

ANEMIA
(See BLOOD DISORDERS)

ANEURYSM
(See also CARDIOVASCULAR CONDITIONS)

Aneurysms are weak spots on the blood vessel wall which balloon out and may eventually rupture. In cases of brain aneurysms, a bursting blood vessel can cause a hemorrhagic stroke, which can result in death or paralysis (with a fatality rate of over 50 percent).

See your physician for treatment immediately if you have, or suspect you have, an aneurysm.

Some essential oils and nutritional supplements support the cardiovascular system. Cypress strengthens capillary and vascular walls. Helichrysum helps dissolve blood clots.

Single Oils:
Helichrysum, sandalwood, Idaho tansy, cypress

Blends:
Aroma Life, Brain Power
Aneurysm blend:
- 5 drops of frankincense
- 1 drop helichrysum
- 1 drop cypress

EO Applications:
  TOPICAL:
    DILUTE 50-50, on affected area 3-5 times daily
  INHALATION:
    DIFFUSION, 15 minutes, 4-6 times daily
  INGESTION:
    CAPSULE, 00 size, 2 times daily

Dietary Supplementation:
Ultra Young, Essential Manna, Rehemogen

ANGINA
(See HEART)

ANOREXIA
(See ADDICTIONS)

While psychotherapy remains indispensable, the inhalation of essential oils may alter emotions enough to effect a change in the underlying psychology or disturbed-thinking patterns which supports this self-destructive behavior. This is accomplished by the ability of fragrance to directly impact the emotional hub inside the brain known as the limbic system. Essential oils such as lemon and ginger when inhaled regularly can combat the emotional addiction that leads anorexics to premature death.

Many people with anorexia believe they don't deserve to be healthy or loved unless they are "slender."

Anorexia nervosa is an eating disorder characterized by total avoidance of food and virtual self-starvation. It may or may not be accompanied by bulimia (binge-purge behavior).

Many anorexics suffer life-threatening nutrient and mineral deficiencies. The lack of magnesium and potassium can actually trigger heart rhythm abnormalities and cardiac arrest. Replacement of calcium, magnesium, potassium, and other minerals is absolutely essential for this condition.

Single Oils:
Tarragon, mandarin, orange, lemon, ginger

Blends:
Christmas Spirit, Valor, Citrus Fresh, Motivation, Brain Power

EO Applications:
  INHALATION:
    DIFFUSION, 15 minutes every 2 hours
    DIRECT, 2-3 times daily, as needed
  TOPICAL:
    NEAT, 1-2 drops on temples and/or back of neck 4 times daily
    COMPRESS, warm, over liver area

Dietary Supplementation:
Ultra Young, Super Cal, Coral Sea, BodyGize, Mineral Essence

ANTHRAX
(See INFECTIONS)

Caused by the bacteria *Bacillus anthracis*, anthrax is one of the oldest and deadliest diseases known. There are three predominant types: the **external** form acquired from contact with infected animal carcasses, the **internal** form is obtained from breathing airborne anthrax spores, and **battlefield anthrax**, which is a far more lethal variety of internal anthrax that was developed for biological warfare. When the airborne variety of anthrax invades and lungs, it is 90 percent fatal unless antibiotics are administered at the very beginning of the infection. Often anthrax goes undiagnosed until it is too late for antibiotics.

External varieties of anthrax may be contracted by exposure to animal hides and wool. While vaccination and antibiotics have stemmed anthrax infection in recent years, new strains have developed that are resistant to all counter measures.

According to Jean Valnet, M.D., thyme oil is effective for killing the anthrax bacillus.[7] Two highly antimicrobial phenols in thyme, carvacrol and thymol, are responsible for this action.

Single Oils:
Thyme, oregano, clove, cinnamon, rosewood

Blends:
Thieves, Exodus II

EO Applications:
  TOPICAL:
    DILUTE 20-80, on hands and exposed skin areas
  INHALATION:
    DIFFUSION, 5 minutes 4-6 times daily to purify air

INGESTION:
CAPSULE, 00 size, 4 times daily

Dietary Supplementation:
Exodus, ImmuneTune, Super C Chewable

Other:
Topical treatments to help prevent contracting or spreading anthrax include Thieves Cleansing Bar Soap, Thieves Household Cleaner, Thieves Spray and Thieves Wipes.

ANTIBIOTIC REACTIONS

Synthetic antibiotic drugs indiscriminately kill both beneficial and harmful bacteria. This can result in yeast infections (including candida), diarrhea, poor nutrient assimilation, fatigue, degenerative diseases, and many other conditions and symptoms.

The average adult has 3-4 pounds of beneficial bacteria permanently residing in the intestines. These beneficial flora:

- Constitute the first line of defense against bacterial and viral infection
- Produce B vitamins
- Maintain pH balance
- Combat yeast and fungus overgrowth
- Aid in the digestive process

Dietary Supplementation:
Royaldophilus, Wolfberry Crisp bars, Berrygize bars, Stevia Select.

During antibiotic treatment, take 5 grams of Stevia Select and 2-3 servings of acidophilus daily on an empty stomach before meals. After completing antibiotic treatment, continue using acidophilus and Stevia Select for 10-15 days.

ANTISEPTIC

Antiseptics prevent the growth of pathogenic microorganisms. Many essential oils have powerful antiseptic properties. Clove and thyme essential oils have been documented to kill over 50 types of bacteria and 10 types of fungi. Other potent antiseptics include, cinnamon/cassia oil, tea tree, oregano, and mountain savory.

Single Oils:
Thyme, clove, oregano, rosemary, manuka, tea tree, mountain savory, eucalyptus (all types), lavandin, cinnamon, cassia, ravensara

Blends:
Purification, Melrose, Christmas Spirit, Thieves, ImmuPower, Raven, R.C.

EO Applications:
TOPICAL:
DILUTE, According to application code (see Appendix A) and apply to affected area 2-10 times daily as needed

Other:
Skin Care: Thieves Bar Soap, Melaleuca Rosewood Bar Soap, Thieves Antiseptic Spray, Thieves Wipes, Rose Ointment

APNEA

Apnea is a temporary cessation of breathing during sleep. It can degrade the quality of sleep resulting in chronic fatigue, lowered immune function, and lack of energy.

Blends:
Clarity, Surrender, Valor

EO Applications:
INHALATION:
DIFFUSION, in the bedroom throughout
the night while sleeping

TOPICAL:
NEAT, 2-4 drops on soles of feet just before bedtime

Dietary Supplementation:
VitaGreen, Super B, Thyromin
Supplementation regimen for apnea:
- Three VitaGreen capsules 2 times daily.
- One Super B 3 times daily with meals.
- Two Thyromin capsules at bedtime.

APPETITE, LOSS OF

Ginger has been shown to stimulate digestion and improve appetite.

Single Oils:
Ginger, spearmint, orange, nutmeg

Blends:
Inner Child, Citrus Fresh, Christmas Spirit

EO Applications:
  INHALATION:
    DIFFUSION, 10 min., 3-5 times daily
    DIRECT, 3-5 times daily, as needed
  INGESTION:
    CAPSULE, 00 size, 1 times daily

Supplements:
Essentialzyme, Polyzyme, ComforTone

ARTERIOSCLEROSIS

This condition is defined as any one of a group of diseases which causes a thickening and a loss of elasticity of arterial walls. It can be caused by inflammation and is frequently an underlying cause of heart attack or stroke.

Single Oils:
Helichrysum, clove, nutmeg, cypress, frankincense

Blends:
Longevity, Aroma Life

EO Applications:
  INGESTION:
  CAPSULE, 00 size, 2 times daily

Dietary Supplementation:
AD&E, Longevity Capsules, Essential Omegas, Chelex, JuvaTone, JuvaPower/Spice, Rehemogen

ARTHRITIS

Osteoarthritis

Osteoarthritis involves the breakdown of the cartilage that forms a cushion between two joints. As this cartilage is eaten away, the two bones of the joint start rubbing together and wearing down. In contrast, rheumatoid arthritis is caused from a swelling and inflammation of the synovial membrane, the lining of the joint.

Natural anti-inflammatories (blue chamomile, wintergreen) combined with cartilage builders (glucosamine/chondroitin) are powerful natural cures for arthritis. The best natural anti-inflammatories include fats rich in omega-3s (like flax seed oil, the key ingredient in Essential Omegas) and essential oils such as nutmeg, wintergreen, German (blue) chamomile, and balsam fir. The best cartilage builders include Type II collagen and glucosamine (contained in BLM powder).

Nutmeg, a source of myristicin, has been researched for its anti-inflammatory effects in several studies. It works by inhibiting pro-inflammatory prostaglandins when taken internally or applied topically. Clove exhibits similar action.

Chamazulene, the blue sesquiterpene in German chamomile, also shows strong anti-inflammatory activity when used both topically and orally.

Methyl salicylate, a major component of wintergreen, is a chemical cousin to the active agent in aspirin and also has strong anti-inflammatory and analgesic properties.

Glucosamine and chondroitin are the two most powerful natural compounds for rebuilding cartilage and are the key ingredients in the supplement BLM.

Single Oils:
Wintergreen/birch, nutmeg, clove, German chamomile, helichrysum, Idaho balsam fir, Douglas fir, white fir, spruce, pine, cypress, peppermint, vetiver, marjoram, rosemary CT cineol, *Eucalyptus citriodora*, basil, oregano, lemongrass, Idaho tansy, black pepper, elemi, lavander

Blends:
PanAway, Relieve It, Aroma Siez, Ortho Ease, Ortho Sport. (PanAway and Relieve It

have cortisone-like action, which give relief of arthritic pain without the cortisone side effects.)

EO Applications:

Dilute 5-10 drops essential oils in 1 tsp. V6 Oil Complex and apply on location. Essential oils can also be applied neat, then followed by application of V6 Oil Complex or AromaSilk Satin Body Lotion.

Dietary Supplementation:

BLM, Essential Omegas, Super Cal, Mega Cal, Coral Seacium, Longevity Capsules, ArthroTune, ImmuneTune, Sulfurzyme.

Supplementation regiment for osteoarthritis:
- BLM: 2-4 capsules, 2 times daily
- Super Cal: 2-3 capsules, 2 times daily
- Essential Omegas: 2 droppers, 3 times daily
- ArthroTune: 2-6 capsules, 3 times daily
- ImmuneTune: 2-3 capsules, 3 times daily

Detoxification of the body and strengthening the joints is important. Cleanse the colon and liver. Rehemogen cleans and purifies the blood which may have toxins blocking nutrient and oxygen absorption into cells Apply oils on location followed by massage oil or AromaSilk Satin Body Lotion.

(see CIRCULATION).

Other:

Regenolone is an excellent companion personal care product to support the joints.

Rheumetoid Arthritis

Rheumatoid arthritis is a painful inflammatory condition of the joints marked by swelling, thickening, and inflammation of the synovial membrane lining the joint. (In contrast, osteoarthritis is characterized by a breakdown of the joint cartilage without any swelling or inflammation.)

Rheumatoid arthritis is classified as an autoimmune disease because it is caused by the body's own immune system attacking the joints.

Other factors can aggravate arthritis such as:
- Deficiencies of minerals and other nutrients
- Microbes and toxins
- Lack of water intake

Essential oils constitute some of the most effective treatments for combating arthritis pain and combating infection in cases where it is present. Peppermint has been studied for its ability to kill pain by blocking substance P and calcium channels.[8]

In cases where arthritis is caused by infectious organisms, such as *Borrelia burgdorferi, (Lyme Disease) Chlamydia,* and *Salmonella,* essential oils may counteract and prevent infection, especially when diffused or applied topically. Highly antimicrobial essential oils include: mountain savory, rosemary, *Melaleuca alternifolia* (tea tree), and oregano. The oils can pass into the bloodstream when applied topically.

Additionally, MSM has been documented to be one of the most effective natural supplements for reducing the pain associated with rheumatism and arthritis. The subject of a number of clinical studies, MSM was used extensively by Ronald Lawrence, M.D., in his clinical practice to successfully treat rheumatism and arthritis. MSM is the key ingredient in the supplement Sulfurzyme.

Also, glucosamine and chondroitin are some of the most powerful natural compounds for reducing inflammation, halting the progression of arthritis and rebuilding cartilage. These are the key ingredients in the supplement BLM.

Single Oils:

Peppermint, wintergreen/birch, oregano, Idaho balsam fir, helichrysum, nutmeg, clove, vetiver, marjoram, cypress, mountain savory, Idaho tansy, valerian,

Blends:
> PanAway, Relieve It, Aroma Siez, Peace & Calming, Sacred Mountain, Melrose

EO Applications:
> **TOPICAL:**
>> DILUTE according to application code (see Appendix A) and apply to affected area 1-3 times daily, as needed
>> COMPRESS, Cold, 1-2 times daily
>
> **INGESTION:**
>> CAPSULE, 00 size, 2 times daily

Dietary Supplementation:
> Sulfurzyme, BLM, Essential Omegas, Super Cal, Coral Sea, Longevity Caps, ArthroTune, Mega Cal

Topical Treatments:
> Regenolone, Peppermint Cedarwood and Morning Start Bar Soap, Ortho Ease, Ortho Sport Massage Oil, Morning Start Bath Gel

ASTHMA

During an asthma attack, the bronchials (air tubes) in the lungs become swollen and clogged with a thick, sticky mucus. The muscles of the air tubes will also begin to constrict or tighten. This results in very difficult or labored breathing. If an attack is severe, it can actually be life-threatening.

Many asthma attacks are triggered by an allergic reaction to pollen, skin particles, dandruff, cat or dog dander, dust mites, and foods such as eggs, milk, flavorings, dyes, and preservatives. Asthma can also be triggered by respiratory infection, exercise, stress, and psychological factors.
(See ALLERGIES)

Single Oils:
> ravansara, Roman chamomile, *Eucalyptus polybractea, Eucalyptus radiata*, Idaho balsam fir, spruce, pine, myrtle, peppermint, thyme, lemon, lavender, juniper, frankincense, marjoram, rose, mountain savory

Blends:
> Melrose, Di-Tone, Purification, Thieves, Raven, R.C., Inspiration, Sacred Mountain

EO Applications:
> **TOPICAL:**
>> NEAT, 2-4 drops to soles of feet
>> 2-3 times daily
>
> **INGESTION:**
>> CAPSULE, 00 size, 2 times daily

Essential oils should not be inhaled for asthma-related problems. The oils should be applied to the soles of the feet or ingested (if they are GRAS – Generally Regarded As Safe)

Dietary Supplementation:
> ImmuGel, VitaGreen, ImmuneTune, Ultra Young, Essentialzyme, Royaldophilus, Carbozyme

ATHLETE'S FOOT
(See FUNGAL INFECTIONS)

ATTENTION DEFICIT DISORDER (ADD and ADHD)

Terry Friedmann, MD has recently completed pioneering studies using essential oils to combat ADD and ADHD. Using twice a day inhalation of essential oils including vetiver, cedarwood, and lavender, Dr. Friedmann was able to achieve clinically significant results in 60 days. Researchers postulate that essential oils mitigate ADD and ADHD through their stimulation on the limbic system of the brain.

Because attention deficit disorder may be caused by mineral deficiencies in the diet, increasing nutrient intake and absorption of magnesium, potassium, and other trace minerals can also have a significant beneficial effect in resolving ADD.

Single Oils:
Vetiver, lavender, sandalwood, cardamom, cedarwood, peppermint, ledum,

Blends:
Brain Power, Joy, Peace & Calming, Clarity, Longevity

EO Applications:
INHALATION:
DIFFUSION, 15 min. 4-8 times daily
DIRECT, 4-8 times daily

Dietary Supplementation:
Mineral Essence, Essential Manna, Wolfberry Crisp, Essential Omegas, Berry Young Juice, Power Meal.

AUTISM
(See Attention Deficit Disorder)

Improving diet can be the key to ameliorating cases of autism. Replacing high glycemic sweeteners (ie. sugar) with low-glycemic sweeteners (ie. agave nectar, Stevia Select) has produced outstanding results in numerous cases of autism.

Autism is a neurologically based developmental disorder that is four times more common in boys than girls. It is characterized by:

- Social ineptness (loner)
- Nonverbal and verbal communication difficulties
- Repetitive behavior (rocking, hair twirling)
- Self injurious behavior (head-banging)
- Very limited or peculiar interests
- Reduced or abnormal responses to pain, noises, or other outside stimuli

Autism is being increasingly linked to certain vaccinations, the MMR being most often cited by researchers. British researcher Andrew Wakefield, MD, suggests single shots for children for measles, mumps and rubella (instead of the combined MMR shot) until further research is done.

Until very recently, children were receiving large doses of mercury (from thimerosal, a vaccine preservative that contains 49.6% mercury) that were well above the limit recommended by the EPA, through vaccination. Some success in reversing autism has resulted through mercury detoxification along with nutritional supplementation.

Some researchers believe that gastrointestinal disorders may be linked to the brain dysfunctions that cause autism in children (Horvath et al., 1998). In fact, there have been several cases of successful treatment of autism using pancreatic enzymes.

Stimulation of the limbic region of the brain may also help treat autism. Aromas from essential oils have a powerful ability to stimulate this part of the brain since the sense of smell (olfaction) is tied directly into the mind's emotional and hormonal centers. As a result the aroma of an essential oil has the potential to exert a powerful influence on disorders such as ADD and autism.

Single Oils:
Vetiver, frankincense, sandalwood, *Eucalyptus globulus*, melissa, cedarwood

Blends:
Valor, Brain Power, Clarity, Peace & Calming

EO Application:
INHALATION:
DIFFUSION, 15 min. 4-6 times daily
DIRECT, 4-6 times daily

Dietary Supplementation:
Essentialzyme, Royaldophilus, Essential Omegas, Polyzyme, ImmuPro, Berry Young Juice, Wolfberry Crisp Bar, Power Meal

BACK INJURIES AND PAIN
(See SPINE INJURIES AND PAIN)

BALDNESS
(see also ALOPECIA AREATA)

Male pattern baldness is often a result of excess conversion of testosterone to dihydrotestosterone through the enzyme 5-alpha reductase. It can also be caused by an inflammatory condition called alopecia areata.

Single Oils:
Fleabane, rosemary, peppermint, black pepper

EO Applications:
  TOPICAL:
  DILUTE 20-80, massage into scalp before retiring. (For this application, fractionated coconut oil is recommended as the diluting oil. It's finer structure is more readily absorbed into the scalp.)

BED WETTING
Blends:
Valor, Acceptance, Harmony

EO Applications:
  INHALATION:
  DIFFUSION, during then night, as needed
  TOPICAL:
  NEAT, 2-4 drops on soles of feet before bedtime

Dietary Supplementation:
Use K&B tincture once in the afternoon and once before bedtime (2 droppers maximum).

BELL'S PALSY
(See NERVE DISORDERS)

BENIGN PROSTATE HYPERPLASIA (BPH)
(See PROSTATE PROBLEMS)

BITES
(See INSECT BITES or SNAKE BITES)

BLADDER INFECTION
(See URINARY/BLADDER INFECTION)

BLEEDING
(See HEMORRHAGING)

BLEEDING GUMS
(See ORAL CARE)

BLISTERS and BOILS
Blisters are created when fluid is trapped under the skin. They can be caused by physical injury (ie. chemical burns, sunburns) or microbial infestation (ie., fungal and viral diseases such as Herpes simplex, athlete's foot, etc.).

Boils (carbuncles are groups of boils) are caused by bacterial infection which creates a pus-filled hair follicle. They are easily treated with antiseptic essential oils including tea tree and clove.

Blisters
Single Oils:
Lavender, sandalwood, melissa, cistus, tea tree, frankincense, lavender, Roman or German chamomile

Blends:
Purification, Inspiration, Melrose

EO Applications:
  TOPICAL:
  DILUTE 50-50, apply to blistered area 3-5 times daily, as needed

Topical Treatments:
Lavaderm.

Boils
Single Oils:
Clove, thyme, oregano, tea tree, cinnamon bark, *Melaleuca ericifolia*, manuka, cassia

Blends:
Purification, Melrose, Exodus II, Thieves

EO Applications:
　TOPICAL:
　　DILUTE 50-50, 2-3 drops on location
　　3-6 times daily

BLOATING
(See also MENSTRUAL CONDITIONS)

Bloating is usually a result of hormonal or mineral imbalances that trigger excess fluid retention in the body. One of the best natural remedies is progesterone, which is added to creams and absorbed transdermally.

Single Oils:
　Tarragon, peppermint, juniper, fennel, clary sage

Blends:
　Di-Tone

EO Applications:
　TOPICAL:
　　NEAT, 2-4 drops on soles of feet 2-3
　　times daily
　INGESTION:
　　Capsules, 00 size, 1 times daily

Dietary Supplementation:
　Estro Tincture, Essentialzyme, Polyzyme, PD80/20, Royaldophilus, Allerzyme

Other:
　Progessence Cream

BLOOD CLOTS
(See also CIRCULATION DISORDERS and CARDIOVASCULAR CONDITIONS)

As people age, the viscosity or thickness of the blood increases and also the tendency of the blood to clot excessively.

If blood clots (also known as embolisms) occur in the brain, they cause strokes; if they obstruct a coronary artery, they cause ischemic heart attacks.

People with diabetes or high blood pressure are far more likely to die from blood clots.

Natural blood thinners, such as clove oil, wintergreen oil, and nutmeg oil can be highly effective. These oils also are some of the most powerful antioxidants known and can slow the formation of oxidized cholesterol and foam cells that are implicated in atherosclerosis. Helichrysum is also effective for preventing blood clot formation and promoting the dissolution of clots.

Foods rich in vitamin E and omega-3 fats are vital for regular use in the diet.

Single Oils:
　Helichrysum, clove, nutmeg, lemon, orange, grapefruit, tangerine, lemon. cistus

Blends:
　Thieves, PanAway, Longevity

EO Applications:
　TOPICAL:
　　DILUTE 50-50, on location 4-6 times
　　daily
　　COMPRESS, warm, 15 min., 2 times
　　daily. Massage equal parts lemon, lavender
　　and helichrysum on location, with or
　　without hot packs.
　INGESTION:
　　CAPSULE, 00 size, 2 times daily between
　　meals (this works especially well with
　　helichrysum and cistus
　　RICE MILK, 2 times daily

Dietary Supplementation:
　AD&E, Essential Omegas, Longevity Caps, Thieves, Essential Manna, Berry Young Juice

Other:
　Dentarome Toothpastes (all varieties) contain clove oil, a natural blood thinner

BLOOD DISORDERS
(See also CIRCULATION DISORDERS and CARDIOVASCULAR CONDITIONS)

Anemia

Anemia is a condition caused from the lack of red blood cells (or a lack of properly functioning ones). Nutritional deficiencies such as the lack of adequate iron or vitamin B12 can contribute to this disorder.

Anemia also may be caused by improper liver function. In such cases, a liver cleanse and liver nutritional support may be effective for rebuilding red blood cell counts.

There can be many different causes of anemia. You should see your physician for proper diagnosis if you suspect anemia.

Single Oils:
Lemon, lemongrass, spikenard, helichrysum

Blends:
Aroma Life, JuvaFlex, Juva Cleanse

EO Applications:
TOPICAL:
NEAT, 2-3 drops on Vita Flex points of feet, or on inside of wrists, 2-3 times daily
INGESTION:
CAPSULE, 00 size, 2 times daily

Dietary Supplementation:
Super B, Master Formula Vitamins, Rehemogen, Mineral Essence, JuvaTone, JuvaPower/Spice, VitaGreen, Chelex

Blood Platelets (Low)

Dietary Supplementation:
Rehemogen
To enhance effects of Rehemogen use with JuvaTone, JuvaPower/Spice

Blood Detoxification

Detoxified blood results in better nutrient and oxygen flow and is the key to begin combating many diseases.

Single Oils:
Helichrysum, German chamomile, Roman chamomile, rosemary, geranium, orange, lemon, cardemom

Blends:
Di-Tone, JuvaFlex, JuvaCleanse, Exodus, EndoFlex

EO Applications:
TOPICAL:
NEAT, 2-3 drops on Vita Flex points of feet, or on inside of wrists, 2-3 times daily
INGESTION:
CAPSULE, 00 size, 2 times daily

Dietary Supplementation:
VitaGreen, Rehemogen, Chelex, JuvaPower/Spice, AlkaLime, Sulfurzyme
Rehemogen helps with most types of blood disorders including toxemia and blood toxicity.
Chelex helps remove heavy metals from the blood system. Use with cardamom and JuvaTone.
MSM (found in Sulfurzyme) purifies the body and blood.

Blood Circulation (Poor)

Single Oils:
Helichrysum, lemongrass, clove, nutmeg, balsam fir, orange, lemon, cistus

Blends:
Citrus fresh, Longevity, R.C., Valor, Thieves

EO Applications:
TOPICAL:
NEAT, 2-3 drops on Vita Flex points of feet, or on inside of wrists, 2-3 times daily
INGESTION:
CAPSULE, 00 size, 2 times daily

Dietary Supplementation:
Super B, Longevity Caps, Wolfberry Crisp
Essential oils when used regularly can improve circulation as much as 20 percent.

BLOOD PRESSURE, HIGH

(Hypertension) (See CARDIOVASCULAR CONDITIONS)

BLOOD PRESSURE, LOW (Hypotension)
(See CARDIOVASCULAR CONDITIONS)

BONE (Bruised, Broken)
Single Oils:
Helichrysum, wintergreen/birch, peppermint, spruce, Idaho balsam fir, white fir, pine, cypress, rosemary, basil, elemi, Idaho tansy, lemongrass, clove, ginger

Blends:
Aroma Siez, PanAway, Peace & Calming, Aroma Life, Relieve It, Melrose, Sacred Mountain

Another blend for bone health and healing:
- 8 drops Idaho balsam fir
- 6 drops helichrysum
- 1 drop oregano
- 1 drop vetiver

EO Applications:
TOPICAL:
NEAT or DILUTE 50-50, 2-4 drops on location, 2-4 times daily as needed
Note: Apply extremely gently if bone break is suspected

Dietary Supplementation:
PD 80/20, Super Cal, Coral Sea, Arthro Plus, Mineral Essence, ArthroTune. Mega Cal, BLM

Other:
Ortho Ease, Ortho Sport, Regenolone, Progessence Cream

Bone Pain (See also ARTHRITIS)
Single Oils:
Wintergreen/birch, spruce, pine, balsam fir, helichrysum

EO Applications:
TOPICAL:
NEAT, 2-4 drops on location, 2-5 times daily as needed

Dietary Supplementation:
Ultra Young, ArthroTune, Essential Manna, BodyGize, Power Meal, Super Cal, Coral Sea, Sulfurzyme. Mega Cal, BLM
Poor bone and muscle development can indicate HGH and/or potassium deficiency.

Broken Bones

A health professional should always be involved in the diagnosis and setting of a broken bone or a suspected broken bone.

Blend:
The following recipe is for a blend which can help speed the bone mending process:
- 10 drops wintergreen/birch
- 3 drops helichrysum
- 2 drops lemongrass
- 3 drops pine
- 4 drops ginger
- 4 drops vetiver

EO Applications:
Prior to casting the broken bone, mix the above oils and very gently apply 2-8 drops (depending on size of area) to break area, neat. If there are any signs of skin sensitivity or irritation, be prepared to apply a small amount of V-6 Oil Complex.

Dietary Supplementation:
ArthroTune, Super Cal, Coral Sea, BLM, AD&E, Mega Cal

BRAIN DISORDERS
(See NEUROLOGICAL DISEASES)

The fragrance of many essential oils exerts a powerful stimulus on the limbic system—a part of the brain located on the margin of the cerebral cortex, including the amygdala, hippocampus, and hypophysis which interact directly with the thalamus and hypothalamus. Acting together, these glands and brain components combined are the seat of memory, emotions, and sexual arousal, They also govern aggressive behavior.

The ability of essential oils to pass the blood-brain barrier gives them enormous therapeutic potential against such neurological diseases like Parkinson's, Alzheimer's, Lou Gehrig's, and MS.

Alzheimer's Disease

Over 4 million Americans suffer from Alzheimer's. Alzheimer's was found to nearly double in subjects with high levels of homocysteine in the Framingham Study. Aluminum continues to be linked to Alzheimer's yet older Americans are urged to get yearly flu shots which contain aluminum as an adjuvant. Pepper, grapefruit and fennel oils have been found to stimulate brain activity.[9] Peppermint oil has been helpful in protecting against stresses and toxins in brain cells.[10]

Dr. Richard Restrick, a leading neurologist in Washington, D.C., stated that maintaining normal synaptic firing would forestall many types of neurological deterioration in the body.

Essential oils high in sesquiterpenes, such as vetiver, cedarwood, patchouly, German chamomile, myrrh, melissa, and sandalwood, are known to cross the blood-brain barrier. The following oils are general cerebral stimulants:

Single Oils:
Cedarwood, vetiver, sandalwood, ginger, nutmeg, myrrh, German chamomile, spikenard, *Eucalyptus globulus*, frankincense, melissa, patchouly, fleabane, helichrysum

Helichrysum increases neurotransmitter activity. Nutmeg is a general cerebral stimulant and also has adrenal cortex-like activity.

Blends:
Brain Power, Valor, Aroma Life

EO Applications:
  TOPICAL:
  NEAT, As needed, apply 1-2 drops directly onto the brain reflex center. These points include the forehead, temples, and mastoids (the bones just behind the ears). Apply oils and mild direct pressure to the brainstem area (center top of neck at base of skull) and work down the spine.
  VITA FLEX, apply 1-2 drops to brain points on feet 1-2 times daily
  RAINDROP Technique once every two weeks. You can also apply 3-6 drops essential oils to a natural bristle brush (essential oils may dissolve plastic bristles). Rub and brush vigorously along the brain stem and spine.

Dietary Supplementation:
JuvaTone, JuvaPower/Spice, VitaGreen, Chelex, AD&E, Power Meal, AminoTech, Essential Omegas, WheyFit, Sulfurzyme

Impaired Concentration

Single Oils:
Basil, lemon, peppermint, bergamot, cardomom, rosemry, clary sage, frankincense

Blends:
Brain Power, Clarity, Harmony, Valor

EO Applications:
  TOPICAL:
  NEAT, apply 1-2 drops to brain reflex centers (see above application), as needed
  INHALATION:
  DIRECT, 2-4 times daily, as needed

Impaired Memory

Single Oils:
Peppermint, rosemary, basil, vetiver, rose, lemon, lemongrass, cardamom

Peppermint improves mental concentration and memory. Dr. Dember conducted a study at the University of Cincinnati in 1994 showing that inhaling peppermint increased mental accuracy by 28 percent.[11]

The fragrance of diffused oils, such as lemon, have also been reported to increase memory retention and recall.

Blends:
Brain Power, Clarity, M-Grain, En-R-Gee

Memory blend Recipe #1:
- 5 drops basil
- 10 drops rosemary
- 2 drops peppermint
- 4 drops helichrysum

Memory blend Recipe #2:
- 4 drops lavender
- 3 drops geranium
- 3 drops rosewood
- 3 drops rosemary
- 2 drops tangerine
- 1 drops spearmint
- 2 drops Idaho tansy

EO Applications:
TOPICAL:
DILUTE 50-50, apply 2-3 drops on temples, forehead, mastoids (bone behind ears) and/or brainstem (back of neck), as needed

INHALATION:
DIRECT, 2-6 times daily, as needed

Dietary Supplementation:
Longevity Caps, Essential Manna, Essential Omegas, Ultra Young, VitaGreen, Mineral Essence

Other:
Vascular cleansing may improve mental function by supporting improved blood flow, boosting distribution of oxygen and nutrients (see VaSCULAR CLEANSING).

Mental Fatigue
Single Oils:
Cardamom, rosemary, vetiver, cedarwood, peppermint, frankincense.

Blends:
Brain Power, Acceptance, Clarity.

EO Applications:
TOPICAL:
NEAT, apply 1-2 drops to brain reflex centers (forehead, temples, mastoids), and/or brain stem (back of neck) as needed

INHALATION:
DIRECT, as needed

Dietary Supplementation:
Essential Omegas, Stevia Select

Stimulate Pineal/Pituitary Gland
Single Oils:
Sandalwood, vetiver, cedarwood, lavender, frankincense.

Blends:
Dream Catcher, Forgiveness, Gathering, Harmony, Humility, 3 Wise Men, ImmuPower
These blends contain frankincense and sandalwood, which help oxygenate the pineal/pituitary gland, thus improving attitude and frequency balance.

Dietary Supplementation:
Ultra Young

Stroke
Two principal kinds of strokes can damage the brain: thrombotic strokes and hemorrhagic strokes. Thrombotic strokes are caused from a blood clot lodging in a cerebral blood vessel and cutting blood supply to a part of the brain. A hemorrhagic stroke is caused by an aneurysm, or a weakness in the blood vessel wall that balloons out and ruptures, spilling blood into the surrounding brain tissue. Strokes are very serious events and if you suspect that you may be susceptible, immediately see a physician.

To reduce your risk of stroke, essential oils can be used topically or as supplements. In particular, the essential oils of clove and nutmeg were found to exert anti-clotting action in clinical trials, and can be used as a preventative measure to reduce the risk of thrombotic stroke.

Thrombotic Strokes
(See BLOOD CLOTS in BLOOD DISORDERS)
Single Oils:
 Helichrysum, cypress, juniper, peppermint, clove, lemon, grapefruit, orange, tangerine, nutmeg, cistus
Blends:
 Thieves, Longevity, ImmuPower, Aroma Life, Clarity, Brain Power
EO Applications:
 TOPICAL:
  DILUTE 50-50, apply 1-3 drops on temples, forehead, mastoids, back of neck and at base of throat just above clavicle notch
  VITA FLEX, apply 1-3 drops on brain points of feet
 INGESTION:
  CAPSULE, 00 size, 2 times daily
  RICE MILK, 2 times daily
Dietary Supplementation:
 Sulfurzyme, Essential Omegas, Essential Manna, Super Cal, Coral Sea
 These supplements are rich in essential minerals, fatty acids, and nutrients necessary for regenerating and rebuilding damaged nerve tissues.

Hemorrhagic Strokes
(See also HEMORRHAGING or BRUISING)
 The essential oil of cypress may help strengthen vascular walls.
Single Oils:
 Cypress, helichrysum
EO Applications:
 INGESTION:
  CAPSULE, 00 size, 2 times daily
  RICE MILK, 2 times daily
Dietary Supplementation:
 Sulfurzyme, Essential Omegas, Essential Manna, Super Cal, Coral Sea

BREASTFEEDING
Dry, Cracked Nipples
Single Oils:
 Lavender, myrrh, geranium, sandalwood, helichrysum
Blends:
 Valor
EO Applications:
 TOPICAL:
  DILUTE 50-50 and massage over breast and on Vita Flex points of the feet

Improve Lactation
Single Oils:
 Geranium, fennel, sage
Blends:
 Joy
EO Applications:
 TOPICAL:
  DILUTE 50-50, massage 2-4 drops over breasts and on Vita Flex points of the feet.

Mastitis (Infected Breast)
Single Oils:
 Roman chamomile, clove, thyme, rosemary, lavender
EO Applications:
 TOPICAL:
  DILUTE 20-80 and massage over breast and on Vita Flex points of the feet.
 Breast blend #1:
 - 8 Roamn Chamomile
 - 8 drops lavender
 - 3 drops cypress
 Breast blend #2:
 - 10 drops tangerine
 - 10 drops lavender
 - 1 tsp V6 Oil Complex
 Massage on the breasts and under armpits twice daily.

BRUISING

(See also BLOOD CLOTS in BLOOD DISORDERS)

Some people bruise easily because the capillary walls are weak and break easily, particularly in the skin. Those who bruise easily may be deficient in vitamin C.

Essential oils can help speed the healing of bruises and reduce the risk of blood clot formation. Oils like cypress help to strengthen capillary walls, while oils like helichrysum help speed the reabsorption of the blood that has collected in the tissue.

Single Oils:

Cypress, helichrysum, white fir, lavender, Roman chamomille, geranium

Blends:

Bruise blend Recipe 1:
- 5 drops helichrysum
- 4 drops lavender
- 3 drops cypress
- 3 drops lemongrass
- 3 drops geranium

Bruise blend Recipe 2:
- 6 drops clove
- 4 drops black pepper
- 3 drops peppermint
- 2 drops marjoram
- 2 drops geranium
- 2 drops cypress

EO Applications:

TOPICAL:

NEAT or DILUTE 50-50, 1-3 drops on bruised area, 2-5 times daily. Helichrysum is especially beneficial in healing bruises when applied neat on location.

COMPRESS, cold, on location, 2-4 times daily, as needed

Dietary Supplementation:

Master Formula Vitamins, VitaGreen, JuvaTone, JuvaPower/Spice, Super C

Regimen:
- Apply 2-3 drops of helichrysum on location neat or put in 2 oz. water and take as a dietary supplement, 2 times daily
- Super C Chewable: 2-6 tablets, 3 times daily.
- Master Formula Vitamin: 2-6 tablets, 3 times daily
- VitaGreen: 2-6 capsules 3 times daily.

BURNS

(See also SKIN DISORDERS and SHOCK)

There are three types of burns:
- First-degree burns only damage the outer layer of the skin. Sunburn is typically a first-degree burn.
- Second-degree burns damage both the outer layer and the underlying layer known as the dermis. It is manifested by blisters.
- Third-degree burns not only destroy or damage skin but can even damage underlying tissues.

Burns can be caused by sunlight, chemicals, electricity, radiation, or heat. Thermal burns are the most common type.

Aloe vera gel (contained in LavaDerm) has been extensively used in the treatment of burns and has been studied for its anti-inflammatory

> ### The Deadly Dehydration of Burns
>
> The reason that burns tend to swell and blister is due to fluid loss from the damaged blood vessels. This is why it is important to keep the burn well hydrated and to drink plenty of water.
>
> In cases of serious burns, fluid loss can become so severe that it sends the victim into shock and requires intravenous transfusions of saline solution to bring up blood pressure.

and tissue-regenerating properties. Helichrysum, lavender, and Idaho balsam fir oils support tissue regeneration and reduce scarring and skin discoloration.

Severe burns can result in dehydration and mineral loss. Inflammation often accompanies burns, so dietary protocols should be used to lessen inflammation.

NOTE: *All burns can be serious, therefore, seek medical attention if necessary. If the burn is large or severe, the individual may go into shock. Inhaling oils may help reduce the shock.* (See SHOCK)

After a burn has started to heal and is drying and cracking, use Rose Ointment or body lotion with a few drops of lavender oil to keep skin soft and to promote faster healing.

Dietary Supplementation:
Essential Omegas, Longevity Capsules, Sulfurzyme, Super Cal, Coral Sea

First-Degree Burns (Sunburn)

The best prevention for sunburn is to avoid prolonged exposure to the sun. When you do go outdoors, always wear sunblock or lotion with an SPF greater than 15—especially during the summer and when you expect to be outdoors for a prolonged period of time.

In the event of a sunburn, lavender essential oil can offer excellent pain-relieving and healing benefits.

Single Oils:
Lavender, Idaho balsam fir, helichrysum, blue cypress, rose, *Melaleuca ericifolia*

Blends:
Gentle Baby, Australian Blue, Melrose, Highest Potential

EO Applications:
TOPICAL:
NEAT or DILUTE 50-50, 1-3 drops on burn location to cool tissue and reduce inflammation. Apply 3-6 times daily or as needed.

Topical Treatments:
LavaDerm Cooling Mist, Tender Tush Ointment, Rose Ointment, Lavender-Rosewood Bar Soap, Peppermint-Cedarwood Bar Soap

For fast relief of first-degree burns, spray burn immediately with LavaDerm Cooling Mist and continue misting as necessary to cool the area. Spray as often as 4-5 times and hour for the first two hours and follow with 2-3 drops of lavender or Idaho balsam fir oil.

Use Lavender-Rosewood Soap or Peppermint-Cedarwood soap only after burn has started to heal (24-48 hours).

Second-Degree Burns (Blisters)
(see also BLISTERS)

Spray burn immediately with LavaDerm Cooling Mist and continue misting when necessary to cool the area. Spray 4-5 times every hour and follow with 2-3 drops of lavender oil.

Thereafter, apply LavaDerm every 15-30 minutes during the first day. (Keep LavaDerm refrigerated.) Apply 2-4 drops of lavender oil as needed immediately after each LavaDerm misting.

On days 2 through 5, mist every hour and follow with 2-4 drops lavender oil.

Continue using cooling mist 3 to 6 times daily until healed. Apply Rose Ointment to keep tissue soft.

Third-Degree Burns

For third-degree burns, seek immediate medical attention and follow the health professional's advice.

Spraying LavaDerm on the burn every few minutes for the first 24 hours will help tissue rehydrate. Applying a few drops of lavender oil after misting, will also help the healing process.

BURSITIS

Bursitis is an inflammation of the bursa, which are small, fluid-filled sacs located near the joints. Bursa act as shock absorbers when muscles or tendons come into contact with bone. As the bursa become swollen, they result in pain, particularly when the affected joint is used.

Bursitis can be caused by injury, infection, or arthritis, and usually involves the joints of the knees, elbows, shoulders, and Achilles tendon. Occasionally bursitis can occur in the base of the big toe. Bursitis may signal the beginning of arthritis.

Single Oils:
Idaho balsam fir, marjoram, basil, elemi, lavender, black pepper, peppermint, wintergreen/birch, Idaho tansy, oregano

Blends:
Relieve It, Sacred Mountain, PanAway.

EO Applications:
  TOPICAL:
  NEAT or DILUTE 50-50, 2-4 drops on affected area/joint 3-5 times daily, or as needed to soothe pain
  COMPRESS, cold, around affected join, 1-3 times daily

Dietary Supplementation:
Essential Omegas, Sulfurzyme, Mega Cal, ArthroTune, AlkaLime, Super Cal, Coral Sea, BLM

Topical Treatment:
Ortho Ease, Ortho Sport Massage Oil, Sacred Mountain Bar Soap, and Peppermint-Cedarwood Bar Soap.

CANCER

NOTE: No cancer treatment should be undertaken without consulting a licensed medical practitioner. The essential oil applications listed here can be used to complement the effectiveness of conventional cancer therapies. These essential oil applications should continue until the cancer is in remission.

Groundbreaking research slated to be published in 2004 at Brigham Young University for the first time identified essential oils which effectively kill cancer cells while being non-toxic to normal cells (non neoplastic cells). Some of the most effective oils studied included sandalwood essential oil which inhibited growth by up to 90% of several different types of cancer cells (cervical, breast, skin and prostate) while having little or no harmful effect on normal cells. Sandalwood showed excellent action even at very small concentrations (100 ppm). Tsuga, thyme, grapefruit, and thyme linalool also showed low normal cell toxicity and strong anticancer action.

Oils rich in limonene, such as lemon, orange, tangerine, and Idaho balsam fir have been shown in clinical studies to have potent anticarcinogenic effects. According to a study at the University of Indiana[12], "monoterpenes would appear to act through multiple mechanisms in the chemoprevention and chemotherapy of cancer." Studies using 1-15 grams a day of limonene in very advanced cancer patients resulted in almost 20% of the patients going into remission.

To enhance the action of essential oils, strong cleansing and nutritional building programs are required. The three programs below can be tailored to fit your particular needs and can have a profound effect on any cancer treatment.

1. Intensive cleanse with Cleansing Trio and JuvaTone.
2. Modified Burrough's Cleanse using cayenne pepper, lemon juice, and agave nectar.

3. The Essentialzyme Ramping Program
(see box on this page).

All cancers are best treated in the early stages by alternating and varying the essential oils used each week, so the cancer cells do not build up a resistance to the treatment.

The following are regarded generally as anti-cancerous oils:

Single Oils:

Helichrysum, lemon, orange, tangerine, ledum, sandalwood, lavender, clove, thyme, Idaho balsam fir, tsuga, frankincense, myrtle

Blends:

ImmuPower, Longevity

When people suffer terminal illness, their minds can be fractured, and they can have difficulty focusing and collecting their thoughts. The Valor, Gathering and Grounding blends promote greater focus and the ability to gather feelings and deal constructively with emotions related to cancer.

Another simple anti-cancer recipe:
- 12 drops frankincense
- 5 drops lavender
- 6 drops helichrysum

EO Applications:

TOPICAL:

NEAT or DILUTE 50-50, 1-3 drops applied directly on skin cancers or cancerous nodes, 2-5 times daily

VITA FLEX, 1-3 drops neat on foot reflex points relevant for internal cancers

RAINDROP Technique, 2-3 times monthly, substituting anti-cancerous oils for the five optional Raindrop oils (see Chapter 5)

INGESTION:

CAPSULE, 00 size, 2 capsules, 2-4 times daily

RETENTION:

RECTAL, 3 times weekly, using 20-80 dilution

> **Essentialzyme Ramping Program for cancer**
>
> This program should be monitored by a health care professional:
>
> **Phase 1:** Start with 3 tablets, 3 times daily. Increase amount by 1 tablet every day until nauseous. At this point, discontinue Essentialzyme for 24-36 hours.
>
> **Phase 2:** Start again with 4 tablets, 3 times daily. Increase daily amount until nausea starts again. Stop and rest for 24-36 hours.
>
> **Phase 3:** Start with 5 tablets, 3 times daily. Increase amount by one tablet every day until nausea starts. Rest for 24-36 hours.
>
> **Phase 4:** Go back to the amount taken before nausea occurred the third time. Continue this amount for 6 weeks.
>
> **Phase 5:** Start enzyme saturation again.

Dietary Supplementation:

ImmuPro, VitaGreen, Super C Chewable, ImmuneTune, Essential Manna, Power Meal, Thyromin, Exodus, Sulfurzyme, Mineral Essence, Essential Omegas, Rehemogen, Berry Young Juice, Royaldophilus

Gary Young's Daily Anti-Cancer Program
- Master Formula: 4-6 tablets daily
- VitaGreen: 8-10 capsules daily
- Super C: 8-10 tablets daily
- ImmuPro: 6-10 tablets at night; 4 morning and afternoon
- Power Meal: 2 scoops, 3 times daily
- WheyFit: 2 scoops daily
- Essentialzyme: 2-6 tablets, 3 times daily according to blood type
- Thyromin: Start 1 before bedtime and increase as needed.
- Exodus: 6-8 capsules daily

- Sulfurzyme: Begin with 1 tsp., 3 times daily and increase to 1-3 Tbsp. daily
- Royaldophilus: 2-3 capsules, 3 times daily for good digestion and assimilation
- Super B 2-4 tablets daily. Super B is a good source of all B vitamins including pantothenic acid (vitamin B5). Many cancer patients evidence a deficiency in vitamin B5

Brain Tumor
Single Oils:
Frankincense, grapefruit, clove, tsuga, blue cypress
EO Applications:
TOPICAL:
NEAT or DILUTE 50-50, if needed, 2-4 drops to temples, forehead, mastoids and back of neck, 2-6 times daily
INGESTION:
CAPSULE, 00 size, 2 capsules, 2-4 times daily
Dietary Supplementation:
ImmuPro, Berry Young Juice, Longevity Caps
Brain Tumor regimen:
- Take 15 to 20 tablets of ImmuPro, 15 capsules of Exodus, and 10 tablets of Super C Chewable daily.
- Maintain a concentrated carrot juice diet. Potassium is critical. Drink plenty of dandelion tea (diuretic) and yellow dock tea (iron), and take milk thistle for the liver.

To increase blood flow to the brain:
- Mix 4 drops frankincense and 5 drops ImmuPower and massage 3-5 drops on the neck 3-5 times daily.
- Mix 15 drops frankincense and 6 drops clove in 1/2 oz. V-6 Mixing Oil or Massage Oil Base and rub 5-7 times daily on the brain stem (spine at base of skull), temples, mastoids (behind the ears), forehead, and crown (top of head).
- Put 10 drops frankincense and 1 drop clove in diffuser. Sit in front of the diffuser and breathe vapors for 1/2 hour, 3 times daily. If you get a headache or feel nauseous, reduce to what is tolerable, but do not quit.
- AlkaLime: Take 1 tsp. in a glass of distilled or purified water 1 hour before or after each meal to help restore pH balance.

Bone Cancer
Single Oils:
Frankincense, sandalwood, clove, tsuga
Blends:
ImmuPower
EO Applications:
TOPICAL:
DILUTE 50-50, massage 4-6 drops on location and on spine 2-4 times daily
NEAT, apply 2-3 drops each of frankincense and ImmuPower along the spine, 3 times daily
INGESTION:
CAPSULE, 00 size, 2 capsules 1-3 times daily
RICE MILK, 4-6 times daily
Bone Cancer blend:
- 15 drops frankincense
- 6 drops clove
- 1 Tbsp. V6 Oil Complex

Massage 4-6 drops on location 3-5 times daily
Dietary Supplementation:
Cleansing Trio. Longevity Caps, Berry Young Juice, Essential Omegas

Breast Cancer
The use of topically applied natural progesterone (20 mg per day) can dramatically reduce the risk of breast cancer. Eighty-five percent of

all breast cancers are ductal cancers, and natural progesterone has been shown to slow the growth of ductal cells that promote cancer growth. In addition, new research indicates that some essential oils can dramatically inhibit cancer growth while leaving normal cells unharmed.

Studies at the Young Life Research Institute of Natural Medicine show that ledum, Idaho balsam fir, tsuga, lavender, clove, and frankincense may be effective in treating breast cancer.

For a cancer preventative, dilute up to 20 drops of either orange, sandalwood, myrtle, or tsuga in 1 tablespoon of olive oil, put in 00-size capsule and take one daily as a dietary supplement.

Lignans in flax seeds have also been shown to prevent breast cancer growth.

Single Oils:
Orange, sandalwood, frankincense, ledum, myrtle, clove, lemon, orange, tangerine, tsuga

Blends:
Brain Power, Present Time

EO Applications:
  TOPICAL:
  DILUTE 50-50, apply 4-10 drops on location daily
  VITA FLEX, apply 1-3 drops to breast Vita Flex points (see location in breast cancer regimen below)
  INGESTION:
  CAPSULE, 00 size, 1 capsule 2-4 times daily
  RICE MILK, 2-4 times daily

Specific breast cancer regimen:
A. Massage 1-3 drops frankincense on breast Vita Flex point on feet, which is on top of the foot at the base of the three middle toes. Continue massaging the Vita Flex areas after applying the oil (see Vita Flex Technique in chapter 4).
B. Layer on location 15 drops frankincense, 10 drops lavender, and 3 drops clove. Apply oils and massage daily for 4 days, then rest for 4 days. Repeat as necessary.
C. Put 6 drops of frankincense and 4 drops ledum in a 00-size capsule, fill remainder with vegetable oil. Take 1-3 capsules daily.
D. Diffuse frankincense and Brain Power for 15 minutes 2-5 times daily.

Dietary Supplementation:
Cleansing Trio, JuvaTone, JuvaPower/Spice, Longevity Caps, Power Meal, ImmuPro, Essential Omegas, AminoTech, WheyFit, Super Cal, Coral Sea, Berry Young Juice, BodyGize

Topical Treatments:
Cel-lite Magic, Progessence Cream

Other:
1. Keep lymphatics open with deep breathing exercise and aerobics.
2. Have a body massage with Cel-lite Magic, once per month to work the lymph nodes in the abdomen and the thoracic region.
3. The soy in BodyGize helps balance estrogen hormones. Take 2-3 Tbsp. BodyGize with water or juice 1-2 times daily.
   Note: ***Do not use for estrogen-receptor positive cancers.***
4. Discontinue use of antiperspirants (not deodorant) and monitor calcium levels.

Cervical Cancer

The use of topically applied natural progesterone creams can dramatically reduce the risk of cervical cancer, especially in postmenopausal women. In addition, new research indicates that some essential oils can significantly inhibit cancer growth while leaving normal cells unharmed.

Single Oils:
Tsuga, thyme, galbanum, patchouly, sandalwood, Douglas fir, hyssop, nutmeg, sage

EO Applications:
 INGESTION:
  CAPSULE, 00 size, 2-4 times daily
 RETENTION:
  TAMPON, 3 times per week

Dietary Supplementation:
(See listing under main Cancer heading)

Colon Cancer

To enhance the action of essential oils, cancer requires strong cleansing and fasting programs. Cancer is best treated in its early stages by alternating and varying the essential oils used each week, so the cancer cells do not build up a resistance to the treatment.

For a cancer preventative, mix up to 20 mg of these essential oils in 1 tablespoon of vegetable oil, and put in 00 size gel caps. Take one per day.

The gastritis associated with *H. pylori* infection is closely associated with gastric cancers.[13] Highly antiseptic oils can kill *Helicobacter pylori* that causes the infection. These oils include oregano, mountain savory, tea tree, and thyme.

Single Oils:
Clove, frankincense, ledum, orange, tsuga, lavender

EO Applications:
 INGESTION:
  CAPSULE, 00 size, 2-4 times daily
  RICE MILK, 2-4 times daily
 Colon Cancer Regimen:
Day 1: Put 10 drops of frankincense, 10 drops tsuga in a vegetable capsule and swallow 3-4 times daily.
Day 2: Mix 16 drops frankincense and 3 drops clove, and put in vegetable capsule. Take orally 3-4 times daily.
Day 3: Mix equal parts frankincense and lavender in a vegetable capsule and take 3-4 times daily.
Day 4: Take frankincense capsules 3-4 times daily.
Days 5-8: Repeat the above 4-day cycle.
Days 9-12: Rest for 4 days.
Day 13: Restart the regimen.

Dietary Supplementation:
EssentialZyme, ComforTone, ICP, Detoxzyme
Supplementation Regimen:
1. Begin with EssentialZyme to digest toxic waste.
2. Take 2 capsules ComforTone, 3 times daily. Increase by one daily until the bowels move. Then begin reducing. If diarrhea occurs, reduce amount of ComforTone used and increase ICP fiber beverage. Drink plenty of purified or distilled water.
3. ICP fiber cleanse: Begin with 1 Tbsp. in water, 3 times daily. Increase to 2 Tbsp. 3 times daily or as needed until bowels are moving regularly.

Hodgkin's Disease

Reed-Sternberg cells are a hallmark trait of lymphatic cancers of this type.

Single Oils:
Clove, lavender, frankincense, cistus

Blends:
Longevity

EO Applications:
 TOPICAL:
  NEAT or DILUTE 50-50 on location 2-4 times daily or as needed
 INGESTION:
  CAPSULE, 00 size, 3-5 times daily

Dietary Supplementation:
(See listing under main Cancer heading)

Leukemia
Single Oils:
Frankincense, clove, lavender.
Blends:
Thieves, Longevity.
EO Applications:
TOPICAL:
VITA FLEX, 1-3 drops on soles of feet 2 times daily
BODY MASSAGE, apply very gently, do not do deep tissue massage.
Dietary Supplementation:
Longevity Caps, Rehemogen, Super C, ImmuPro, ImmuneTune, VitaGreen, Berry Young Juice, Longevity Caps
Supplementation regimen:
Take the following daily, for 30-40 days:
- ImmuPro: 10 tablets before retiring; 2-4 tablets morning and afternoon
- Rehemogen: 3 droppers, 3 times daily
- Super C: 12 tablets daily
- ImmuneTune: 15 capsules daily
- VitaGreen: 9 capsules daily
- Longevity Caps: 3 capsules 3 times daily
- Fresh carrot juice: 1/2 gallon daily

Liver Cancer
Cleansing is extremely important since an optimally functioning liver is necessary to rid the body of toxins. Anger and hate affect the liver and cause extreme toxicity, eventually triggering disease.
Single Oils:
Frankincense, lavender, lemon, orange, tangerine, thyme
Blends:
JuvaFlex, JuvaCleanse
EO Applications:
TOPICAL:
NEAT or DILUTE 50-50 if needed, 2-6 drops over liver area 2-4 times daily
COMPRESS, warm, over liver area nightly
VITA FLEX, massage 1-3 drops on liver Vita Flex points of feet
INGESTION:
CAPSULE, 00 size, 3-5 times daily
RICE MILK, 3-5 times daily
Liver Cancer blend:
- 30 drops frankincense
- 20 drops lavender
- 10 drops tsuga
- 10 drops ledum
- 4 tablespoons castor oil

Apply 20-30 drops of this mixture over the liver area, then cover with a warm moist towel for 20 minutes as a compress, 5 nights per week.

Also, fill 00-size capsules with this mixture and take 1 capsule 3-5 times daily

Supplements:
JuvaTone, JuvaPower/Spice, Essential Omegas, Berry Young Juice, alpha lipoic acid, Ultra Young

Lung Cancer
Single Oils:
Ledum, orange, frankincense, Idaho balsam fir, ravensara, sage
Blends:
Raven, R.C., Longevity, ImmuPower
Lung cancer blend #1:
- 4 drops frankincense
- 3 drops sage
- 3 drops myrrh
- 3 drops clove
- 2 drops ravensara
- 2 drops hyssop

Lung cancer blend #2:
- 6 drops R.C.
- 5 drops clove
- 4 drops myrrh
- 5 drops frankincense
- 2 drops sage

EO Applications:
  INHALATION:
    DIFFUSION, 15 minutes 3-5 times daily
  INGESTION:
    CAPSULE, 00 size, 1 capsule 3 times daily
  RETENTION:
    RECTAL, nightly, retain for 8 hours
  Lung Cancer Regimen:

Day 1: Diffuse frankincense and R.C. for 1 hour three times a day. Make a rectal implant by diluting 10 drops of each of these two oils with 1 tbsp V6 Oil Complex and retain overnight.

Day 2: Same as day 1, using frankincense and R.C. in rectal implant.

Day 3: Same as day 1, using frankincense and lavender in rectal implant.

Day 4: Same as day 1, using 20 drops frankincense in a rectal implant.

Rest 2 days before continuing. If no improvement is detected, omit rest days and begin again.

Alternate oils for retention enema use (add any one of the following oils to 1 teaspoon of olive oil):

- *Eucalyptus globulus*: 10 drops
- Frankincense: 10 drops
- Peppermint and frankincense: 5 drops
- Idaho balsam fir: 20 drops
- Cypress: 10 drops

Diffuse regularly during the day the same oil combinations (neat) that are used in the retention enema for that night.

Rub ImmuPower up the spine, daily. Apply warm compress on back and chest twice daily.

Dietary Supplementation:

Super C, ImmuPro, Super Cal, Coral Sea, Berry Young Juice, alpha lipoic acid, Essential Manna, K & B

Supplementation regimen:

Take 10 to 20 Super C Chewable daily, dandelion tea, raw lemon juice, red clover tea, and K & B.

If edema is a problem, include: Super Cal, Coral Sea, Essential Manna, Berry Young Juice, Mega Cal, or organic bananas.

Lymphoma (Cancer of Lymph Nodes)

Both Hodgkin's disease and non-Hodgkin's disease are characterized by swollen lymph gland nodes, generally first appearing on the neck, armpit or groin.

Lymphoma may be caused from petrochemical pollution in the air and water. After prolonged exposure, toxins such as benzene, styrene, and toluene begin to accumulate in the lymphatic system, eventually triggering cellular mutations and cancer.

Symptoms for non-Hodgkin's lymphoma
- Generally ill, loss of appetite, loss of weight, fever, and night sweats

Symptoms of Hodgkin's lymphoma
- Fever, fatigue, weakness, itching

Single Oils:
Frankincense, myrrh, clove, sage, sandalwood, lavender

Blends:
ImmuPower

Recipe 1:
- 10 drops frankincense
- 5 drops clove or myrrh
- 3 drops sage

Recipe 2: (for massage):
- 15 drops frankincense
- 6 drops clove

EO Applications:
  TOPICAL:
    NEAT or DILUTE 50-50 if needed, 2-4 drops on swollen nodes 2 times daily. Rub along spine 2-3 times daily

BODY MASSAGE, 2-3 times weekly
RAINDROP Technique, 2 times monthly
RETENTION:
RECTAL, nightly, will bring faster results than topical applications

Dietary Supplementation:

ImmuPro, ImmuneTune, Super C, Vita-Green, Cleansing Trio

Supplementation regimen
- ImmuneTune: 4 capsules, 3 times daily
- Super C: 6 tablets, 3 times daily
- VitaGreen: 6 capsules, 3 times daily
- ImmuPro: 3 tablets, 4 times daily.

Follow this program for one month, then gradually reduce. If lymphoma goes into remission, continue program for another month, then gradually reduce. It is best to eat a total vegetarian diet. O-blood types, who need more protein, should eat fresh stream trout or wild Arctic salmon.

Melanoma (Skin Cancer)

Melanoma is the most lethal form of skin cancer. It tends to aggressively spread and metastasize, quickly colonizing the lymph nodes and internal organs. It has a high rate of fatality.

A sudden change in the appearance of an old mole or the appearance of red lesions, may indicate melanoma. If you suspect that you have melanoma or any skin cancer, you should immediately contact your physician.

Single Oils:

Sandalwood, orange, blue cypress, tangerine, myrrh, lavender, Idaho tansy, tsuga, tea tree, lemongrass

Blends:

Longevity, Release, JuvaFlex, JuvaCleanse, EndoFlex, Purification, Thieves

Melanoma blend:
- 3 drops lavender
- 4 drops frankincense

EO Applications:
TOPICAL:
NEAT, apply 2-5 drops on location 3-5 times daily
INGESTION:
CAPSULE, 00 size, 2 times daily
RICE MILK, 2-4 times daily

Dietary Supplementation:
ImmuPro, Essential Omegas

Ovarian Cancer

Single Oils:

Sandalwood, lemon, orange, blue cypress, myrrh, frankincense, geranium

Blends:

Protec, Longevity, ImmuPower

EO Applications:
TOPICAL:
NEAT, 3-5 drops up the spine, on the feet, just below the navel and on the throat. Do this application 1-2 times daily
INGESTION:
CAPSULE, 00 size, 3 times daily
RICE MILK, 2-4 times daily
RETENTION:
TAMPON, nightly

Daily Regimen for Ovarian Cancer:
- Mix the blend below and use in alternating rectal and vaginal retention. Use vaginal retention with tampon one night and rectal retention the second night, and so on.
- 15 drops frankincense
- 5 drops myrrh
- 6 drops geranium
- 1 Tbsp. V-6 Oil Complex
- Rub 3-4 drops ImmuPower up the spine, on the feet, and on the throat, daily.
- Rub 1/2 tsp. Protec topically over each of the following locations: abdomen, ovaries, the reproductive Vita Flex points on hands and feet.

- Use Protec for nightly vaginal retention. Start with 1/2 tsp. and build up to 1 Tbsp. If irritation occurs, discontinue for 3 days and start again with a smaller amount.

To increase Protec's strength, add extra oils and use in alternating applications:
- *NIGHT 1: Add 3 to 4 drops of frankincense.*
- *NIGHT 2: Add 3 to 4 drops of clove.*
- *NIGHT 3: Add 3 to 4 drops of myrrh.*

Dietary Supplementation:
ImmuPro, BodyGize, Essential Omegas, alpha lipoic acid, ArthroTune

Prostate Cancer

Many prostate cancers may be testosterone-dependent, so it may be necessary to avoid taking anything that can raise testosterone levels, such as DHEA or androstenedione. Research by Dr. John Lee, MD, suggests that a quality progesterone cream may be the most potent therapy for preventing prostate cancer. Neurogen and Progessence creams provide natural progesterone.

Single Oils:
Orange, tangerine, ledum, Idaho balsam fir, frankincense, myrrh, cumin, sage, tsuga

Blends:
Protec, Mister, Longevity, Juva Cleanse

EO Applications:
TOPICAL:
DILUTE 50-50, 1-3 drops between the rectum and scrotum 1-3 times daily
VITA FLEX, 1-3 drops, neat. on reproductive points on feet (sides of ankles)
INGESTION:
CAPSULE, 00 size, 3 times daily
RICE MILK, 2-4 times daily
RETENTION:
RECTAL, nightly

Prostate blend Regimen:
The blend below helped to reduce PSA (prostate specific antigen) counts over 70 percent in a 2 months period:
- 10 drops frankincense
- 5 drops myrrh
- 3 drops sage

1. Mix the above oils in 1 Tbsp. V-6 Oil Complex for rectal retention, nightly
2. Rub 1-3 drops of the above blend, neat, on the Vita Flex reproductive points (ankles) on both feet, 2 times daily.
3. Dilute the blend 50-50 and apply 2-4 drops on the area between the rectum and scrotum 2 times daily.

Also, use Protec for nightly rectal retention. Start with 1/2 tsp. and build up to 1 Tbsp. If irritation occurs, discontinue for 3 days and start again with a smaller amount.

To increase Protec's strength, add extra oils and use for alternating applications:
- *NIGHT 1: Add 3 to 4 drops of frankincense.*
- *NIGHT 2: Add 3 to 4 drops of clove.*
- *NIGHT 3: Add 3 to 4 drops of tsuga.*

Dietary Supplementation:
Super B, ProGen, ImmuPro, Cleansing Trio, JuvaTone, JuvaPower/Spice

Topical Treatments:
Neurogen and Progessence creams. Apply 1/2 tsp 2 times daily to the area between the scrotum and the rectum.

Uterine Cancer

Environmental pollutants become lodged in tissues, such as the breasts, thyroid, ovaries, and uterus. Many chemicals mimic or imitate our natural hormones and can fit the hormone receptors, thus tricking and over-stimulating these organs. This can become a major source of cancer of the breast, uterus, ovaries, and lymph nodes.

(Same program as OVARIAN CANCER)

CANDIDA
(See FUNGAL INFECTIONS)

CANKER SORES
(See also COLD SORES)

These are technically known as aphthous ulcers and are not regarded as an infectious disease and are not caused by the Herpes virus.

Canker sores tend to occur because of stress, illness, weakened immune system, and injury caused by such things as hot food, rough brushing of teeth, or dentures. They appear under the tongue more commonly than cold sores.

Single Oils:
Melissa, clove, lavender, niaouli, sandalwood

Blends:
Thieves, Australian Blue

Topical/Oral Treatments
Thieves Antiseptic Spray, Fresh Essence Plus

EO Applications:
TOPICAL:
NEAT, 1 drop applied gently with fingertip to canker sore 4-8 times daily
ORAL:
GARGLE, 2-4 times daily
INGESTION:
SYRUP, Maple, 2-4 times daily

Dietary Supplementation:
ImmuPro, goldenseal root powder

CARBON MONOXIDE POISONING

Almost everyone who lives in a large metropolitan area will suffer varying degrees of subtle carbon monoxide poisoning. The more polluted or stagnant the air, the more likely that carbon monoxide levels in the blood may be elevated.

IMPORTANT: Anyone who has suffered serious carbon monoxide poisoning should be immediately exposed to fresh air while a doctor, paramedic, or other emergency health professional is summoned.

Singles:
Ravansara, *Eucalyptus radiata*, myrtle

Blends:
Longevity, R.C., Purification, Inspiration, Valor, Sacred Mountain

EO Applications:
Re-oxygenation regimen
(perform every 3-4 hours)
- Massage Valor on the bottom of feet.
- Apply Purification on the spine and back, Raindrop style
- Diffuse Purification, rub 2-4 drops on the feet.
- Massage 2-4 drops of R.C., Purification, Inspiration, or Sacred Mountain, and massage on the lung Vita Flex areas on bottom of the feet and on top of the feet at the base of the toes.

Dietary Supplementation:
Master Formula Vitamins, VitaGreen, Super B, Super C Chewable

CARDIOVASCULAR CONDITIONS
(See also BLOOD CLOTS, BLOOD DISORDERS, HEART, DIABETES, ORAL CARE)

Hardening of the Arteries

Singles:
Helichrysum, lavender, cypress, cistus

Blends:
Aroma Life, Longevity.

EO Applications:
TOPICAL:
BODY MASSAGE, 2 times weekly
INGESTION:
CAPSULE, 00 size, 3 times daily

Dietary Supplementation:
Essential Omegas, Longevity Caps, Wolfberry Crisp, mega Cal, AD&E

Blood Pressure, High (Hypertension)
Single Oils:
Lavender, marjoram, rosemary, ylang ylang, cypress, rosemary, jasmine absolute

Blends:
Aroma Life, Aroma Siez, Peace & Calming, Citrus Fresh, Joy

EO Applications:
 TOPICAL:
 DILUTE 20-80, full body massage daily
 INHALATION:
 DIFFUSION, 20 minutes, 3 times daily
 INGESTION:
 CAPSULE, 00 size, 1-2 times daily

Additional essential oil regimens:
1. For 3 minutes, massage 1-2 drops each of Aroma Life and ylang ylang on the heart Vita Flex point and over the heart and carotid arteries alon the neck. Blood pressure will begin to drop within 5 to 20 minutes. Monitor the pressure and reapply as required. Lemon and helichrysum can also be used.
2. Inhalation of jasmine reduces anxiety and therefore, lowers blood pressure.

Dietary Supplementation:
HRT, CardiaCare, Essential Manna, ImmuPro, ImmuneTune, Super B, Stevia, Mineral Essence, Super Cal, Coral Sea,
Supplementation regimen:
1. Increase intake of magnesium which acts as a smooth-muscle relaxant and acts as a natural calcium channel blocker for the heart, lowering blood pressure and dilating the heart blood vessels. Mineral Essence, Essential Manna, and Super Cal are good sources of magnesium.
2. Take 20 mg daily of vitamin B3 (niacin) an excellent vasodilator (found in Super B).
3. Use therapeutic-grade Hawthorne berry extracts. Hawthorne berry (contained in HRT tincture provides powerful cardio-vascular support.
4. Do a colon and liver cleanse.

Blood Pressure, Low (Hypotension)
Single Oils:
Sage, pine, rosemary

Blends:
Aroma Life, EndoFlex, Joy

EO Applications:
 TOPICAL:
 DILUTE 20-80, full body massage daily
 INHALATION:
 DIFFUSION, 20 minutes, 3 times daily
 INGESTION:
 CAPSULE, 00 size, 1-2 times daily

Additional essential oil regimens:
1. Use 1-2 drops each of Aroma Life and rosemary on heart Vita Flex points; for massage, dilute with few drops of V6 Oil Complex.
2. Place 3 drops each of Aroma Life and rosemary in a capsule and take 2 times daily

High Cholesterol
Helichrysum lowers and regulates cholesterol and reduces blood clotting. Aroma Life regulates and lowers blood pressure and breaks down plaque on the blood vessel walls.

Single Oils:
Rosemary, clove, German and Roman chamomile, spikenard, helichrysum, geranium, fennel

Blends:
Aroma Life, Longevity, JuvaFlex, JuvaCleanse, Di-Tone, EndoFlex, ImmuPower

Cholesterol reducing blend:
- 2 to 5 drops rosemary
- 5 drops Roman chamomile
- 3 drops helichrysum
- 5 drops allium cepa

EO Applications:
  TOPICAL:
    NEAT or DILUTE 50-50 if needed, 2-4 drops at pulse points where arteries are close to the surface (wrists, inside elbows, base of throat), 2-3 times daily. Also rub 6-10 drops along spine 3 times daily
    BODY MASSAGE, 2 times weekly
  INGESTION:
    CAPSULE, 00 size, 3 times daily
    RICE MILK, 1-2 times daily

Dietary Supplementation:
CardiaCare, JuvaPower/Spice, VitaGreen, Super C Chewable, Super Cal, Coral Sea, Longevity Caps, Mineral Essence, Essential Omegas, ICP, Polyzyme, Essentialzyme
Supplementation regimens:
1. Do a colon and liver cleanse using the Cleansing Trio, JuvaTone, JuvaPower/Spice, and JuvaFlex and JuvaCleanse. JuvaTone is particularly useful for high cholesterol. ICP helps break down plaque.
2. Mix 25 drops of HRT in 6 ounces of distilled water, and drink 3 times daily. Supports blood system and circulation deficiency.
3. Magnesium acts as a smooth muscle relaxant and supports the cardiovascular system. It acts as a natural calcium channel blocker for the heart, lowering blood pressure and dilating the heart blood vessels (*Dr. T. Friedmann*). Mineral Essence, Super Cal and Mega Cal are good sources of magnesium.

Phlebitis (Inflammation of Veins)
Single Oils:
  Helichrysum, German chamomile, nutmeg, Roman chamomile, geranium, lavender, cistus
Blends:
  Longevity, Aroma Life
EO Applications:
  TOPICAL:
    NEAT, 2-4 drops on location 2-4 times daily
    COMPRESS, cold on location 2-4 times daily
Dietary Supplementation:
  Essential Omegas, Longevity Caps

CARPAL TUNNEL SYNDROME
(See NERVE DISORDERS)

CATARACTS/GLAUCOMA
(See EYE DISORDERS)

CELLULITE

Cellulite is one of the harder types of fats to dissolve in the body. Cellulite is an accumulation of old fat cell clusters that solidify and harden as the surrounding tissue loses its elasticity.

Excess fat is undesirable for two reasons:
1. The extra weight puts an extra load on all body systems, particularly the heart and cardiovascular system, as well as the joints (knees, hips, spine etc).
2. Toxins and petrochemicals (pesticides, herbicides, metallics) tend to accumulate in fatty tissue. This can contribute to hormone imbalance, neurological problems, and a higher risk of cancer.

Essential oils such as ledum, tangerine and grapefruit may help reduce fat cells. Cypress enhances circulation to support the elimination of fatty deposits. The essential oils of lemongrass and spearmint also may help fat metabolism. Cel-Lite Magic Massage Oil contains many of these oils and may help reduce cellulite deposits.

Cellulite is slow to dissolve, so target areas should be worked for a month or more in conjunction with weight training, a weight loss program, and drinking purified water—one-and-a-half times the body weight in ounces each day. Be patient. You should begin to see results in 4 to 6 weeks when using the oils in combination with a muscle-building and weight-loss regimen.

Single Oils:

Rosemary, cypress, fennel, grapefruit, lemon, tangerine, juniper, spearmint, lemongrass

Blends:

EndoFlex, Citrus Fresh

Cellulite blend #1:
- 5 drops rosemary
- 10 drops grapefruit
- 2 drops cypress

Cellulite blend #2:
- 10 drops grapefruit
- 5 drops lavender
- 3 drops helichrysum
- 3 drops patchouly
- 4 drops cypress

Cellulite blend #3: (Bath):
- 5 drops juniper
- 3 drops orange
- 3 drops cypress
- 3 drops lemon

Mix the above recipe together with 2 tablespoons Epsom salts or Bath Gel Base and dissolve in warm bath water. Massage with Cel-Lite Magic after bath.

EO Applications:

TOPICAL:

DILUTE 50-50, massage 3-6 drops vigorously on cellulite locations at least 3 times daily, especially before exercising.
BATH SALTS, 2-4 times weekly

Apply 3-5 drops of grapefruit, neat, 1-2 x daily to increase fat-reducing action in areas of fat rolls, puckers, and dimples.

Dietary Supplementation:

Thyromin, ThermaBurn, ThermaMist, Essential Omegas, Power Meal, Wheyfit, AminoTech

Thyromin, ThermaBurn, and ThermaMist balance and boost metabolism.

Topical Treatments:

Cel-Lite Magic Massage Oil

CEREBRAL PALSY
(See MUSCLES, NEUROLOGICAL DISORDERS)

CHEMICAL SENSITIVITY REACTION

Environmental poisoning and chemical sensitivity are becoming a major cause of discomfort and disease. Strong chemical compounds, such as insecticides, herbicides, and formaldehyde found in paints, glues, cosmetics, and finger nail polish, enter the body easily. Symptoms include indigestion, upper and lower gas, poor assimilation, poor electrolyte balance, rashes, hypoglycemia, allergic reaction to foods and other substances, along with emotional mood swings, fatigue, irritability, lack of motivation, lack of discipline and creativity.

Single Oils:

Frankincense, sandalwood

Blends:

Purification, Clarity, Brain Power, JuvaFlex, JuvaCleanse, M-Grain

EO Applications:

TOPICAL:

DILUTE 50-50, on affected areas, 2-4 times daily

INGESTION:

CAPSULE, 00 size, 1-3 times daily

Dietary Supplementation:
ImmuPro, ImmuneTune, Exodus, Rehemogen, Chelex, JuvaTone, JuvaPower/Spice

Cleansing Trio

For headache relief:
- 4 Essentialzyme
- 1/8 tsp M-Grain diluted 50/50 in vegetable oil

Drink 2-3 large glasses of water immediately after using these products.

(See also VASCULAR CLEANSING)

Toxic Chemical Absorption

Handling refuse or any type of contaminant without protective gloves may cause discoloration of hands, as well as chemical exposure.

Use good rubber gloves and change them often or at least wash them out with strong soap, rinse well, and dry well. If hands become discolored through chemical absorption, soak them in a solution of 3 percent hydrogen peroxide, available at most drug stores. This helps remove chemicals from the skin.

Single Oils:
Lavender, lemon

Blends:
Purification

EO Applications:
TOPICAL:
NEAT, rub 3-7 drops lavender, lemon or Purification on hands, then cover with clean cotton gloves or wrap lightly with cotton bandage all night.

CHICKEN POX (Herpes Zoster)
(See also COLD SORES, BLISTERS)

Chicken pox (also known as shingles, *Varicella Zoster*, or *Herpes zoster*) is caused by a virus that is closely related to the Herpes simplex virus. This virus is prone to hiding along nerves under the skin and may cause recurring infection through life.

When *Herpes zoster* infection occurs in children it is known as chicken pox; when infection occurs or reoccurs in adults, it is known as shingles.

A childhood bout with chicken pox may leave the virus dormant in sensory (skin) nerves. If the immune system is taxed by severe emotional stress, illness, or long-term use of corticosteroids, the dormant viruses may become active and start to infect the pathway of the skin nerves.

Single Oils:
Lavender, tea tree, sandalwood, niaouli, melissa, clove

Blends:
Australian Blue, Thieves

EO Applications:
TOPICAL:
Add 20 drops of essential oils (using any of the above oils) to 1 tablespoon of calamine lotion or V6 Oil Complex and lightly dab on spots (lesions)

Dietary Supplementation:
ImmuPro, Essential Omegas

Topical Treatments:
Thieves Antiseptic Spray, Ortho Ease, LavaDerm Cooling Mist, Shower Mate with Filter (filled with lavender oil and Epsom salts), Lavender-Rosewood Bar Soap, Melaleuca Geranium Bar Soap

Shingles

Shingles is a short-lived viral infection of the nervous system that starts with fatigue, fever, chills, and intestinal upset. The affected skin areas become sensitive and prone to blistering. One attack usually provides immunity for life. However, for many people, particularly the elderly, pain can persist for months, even years.

NOTE: Occurrences of shingles around the eyes or on the forehead can cause blindness. Consult an ophthalmologist (eye doctor) immediately if such outbreaks occur.

Single Oils:

Elemi, Idaho tansy, tea tree, ravensara, oregano, mountain savory, blue cypress, sandalwood, thyme, peppermint, tamanu (a fatty acid oil)

Blends:

Thieves, Australian Blue, Exodus II

Shingles blend #1:
- 10 drops German chamomile
- 5 drops lavender
- 4 drops sandalwood
- 2 drops geranium

Shingles blend #2:
- 10 drops sandalwood
- 5 drops blue cypress
- 4 drops peppermint
- 2 drops ravensara

EO Applications:

TOPICAL:

DILUTE 50-50, apply 6-10 drops on affected

area, back of neck and down the spine 1-3 times daily.

COMPRESS, alternating warm and cold, on spine, 1-3 times daily

Shingles regimen:

A. Layering in Raindrop Technique style, apply 3-4 drops each of oregano, mountain savory and thyme along the spine

B. Apply 15-20 drops V6 Oil Complex to the spine, massage briefly over the other oils, then cover the skin with a dry towel and apply a warm pack for 15-20 minutes).

NOTE: Be cautious about warming. If the back becomes too hot, remove the warm pack immediately and add more V6 Oil Complex to cool.

C. Remove the warm pack and towel, then layer 4-8 drops each of tea tree, elemi and peppermint along the spine

D. Put the dry towel back over the skin and apply an ice pack for 30 minutes.

Dietary Supplements:

ArthroTune, Super Cal, AD&E, Essential Omegas, Sulfurzyme

CHOLECYSTITIS
(See GALLBLADDER INFECTION)

Inflammation of the gallbladder due to obstruction of the gallbladder (bile) outlet with symptoms ranging from mild edema and congestion to severe infection and perforation.

CHOLERA

Cholera is an acute diarrheal disease caused by an interotoxin produced by a gram negative bacteria called *Vibrio cholerae*. Severe cases are marked by vomiting, muscle cramps and constant watery diarrhea which can result in serious fluid loss, saline depletion, acidosis and shock. The disease is typically found in India and Southeast Asia and is spread by feces-contaminated water and food. If you suspect cholera, you should immediately seek professional medical advice.

A recent study shows that lemon—freshly squeezed juice, peel, and essential oil—act as a biocide against *Vibrio cholerae* with no harmful side effects.[14]

Single Oils:

Lemon, clove, thyme, rosemary, oregano

EO Applications:

INGESTION:

CAPSULE, 00 size, 3 times daily with meals

CHOLESTEROL
(See CARDIOVASCULAR CONDITIONS)

CHRONIC FATIGUE SYNDROME
(See EPSTEIN-BARR VIRUS)

CIRCULATION DISORDERS
(See also BLOOD CLOTS, BLOOD DISORDERS and CARDIOVASCULAR CONDITIONS)

Good circulation is undoubtedly the foundation of good health; however, sluggish or inadequate circulation can result in tissue toxicity, starvation, and eventually, cellular death. The damage that poor or inadequate circulation can cause is best illustrated in the gangrene that often develops in the legs and arms of many advanced diabetic patients. Because the blood cannot efficiently circulate through these areas, parts of the tissues literally rot away.

Niacin (nicotinic acid) is effective for dilating blood vessels and increasing circulation. The amino acid L-arginine and cayenne pepper have similar properties.

Essential oils may be extremely useful for promoting circulation. Myrtle, lemon, and cypress have been used to strengthen and dilate capillaries and increase circulation. Helichrysum, clove and citrus oils are natural blood thinners, balancing the viscosity or thickness of the blood, and they amplify the effects of cypress. Marjoram relaxes muscles and dilates blood vessels, while nutmeg acts as a circulatory stimulant and anti-inflammatory. Goldenrod is a vein decongestant.

Single Oils:
Goldenrod, helichrysum, marjoram, cypress, myrtle, orange, grapefruit, clove, peppermint, geranium, nutmeg, cistus

Blends:
Aroma Life, Pan Away, En-R-Gee, Longevity, Citrus Fresh, Di-Tone, Harmony

EO Applications:
TOPICAL:
DILUTE 50-50, 2-4 drops on affected area 2-3 times daily. Also apply over carotid arteries and pulse points, wherever arteries are close to the skin surface.

BODY MASSAGE, 2-3 times weekly, start at feet and work up to heart

INGESTION:
CAPSULE, 0 size, 2 times daily

Dietary Supplementation:
Super B, Cel-Lite Magic, HRT, CardiaCare, VitaGreen, Longevity Caps, Rehemogen, and JuvaTone, JuvaPower/Spice

Circulation support regimen:
1. Put 25 drops HRT in 1 oz. distilled water and take 3 times daily
2. Rub 2-4 drops Aroma Life on the carotid arteries and pulse points, wherever an artery comes close to the skin, 2 times daily
3. Apply 2-4 drops Harmony over areas of poor circulation, 1-3 times daily as needed
4. Take 1/4 tsp of cayenne pepper with a full glass of pure water daily. Avoid using at bedtime.

To Improve Circulation
Blends:
Circulation blend #1:
- 5 drops basil
- 8 drops marjoram
- 10 drops cypress
- 3 drops peppermint

Circulation blend #2:
- 3 drops basil
- 2 drops peppermint
- 4 drops cypress
- 8 drops marjoram
- 10 drops wintergreen/birch

EO Applications:
TOPICAL:
DILUTE either of the above recipes in 1 tsp V6 Oil Complex and massage on location, 1-3 times daily

Varicose Veins (Spider Veins)

The blue color of varicose veins is congealed blood in the surrounding tissue from hemorrhaging of capillaries around the veins. This blood has to be dissolved and re-absorbed.

Helichrysum helps dissolve the coagulated blood in the surrounding tissue.

Cypress strengthens capillary walls.

Single Oils:

Helichrysum, cypress, wintergreen/birch, basil, peppermint, lemon, lavender

Blends:

Citrus Fresh, Aroma Life, Aroma Siez

Varicose vein blend #1:
- 3-4 drops basil
- 1 drop wintergreen/birch
- 1 drop cypress
- 1 drop helichrysum

Varicose vein blend #2:
- 2 drops helichrysum
- 2 drops of cypress.

EO Applications:

TOPICAL:

NEAT, apply 2-4 drops on location, massaging toward the heart, 3-6 times daily

Nightly Varicose Vein Regimen (legs):

A. Apply 1-3 drops varicose vein blend #1, neat on location. Rub very gently towards heart with smooth strokes along the vein, then up and over the vein until the oil is absorbed. Repeat with blend #2.

B. Apply 6 drops tangerine and 6 drops cypress to the area. Gently massage until absorbed.

C. Do the lymphatic pump procedure described in Chapter 6.

D. Follow with a soft massage of the whole leg using 10-15 drops of Aroma Life, diluted 50-50

E. Wrap and elevate the leg. It is best to do this at night before retiring and to gradually elevate the foot off the bed, an inch more each night, until it is 4 inches higher than the head.

F. Wear support hose during the daytime. It may take up to a year to achieve desired results.

Dietary Supplementation:

VitaGreen, Super B, Longevity Caps

Topical Treatment:

OrthoEase, Cel-Lite Magic, Thieves Spray

COLD SORES (Herpes Simplex Type 1)

Cold sores are also known as *Herpes labialis*. Diets high in the amino acid lysine can reduce the incidence of herpes. Conversely, the amino acid arginine can worsen herpes outbreaks.

Studies have shown neat applications of melissa to be effective against Herpes Simplex type I and Herpes Labialis. The healing period was shortened, the spread of infection prevented, and symptoms such as itching, tingling and burning were lessened.[15,16]

Peppermint and tea tree oils have also been studied for positive effects on the pain of herpes.[17,18]

Single Oils:

Melissa, tea tree, peppermint, lavender, sandalwood, mountain savory, ravensara, oregano, thyme

Blends:

Thieves, Melrose, Purification

EO Applications:

TOPICAL:

NEAT, apply one drop as soon as a cold sore starts. Repeat 5-10 times daily. DILUTE 50-50, dilution in V6 Oil Complex will help to reduce discomfort or drying of the skin when applying essential oils to an open sore.

Dietary Supplementation:
  ImmuPro, Super C, Longevity Caps, VitaGreen, ImmuneTune, Stevia, Cleansing Trio, JuvaTone, JuvaPower/Spice

Topical Treatments:
  Thieves Antiseptic Spray, Thieves Lozenges, ImmuGel
  Apply ImmuGel with 1 drop each of sandalwood and tea tree.

COLDS
(See also INFECTION, SINUS INFECTIONS, THROAT INFECTIONS, and LUNG INFECTIONS)

The best treatment for a cold or flu is prevention. Because many essential oils have strong antimicrobial properties, they can be diffused to prevent the spread of airborne bacteria and viruses. Antiviral essential oils (such as basil, hyssop, rosemary, tea tree, clove, oregano and thyme) and blends (such as Thieves, Purification, R.C., Raven, and Sacred Mountain (as well as many of the oils in the Oils of Ancient Scripture kit) are very effective as preventative aids in avoiding colds as well as in helping the body defenses fight colds, once an infection has started. ImmuPro tablets are a powerful immune stimulant that can also increase infection resistance.

Single Oils:
  Peppermint, thyme, bay laurel, oregano, rosewood, *Eucalyptus radiata*, tea tree, ravensara, rosemary, mountain savory

Blends:
  Melrose, Thieves, Australian Blue, Purification, ImmuPower, Sacred Mountain, Exodus II, Raven, R.C., Christmas Spirit
  Cold blend #1:
  - 2 drops lemon
  - 4 drops Eucalyptus radiata
  - 5 drops rosemary
  - 4 drops peppermint
  - 3 drops cypress

  Cold blend #2:
  - 5 drops rosemary
  - 4 drops R.C.
  - 4 drops frankincense
  - 1 drops oregano
  - 2 drops peppermint

EO Applications:
  INHALATION:
    DIRECT, 3-5 times daily, or as needed
    VAPOR, 2-3 times daily, as needed
  INGESTION:
    SYRUP, 3-6 times daily
  ORAL:
    GARGLE, 3-6 times daily
  TOPICAL:
    DILUTE 50-50, massage 1-3 drops on each of the following areas: forehead, nose, cheeks, lower throat, chest and upper back, 1-3 times daily
    VITA FLEX, massage 1-3 drops on Vita Flex points on the feet, 1-2 times daily
    RAINDROP Technique, 1-2 times weekly
    BATH SALTS, (see below)
    Bath blend for relief of cold symptoms:
    - 2 drops Eucalyptus radiata
    - 6 drops frankincense
    - 3 drops helichrysum
    - 6 drops spruce
    - 15 drops ravensara
    - 1 drop wintergreen or birch

  Stir above essential oils into 1/2 cup Epsom salt or baking soda, then add the mixture to hot bath water while tub is filling. Soak in hot bath until water cools.

Dietary Supplementation:
  ImmuPro, Thieves Lozenges, Super C, Super C Chewables, Longevity Caps, VitaGreen, ImmuneTune, Royaldophilus, Rehemogen, Power Meal, Exodus

Oral Treatment:
Thieves Antiseptic Spray

Congestive Cough
Single Oils:
Eucalyptus globulus, goldenrod, ledum, spruce, ravensara, cedarwood, marjoram, hyssop

Blends:
Thieves, Melrose, Peace & Calming, Raven, R.C., Idaho balsam fir

EO Applications:
  INGESTION:
   SYRUP, 2-4 times daily
  INHALATION:
   DIRECT, 3-6 times daily, as needed
   VAPOR, 1-3 times daily, as needed
  ORAL:
   GARGLE, 4-6 times daily
  TOPICAL:
   COMPRESS, warm, 1-2 times daily over chest, over throat and on upper back

Dietary Supplementation:
ImmuPro, Super C, Super C Chewables, Exodus, Thieves lozenges, Thieves Antiseptic Spray

Other:
Gargle 3-6 times daily with Fresh Essence Plus mouthwash

Excess Mucus
(See MUCUS)

Head Cold / Sinus Congestion
(See also SINUS INFECTIONS)

Single Oils:
Ledum, German chamomile, *Eucalyptus radiata*, frankincense, pine, Idaho balsam fir, peppermint, rosemary, ravensara, lemon

Blends:
R.C., Raven, Melrose, Sacred Mountain, Christmas Spirit

EO Applications:
  INHALATION:
   DIRECT, 3-5 times daily, or as needed
   VAPOR, 2-3 times daily, as needed
  INGESTION:
   SYRUP, 3-6 times daily
  ORAL:
   GARGLE, 3-6 times daily
  TOPICAL:
   DILUTE 50-50, massage 1-3 drops on each of the following areas: forehead, nose, cheeks, lower throat, chest and upper back, 1-3 times daily
   VITA FLEX, massage 1-3 drops on Vita Flex points on the feet, 1-2 times daily
   RAINDROP Technique, 1-2 times weekly
   BATH SALTS, daily

COLITIS, Ulcerative

Also known as ileitis or proctitis, ulcerative colitis is marked by the inflammation of the top layers of the lining of the large intestine (colon) It is different from both irritable bowel syndrome (which has no inflammation) and Crohn's disease (which occurs deeper in the colon wall).

The inflammation and ulcerous sores that are characteristic of ulcerative colitis occur most frequently in the lower colon and rectum and occasionally throughout the entire colon.

Symptoms include: fatigue, nausea, weight loss, loss of appetite, bloody diarrhea, loss of body fluids and nutrients, frequent fevers, abdominal cramps, arthritis, liver disease, skin rashes

Single Oils:
Peppermint, spearmint, tarragon, anise, fennel

Blends:
Di-Tone, Thieves

EO Applications:

INGESTION:
CAPSULE, 00 size, 2-3 times daily
SYRUP, 3-4 times daily
TOPICAL:
DILUTE 50-50, massage 4-6 drops over lower abdomen area 2-4 times daily

Dietary Supplementation:
Royaldophilus, ICP, ComforTone, AlkaLime, Polyzyme, Essential Omegas, Detoxzyme, Mega Cal

COLITIS, Viral

In cases where colitis is caused by a virus rather than a bacteria, the following treatments are recommended:

Single Oils:
Blue cypress, melissa, oregano, cumin, tea tree, lemongrass, tarragon, niaouli, thyme, Roman chamomile, German chamomile, rosemary, peppermint, clove, cinnamon

Blends:
Thieves, Longevity, Di-Tone, Melrose, Purification, 3 Wise Men

EO Applications:
INGESTION:
CAPSULE, 00 size, 2-3 times daily
TOPICAL:
DILUTE 50-50, massage 4-6 drops over colon area 2-4 times daily
VITA FLEX, 1-3 drops on colon Vita Flex points
RAINDROP Technique, 1-2 times weekly
COMPRESS, warm, diluted 20-80, using equal parts helichrysum and Di-Tone over colon area
RETENTION:
RECTAL, use the formula below in a rectal implant 3 times weekly

Viral colitis retention blend:
- 2 drops oregano
- 2 drops thyme
- 3 drops Purification
- 2 drops Roman chamomile
- 2 drops clove or cinnamon
- 2 drops Di-Tone

Mix above oils with 1 tablespoon V6 Advanced Oil Complex

Dietary Supplementation:
Polyzyme, ImmuPro, VitaGreen, Master Vitamin Formula

Colon and Liver Cleanse:
Cleansing Trio, JuvaTone, JuvaFlex, JuvaCleanse

Take Polyzyme, along with ComforTone. Wait about 2 weeks or more before adding ICP. Start with a small amount of the ICP and increase slowly. If any discomfort is experienced, reduce the amount taken.

COMA

Single Oils:
Frankincense, vetiver, sandalwood, cypress, black pepper, peppermint, Idaho balsam fir

Blends:
Trauma Life, Hope, Valor, Surrender

EO Applications:
INHALATION:
DIFFUSION, 15 minutes, 4-7 times daily
TOPICAL:
DILUTE 50-50, 3-5 drops on temples, neck and shoulders

Dietary Supplementation:
Mineral Essence, Ultra Young

CONFUSION

Single Oils:
Peppermint, lemon, rosemary, basil, cardamom

Blends:
Clarity, Brain Power, M-Grain, Legacy, Gathering

Dietary Supplementation:
Mineral Essence, Super Cal, Coral Sea, Super B, Ultra Young.

CONGESTIVE HEART FAILURE
(See HEART)

Coenzyme Q10 is one of the most effective supplements for supporting the heart muscle.
Single Oils:
Helichrysum, cypress, goldenrod
Blends:
Aroma Life, Longevity
Dietary Supplementation:
HRT, CardiaCare, Super Cal, Coral Sea, Mineral Essence, Essential Omegas

CONNECTIVE TISSUE TRAUMA
(Ligaments, Tendons)

Tendonitis, (often called Tennis Elbow and Golfer's Elbow), is a torn or inflamed tendon. Tenosynovitis, sometimes called "Trigger Finger," is an inflamed tendon being restricted by its sheath (particularly thumbs and fingers). Repetitive use or infection may be the cause.

Super Cal, Coral Sea, and BLM provide critical nutrients for connective tissue repair. Sulfurzyme, an outstanding source of organic sulfur, equalizes water pressure inside the cells and reduces pain.

PanAway reduces pain and lemongrass promotes the repair of connective tissue. Lavender with lemongrass, and marjoram with lemongrass work well together for inflamed tendons.

When selecting oils for injuries, think through the cause and type of injury and select appropriate oils. For instance, tendonitis could encompass muscle damage, nerve damage, ligament strain/tear, inflammation, infection, and possibly an emotion. Therefore, select an oil or oils for each potential cause and apply in rotation or prepare a blend to address multiple causes. The emotional distress may be anger or guilt.

The oils in Ortho Sport and Ortho Ease Massage Oils reduce pain and promote healing.
Single Oils:
Basil, lemongrass, marjoram, helichrysum, wintergreen/birch, cypress, peppermint, rosemary, *Eucalyptus radiata*
Blends:
PanAway, Aroma Life, R.C., Relieve It, Release, Citrus Fresh

The following lists show singles and blends best suited to the specific trouble spots involved with connective tissue:

BONE:
Wintergreen/birch, spruce, Idaho balsam fir, PanAway, Relieve It

MUSCLE:
Basil, marjoram, lavender, Relieve It, PanAway

LIGAMENT:
Lemongrass, helichrysum, lavender, PanAway, Relieve It, elemi, Idaho tansy
TENDONS:
Lavender, lemongrass, marjoram

> **How to Speed Healing**
>
> With any damaged tissue, circulation should be increased to promote healing. The essential oil of cypress can increase circulation.
>
> Anytime there is tissue damage, there is always inflammation which should be addressed first.

SPASMS:
Aroma Siez with Ortho Ease or Ortho Sport Massage Oils

EO Applications:
TOPICAL:
NEAT or DILUTE 50-50 as required. Gently massage 4-6 drops on affected areas 2-4 times daily. For swelling, elevate and apply ice packs
COMPRESS, cold, 2-4 times daily

Dietary Supplementation:
Master Formula, ArthroTune, Super Cal, Super B, Super C, VitaGreen, Longevity Caps, Mineral Essence, Sulfurzyme (capsules or powder)

Topical Treatment:
Ortho Ease, Regenolone, Neurogen, Ortho Sport Massage Oils

Knee Cartilage Injury
Single Oils:
Peppermint, Idaho balsam fir, Douglas fir, wintergreen/birch, white fir

Blends:
Cartilage blend:
- 9 drops lemongrass
- 10 drops marjoram
- 12 drops ginger

Sprain/Torn Ligament
NOTE: For sprains, use cold packs. For any serious sprain or constant skeletal pain, always consult a health care professional. Any time there is tissue damage, there is always inflammation. Reduce this first.

Single Oils:
Idaho tansy, valerian, vetiver,

Blends:
PanAway
Sprain blend:
- 5 drop lemongrass
- 15 drops Aroma Siez

Tendonitis
Tendonitis blend #1:
- 8 drops vetiver
- 8 drops valerian
- 4 drops Idaho tasny

Tendonitis blend #2 (for pain relief):
- 10 drops rosemary
- 10 drops *Eucalyptus radiata*
- 10 drops peppermint

Topical Treatment:
Ortho Ease, Regenolone, Neurogen, Mega Cal, BLM

CONSTIPATION
(see also DIVERTICULOSIS and DIVERTICULITIS)

The principle causes of constipation are inadequate fluid intake and low fiber consumption. Constipation can eventually lead to diverticulosis and diverticulitis, conditions common among older people. Certain essential oils have demonstrated their ability to improve colon health through supporting intestinal flora, stimulating intestinal motility and peristalsis, fighting infections and eliminating parasites.

Single Oils:
Ginger, peppermint, fennel, tarragon, anise seed.

Blends:
Di-Tone

EO Applications:
INGESTION:
CAPSULE, 00 size, 2-3 times daily
RICE MILK, 2-4 times daily

Dietary Supplementation:
Essentialzyme, Cleansing Trio, AlkaLime, Polyzyme, Royaldophilus, BodyGize, Longevity Caps, Wolfberry Crisp, BerryGize Bar, Power Meal

Regimen:
- Essentialzyme: 3 to 6 capsules, 3 times daily

- AlkaLime: 1 Tbsp. in water, 2 times daily before or after meals
- ComforTone: Start with 1 capsule and increase next day to 2 capsules. Continue to increase 1 capsule each day until bowels start moving.
- ICP: One week after beginning ComforTone, start with 1 Tbsp., 2 times daily and then increase to 3 times daily, up to 2 Tbsp., 3 times daily.
- Drink aloe vera juice, water, prune juice, unsweetened pineapple juice, and other raw fruit and vegetable juices, regularly.

CONVULSIONS
(See also BRAIN DISORDERS)

Monitor diet. Discontinue sugar and dairy products, fried and processed foods.

Blends:
Brain Power, Valor

Dietary Supplementation:
Master Formula, Mighty Vites, Ultra Young

EO Applications:
  INHALATION:
    DIRECT, 4-6 times daily
    DIFFUSION, 20 minutes, 2-3 times daily
  TOPICAL:
    NEAT, apply 2-4 drops at base of skull, across the neck and top of spine (C1-C6 vertebrae) and on bottom of feet (for relief only)

CORNS
(See FOOT PROBLEMS)

COUGHS
(See LUNG INFECTIONS and COLDS)

CRAMPS (Abdominal)
(See DIGESTIVE PROBLEMS)

CRAMPS (Muscle)
(See MUSCLES)

CROHN'S DISEASE

Crohn's disease creates inflammation, sores, and ulcers on the intestinal wall. These sores occur deeper than ulcerative colitis. Moreover, unlike other forms of colitis, Crohn's disease can also occur in other areas of the body including the large intestine, appendix, stomach, and mouth.

Symptoms include:
- Abdominal cramping
- Lower right abdominal pain
- Diarrhea
- A general sense of feeling ill

Attacks may occur once or twice a day for life. If the disease continues for years, it can cause deterioration of bowel function, leaking bowel, poor absorption of nutrients, loss of appetite and weight, intestinal obstruction, severe bleeding, and increased susceptibility to intestinal cancer.

Some researchers believe that Crohn's disease is caused by an overreacting immune system and is actually an autoimmune disease (where the immune system mistakenly attacks the body's own tissues). MSM has been extensively researched for its ability to treat many autoimmune diseases, and is the subject of research by University of Oregon researcher Stanley Jacobs. (MSM is a key ingredient in Sulfurzyme).

Single Oils:
Peppermint, nutmeg

Blends:
Di-Tone

EO Applications:
  INGESTION:
    CAPSULE, 00 size, 3 times daily
    RICE MILK, 2-4 times daily
  TOPICAL:
    RAINDROP Technique, 1-2 times weekly, using ImmuPower

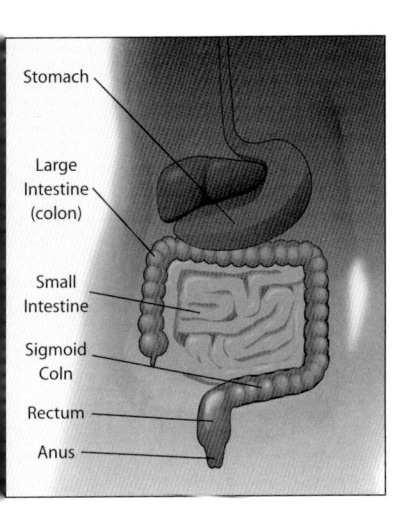

Stomach
Large Intestine (colon)
Small Intestine
Sigmoid Coln
Rectum
Anus

Dietary Supplementation:
Sulfurzyme, Polyzyme, Royaldophilus, ImmuGel, AlkaLime, ICP, VitaGreen, Cleansing Trio, Power Meal, and Mineral Essence

Regimen for Crohn's disease:
- Polyzyme: 1-2 capsules, 3 times daily.
- Royaldophilus: 2-4 capsules, 3 times daily. Empty capsules and add to water or yogurt if needed.
- ImmuGel: 1/2 tsp., 5 times daily.

Each phase lasts 1 week and should be added to the previous phases.

Phase I: Take Polyzyme in yogurt or liquid acidophilus, and charcoal tablets. Do not use ICP, ComforTone, or Essentialzyme.

Phase II: Add AlkaLime if no diarrhea, and BodyGize.
Raw juices (5 oz. celery and 2 oz carrot).

Phase III: VitaGreen

Phase IV: (Start only after a week with no sign of bleeding).

- ComforTone (1 capsule morning and night) until stools loosen.
- ICP: Start with 1 level tsp., 2 times daily and gradually increase.
- Essentialzyme: Start 1 tablet, 3 times daily. If irritation occurs, discontinue Cleansing Trio for a few days and start again.
- Mineral Essence: Start the second week: 1 dropper, 2 times daily.

CUSHING'S DISEASE
(See ADRENAL GLAND IMBALANCE)

CUTS
(See WOUNDS, SCRAPES AND CUTS)

CYST (Ganglion)
Singles:
Oregano, thyme
EO Applications:
TOPICAL:
NEAT, 2 drops oregano first day, 2 drops thyme second day, apply on location as often as needed

CYSTITIS
(See URINARY TRACT/BLADDER INFECTION)

DANDRUFF
(See HAIR AND SCALP PROBLEMS)

DECONGESTANTS
(See MUCUS)

DENTAL PROBLEMS
(See ORAL CARE)

DEODORANT
(See FUNGAL INFECTIONS)

Excessive body odor indicates putrefaction in the system and possibly poor digestion from the lack of enzymes in the digestive tract. It can also be caused by hormone imbalances and candida infections.

The essential oils of lavender, lavandin, citronella, geranium, and melaleuca inhibit proliferation of odor-causing bacteria on the skin.

Single Oils:
Lavender, geranium, bergamot, cypress, blue cypress, *Eucalyptus globulus*, myrtle

Blends:
Aroma Siez, Dragon Time, EndoFlex, Joy, Mister, R.C., Melrose

EO Applications:
TOPICAL:
DILUTE 50-50, apply 2-4 drops under arms or on the skin. Put 2 drops on a washcloth when washing.
BATH SALTS, daily

Deodorant Powder Recipe:
- 4 ounces of unscented talcum powder
- 2 ounces of baking soda
- 3 drops lavender oil or geranium oil

Mix well. Use under arms, on the feet (or in shoes).

Topical Treatment:
Aromaguard Deodorant, Fresh Essence Plus, Progessence Cream, Thieves Antiseptic Spray

DEPRESSION
(See also INSOMNIA)

Diffusing or directly inhaling essential oils can have an immediate positive impact on mood. Olfaction is the only sense that can have direct effects on the limbic region of the brain. Studies at the University of Vienna[19] have shown that some essential oils and their primary constituents (cineol) can stimulate blood flow and activity in the emotional regions of the brain.

Clinical studies at the Department of Psychiatry at the Mie University of Medicine showed that lemon not only reduced depression but reduced stress when inhaled.[20]

Single Oils:
Jasmine absolute, lemon, sage, frankincense, peppermint

Blends:
Joy, Valor, Passion, Hope

EO Applications:
INHALATION:
DIFFUSION, 20 minutes, 3 times daily
DIRECT, 4-6 times daily

Dietary Supplementation:
Essential Omegas, AD&E, Vitagreen, Royaldolphus

Postpartum Depression
Single Oils:
Vetiver, lemon, cedarwood, sandalwood, St. John's wort

Blends:
Trauma Life, Joy, Peace & Calming

EO Applications:
INHALATION:
DIFFUSION, 20 minutes, 3 times daily
DIRECT, 4-6 times daily
TOPICAL:
NEAT, 2-4 drops on temples and/or back of neck 2-4 times daily, as needed

Dietary Supplementation:
Ultra Young

DERMATITIS
(see Eczema/Dermatitis in SKIN DISORDERS)

DIABETES (Blood Sugar Imbalance)
Diabetes is the leading cause of cardiovascular disease and premature death in westernized countries today. Diabetes causes low energy and persistently high blood glucose.

Type I Diabetes usually manifests by age 30 and is often considered to be genetic. Type II Diabetes generally manifests later in life and may have a nutritional origin.

Single Oils:

Coriander, cinnamon, fennel, dill, cypress, rosemary, clove

Blends:

Thieves, EndoFlex, JuvaFlex, JuvaCleanse, Di-Tone

EO Applications:
INGESTION:

CAPSULE, 0 size, 3 times daily

Dietary Supplementation:

VitaGreen, Stevia, Master His/ Hers, Essentialzyme, Carbozyme, Super B, BodyGize, Power Meal, Longevity Caps, Mineral Essence, Sulfurzyme, Wolfberry Crisp Bars

Regimen for diabetes:

- BodyGize and Power Meal, at least one serving of each daily
- VitaGreen: 8 to 16 capsules daily.
- Sulfurzyme: 1 to 4 Tbsp. daily.
- Mix equal amounts of Thieves, coriander, fennel and dill and massage this blend on pancreas Vita Flex points of the feet 2-4 times daily. Alternatively, this same blend can be applied in a warm compress over pancreas area.
- Cleansing Trio, JuvaTone, JuvaFlex, JuvaCleanse, JuvaCleanse. Use these as recommended to help the body detoxify.

VitaGreen is high in plant protein, which helps balance blood glucose. The MSM/sulfur found in the Sulfurzyme promotes insulin production.

Essentialzyme supports enzyme production, which helps keep the pancreas from premature wasting and enlargement, a condition linked to diabetes and premature aging.

Super B is a good source of B vitamins to support pancreas function.

The Stevia leaf extract is one of the most health-restoring plants known. It is a natural sweetener, has no calories, and does not have the harmful side effects of processed sugar or sugar substitutes. Stevia increases glucose tolerance and helps normalize blood sugar fluctuations.

Wolfberry balances the pancreas and is a detoxifier and cleanser. Diabetes is not common in certain regions of China, where wolfberry is consumed regularly.

An East Indian herbal formula was shown in a *Journal of the National Medical Association* study to possess hypoglycemic activity. The herbs are: *Cinnamomum tamale, Pterocarpus marsupeum, Momordica charantia, Azardichta indica, Tinospora cordifolia, Aegle marmelose, Gymnema sylvestre, Syzygium cumini, Trigonella foenum graecum*, and *Ficus racemosa*.

DIGESTION PROBLEMS

Any of the following indicate that the digestive system is not digesting properly:

- Rumbling or gurgling sounds in the abdomen.
- Heartburn (may be a possible indication of candida).
- Constipation and/or diarrhea.
- Constant hunger or fatigue after eating.
- Food intolerance or food allergies.
- Intestinal parasites.

Poor bowel function is linked to enzyme deficiency, low fiber, insufficient liquid, bad diet, and stress.

Cramps (Stomach)
Single Oils:

Rosemary, ginger, basil, peppermint

EO Applications:
INGESTION:

CAPSULE, 0 size, 2 times daily
RICE MILK, 1-3 times daily
TOPICAL:
DILUTE 50-50, apply 6-10 drops over stomach area 2 times daily
COMPRESS, warm, 1-2 times daily
VITA FLEX, 1-3 drops on stomach Vita Flex points of feet

Diarrhea
Single Oils:
Peppermint, nutmeg, ginger, oregano, mountain savory, clove, lemon
Blends:
Di-Tone, Thieves
Diarrhea detox blend:
- 4 drops lemon
- 3 drops mountain savory
- 2 drops oregano

EO Applications:
INGESTION:
CAPSULE, 0 size, 2 times daily
RICE MILK, 1-3 times daily
TOPICAL:
DILUTE 50-50, apply 6-10 drops over stomach area 2 times daily
COMPRESS, warm, 1-2 times daily
VITA FLEX, 1-3 drops on stomach Vita Flex points of feet

Dietary Supplementation:
Royaldophilus, Essential Omegas, ComforTone, ICP, Essentialzyme, JuvaTone, JuvaPower/Spice

A maintenance dosage of ComforTone has protected travelers going to other countries from diarrhea and other digestive discomforts.

Nutmeg has been shown to have powerful action against diarrhea in a number of medical studies.[21,22]

Gas, Flatulence
Single Oils:
Peppermint, tarragon, nutmeg, anise seed, fennel, ledum, carrot seed
Blends:
Di-Tone
EO Applications:
INGESTION:
CAPSULE, 0 size, 2 times daily
TOPICAL:
DILUTE 50-50, apply 6-10 drops over stomach area twice daily
COMPRESS, warm, 1-2 times daily
VITA FLEX, 1-3 drops on stomach Vita Flex points of feet

Dietary Supplementation:
Essentialzyme, Polyzyme, AlkaLime, mega Cal, Royaldophilus, Coral Sea, Super Cal

Heartburn
Lemon juice is one of the best remedies for heartburn. Mix the juice of 1/2 squeezed lemon in 8 oz. water and slip slowly upon awakening each morning.

By ingesting lemon juice and/or essential oils the stomach stops excreting digestive acids. Therefore alleviating heartburn or other stomach ailments.

Single Oils:
Peppermint, ginger, spearmint, lemon
Blends:
Di-Tone, EndoFlex, JuvaFlex, JuvaCleanse
Heartburn blend:
- 2 drops basil
- 1 drop Idaho tansy
- 8 drops sage
- 3 drops sandalwood

EO Applications:
INGESTION:
CAPSULE, 0 size, 2 times daily

TOPICAL:
    DILUTE 50-50, apply 6-10 drops over stomach area twice daily
    COMPRESS, warm, 1-2 times daily
    VITA FLEX, 103 drops on stomach Vita Flex points of feet

Dietary Supplementation:
ICP, ComforTone, Essentialzyme, Juva Power, Polyzyme, Detoxzyme, Alkalime

Hiccups
(See HICCUPS)

Indigestion
Singles:
Peppermint, nutmeg, fennel, ginger, cumin, spearmint, orange, grapefruit

Blends:
Di-Tone

EO Applications:
  INGESTION:
    CAPSULE, 0 size, 2 times daily
    RICE MILK, 1-3 times daily, as needed
  TOPICAL:
    DILUTE 50-50, apply 6-10 drops over stomach area twice daily
    VITA FLEX, 1-3 drops on stomach Vita Flex points of feet

Dietary Supplementation:
Stevia, ICP, ComforTone, Essentialzyme, Polyzyme, Carbozyme, Lipozyme, Stevia Polyzyme, Essentialzyme or Detoxzyme taken before eating helps with digestion and upset stomach. When heaviness is felt in the stomach, Polyzyme is a beneficial companion to Di-Tone.

Nausea
(See NAUSEA)

Ulcers, Stomach
Ulcers may be caused by *Helicobacter pylori* (bacteria). Several gastroduodenal diseases include gastritis and gastric or peptic ulcers.

Single Oils:
Clove, cinnamon, tea tree, oregano, thyme

Blends:
Thieves, R.C., Exodus II, Legacy

EO Applications:
  INGESTION:
    CAPSULE, 0 size, 1 capsule 3 times a day for 20 days

DIPTHERIA

An acute infectious disease caused by toxigenic strains of *Corynebacterium diphtheriae,* acquired by contact with an infected person or carrier. It is usually confined to the upper respiratory tract, and characterized by the formation of a tough false membrane attached firmly to the underlying tissue that will bleed if forcibly removed. In the most serious infections the membrane begins in the tonsil area and may spread to the uvula, soft palate and pharyngeal wall, followed by the larynx, trachea, and bronchial tree where it may cause life-threatening bronchial obstructions.

Single Oils:
Goldenrod, thyme, clove, *Eucalyptus radiata*

EO Applications:
  INHALATION:
    DIRECT, 6-8 times daily
  INGESTION:
    CAPSULE, 00 size, 2 times daily

DISINFECTANT
(See ANTISEPTIC)

DIVERTICULOSIS/DIVERTICULITIS

Diverticulosis is one of the most common conditions in the U.S. It is caused by a lack of fiber in the diet. Diverticulosis is characterized by small, abnormal pouches (diverticula) that bulge out through weak spots in the wall of the intestine. It is estimated that half of all Americans from age 60 to 80 have diverticulosis.

Symptoms:
- Cramping
- Bloating
- Constipation

One of the easiest ways to resolve this condition is by increasing fiber intake to 20-30 grams daily. Peppermint oil stimulates contractions in the colon.

While diverticulosis involves the condition of merely having colon abnormalities, diverticulitis occurs when these abnormalities or diverticula become infected or inflamed. Diverticulitis is present in 10 to 25 percent of people with diverticulosis.

Symptoms:
- Tenderness on lower left side of abdomen
- Fever and chills
- Constipation
- Cramping

Many of these symptoms are similar to those of irritable bowel syndrome.
(See also IRRITABLE BOWEL SYNDROME)

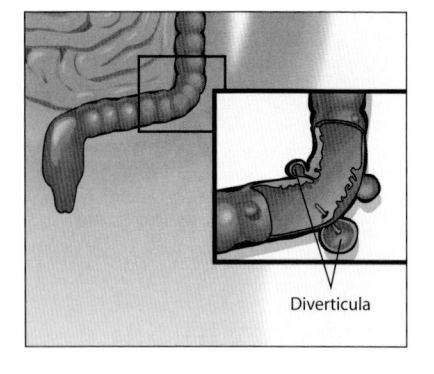

Diverticula

Single Oils:
Patchouly, anise seed, tarragon, rosemary, fennel, peppermint, mountain savory, oregano, thyme, nutmeg, frankincense

Blends:
Di-Tone. Melrose
Recipe 1:
- 15 drops Di-Tone
- 5 drops Melrose

Recipe 2:
- 10 drops Di-Tone
- 15 drops frankincense

EO Applications:
  INGESTION:
    CAPSULE, enteric coated, 0 size, 2-3 times daily
    SYRUP, 2-3 times daily
  TOPICAL:
    DILUTE 50-50, 3-5 drops on lower abdomen 2 times daily
    VITA FLEX, 2-4 drops on intestinal Vita Flex points on feet, 2-3 times daily
    COMPRESS, warm, 2 times daily
  RETENTION:
    RECTAL, nightly before retiring, retain overnight

Dietary Supplementation:
ICP, Essential Manna, products in the Cleansing Trio, Mineral Essence, Stevia, Stevia Select, ImmuPro, ImmuneTune, Essential Omegas, Exodus, Juva Power Royaldophilus, Comfortone, Immugel,

DIZZINESS
Single Oils:
Cypress, tangerine, peppermint, basil, cardamom, frankincense

Blends:
Aroma Life, Clarity, Brain Power, Thieves
  EO Applications:
    INHALATION:

DIRECT, 1-2 minutes, as needed
TOPICAL:
NEAT, 1-3 drops on temples, back of neck and shoulders, as needed
VITA FLEX, 1-3 drops on brain Vita Flex points of feet, as needed
Dietary Supplementation:
VitaGreen, Essential Manna
Topical Treatment:
Cel-Lite Magic Massage Oil
If blood circulation is a factor, see CIRCULATION.

DYSENTERY
Single Oils:
Lemon, mountain savory, oregano, peppermint
Blends:
Thieves, Di-Tone
Mix Thieves with 5 drops of peppermint and take orally.
EO Applications:
INGESTION:
CAPSULE, 00 size, 3 times daily
Dietary Supplementation:
Polyzyme, Detoxzyme, ImmuPro, Royaldophilus, Essentialzyme, ICP, Mineral Essence, Juva Power

DYSPEPSIA
(See DIGESTIVE PROBLEMS)

EAR PROBLEMS
Ear Ache
Single Oils:
Thyme, lavender, tea tree, rosemary, helichrysum, Roman chamomile, ravensara, peppermint, *Eucalyptus radiata*
Blends:
Melrose, Purification, PanAway, Thieves (diluted), Immupower

Other:
Thieves Antiseptic Spray
EO Applications:
TOPICAL:
DILUTE 50-50 in warm olive or fractionated coconut oil. Apply 2 drops to a cotton swab. Using the swab, apply traces to the skin AROUND the opening of the ear, but not in it. Put 2-3 drops of the diluted essential oil on a piece of cotton and place it carefully over the ear opening. Leave in overnight. Additional relief may be obtained by placing a warm compress over the ear
VITA FLEX, massage 1-2 drops on ear lobes and on ear Vita Flex points of the feet
CAUTION: Never put essential oils directly into the ear. Ear pain can be very serious. Always seek medical attention if pain persists.
Dietary Supplementation:
Super C, Longevity Caps, ImmuPro, VitaGreen, ImmuneTune, Rehemogen, Cleansing Trio, JuvaTone, JuvaPower/Spice

Ear Mites
Single Oils:
Eucalyptus radiata, tea tree
Blends:
Purification
EO Applications:
TOPICAL:
DILUTE 50-50 in warm olive oil. Apply 2 drops to a cotton swab. Using the swab, apply traces to the skin AROUND the opening of the ear, but not in it. Put 2-3 drops of the diluted essential oil on a piece of cotton and place it carefully over the ear opening. Leave in overnight. Additional relief may be obtained by placing a warm compress over the ear

VITA FLEX, massage 1-2 drops on ear lobes and on ear Vita Flex points of the feet

CAUTION: Never put essential oils directly into the ear. Ear pain can be very serious. Always seek medical attention if pain persists.

Perforated Eardrum
Single Oils:
Lavender
Blends:
Melrose
EO Applications:
  TOPICAL:
   DILUTE 50-50 in warm olive oil. Apply 2 drops to a cotton swab. Using the swab, apply traces to the skin AROUND the opening of the ear, but not in it. Put 2-3 drops of the diluted essential oil on a piece of cotton and place it carefully over the ear opening. Leave in overnight.

CAUTION: Never put essential oils directly into the ear. Ear pain can be very serious. Always seek medical attention if pain persists.

ECZEMA
(See ECZEMA/PSORIASIS in SKIN DISORDERS)

EDEMA (Swelling)
(See also KIDNEY DISORDERS, WATER RETENTION)

Swelling--particularly around the ankles--is noticeable when fluids accumulate in the tissue. This puffiness under the skin and around the ankles is more apparent at the end of the day when fluids settle to the lowest part of the body. A potassium deficiency can make swelling worse, so the first recourse is to increase potassium intake.

Single Oils:
Ledum, German chamomile, cedarwood, wintergreen/birch, peppermint, lavender, clove, grapefruit, juniper, orange, fennel, geranium
Blends:
Aroma Life, EndoFlex, DiTone
Edema blend #1:
- 10 drops tangerine
- 5 drops cypress
- 10 drops lemon or 3 drops juniper

Edema blend #2:
- 10 drops wintergreen or birch
- 6 drops fennel
- 2 drops idaho tansy
- 3 drops patchouly
- 10 drops tangerine

EO Applications:
  TOPICAL:
   DILUTE 50-50, massage 3-5 drops into affected area 2-3 times daily
   COMPRESS, cold, 1-2 times daily
   VITA FLEX, massage 1-3 drops on bladder Vita Flex point on foot
  INGESTION:
   CAPSULE, 0 size, 2 times daily

Morning and Evening Edema regimen:
Morning blend:
- 10 drops tangerine
- 10 drops cypress

Evening blend:
- 8 drops geranium
- 5 drops cypress
- 5 drops helichrysum

Dilute each blend 50-50 in vegetable or massage oil and rub 6-10 drops on legs working from the feet up to the thighs. Do this for one week

Dietary Supplementation:
Essential Manna, nutmeg oil, Super Cal, Super C, K & B, Master Formula Vitamins

EMOTIONAL TRAUMA

The effect of heavy emotional trauma can disrupt the stomach and digestive system. (See DIGESTION)

Single Oils:
Idaho balsam fir, frankincense, lavender, lemon, German chamomile, *Citrus hystrix*, rose, galbanum, valerian

Blends:
Present Time, Valor, Release, Peace & Calming, Trauma Life, Sacred Mountain, White Angelica, Christmas Spirit, 3 Wise Men, Citrus Fresh

Dietary Supplementation:
Royaldophilus, JuvaTone, JuvaPower/Spice

EO Applications:
INHALATION:
DIRECT, 3-4 times daily, as needed
TOPICAL:
NEAT, apply 1-2 drops to crown of head and forehead as needed. Best if applied in a quiet, darkened room
VITA FLEX, massage 1-3 drops on heart Vita Flex points, 2-3 times daily
INGESTION:
SYRUP, 1-2 times daily

Additional regimens:
Place 1-3 drops of Release over the thymus and rub in gently. Apply up to 3 times daily as needed.
Blend equal parts frankincense and Valor and apply 1-2 drops neat on temples, forehead, crown and back of neck before retiring. Use for 3 nights.

ENDOCRINE SYSTEM

The endocrine system encompasses the hormone-producing glands of the body. These glands cluster around blood vessels and release their hormones directly into the bloodstream. The pituitary gland exerts a wide range of control over the hormonal (endocrine) system and is often called the master gland. Other glands include the pancreas, adrenals, thyroid and parathyroid, ovaries, and testes. The limbic system lies along the margin of the cerebral cortex (brain) and is the hormone-producing system of the brain. It includes the amygdala, hippocampus, pineal, pituitary, thalamus, and hypothalamus.

Essential oils increase circulation to the brain. This better enables the pituitary and other glands to secrete neural transmitters and hormones that support the endocrine and immune systems.

The thyroid is one of the most important glands for regulating the body systems. The hypothalamus plays an even more important role, since it not only regulates the thyroid, but the adrenals and the pituitary gland as well.

The following oils are endocrine supportive:

Single Oils:
Fleabane, helichrysum, lemon verbena, nutmeg, clove, rosemary, spearmint, spruce

Blends:
EndoFlex, En-R-Gee, Humility

EO Applications:
INGESTION:
CAPSULE, 0 size, 2 times daily
INHALATION:
DIRECT, 3 times daily
DIFFUSION, 15 minutes 3 times daily
TOPICAL:
VITA FLEX, massage 1-3 drops on Vita Flex points for the glands on feet

Additional regimen:
Place 1-2 drops of EndoFlex on the tongue, the roof of the mouth, the thyroid and adrenals, and the Vita Flex points for these glands on the feet.

Dietary Supplementation:
Thyromin, Ultra Young, PD 80/20, Ultra Young+

EPILEPSY
Single Oils:
Clary sage, jasmine absolute
Blends:
Valor, Brain Power
EO Applications:
   INHALATION:
   DIRECT, 4 times per day as needed.
   TOPICAL:
   DILUTE 50-50, apply 1-3 drops on back of neck and behind ears 2-3 times daily
   VITA FLEX, massage 2-4 drops on brain Vita Flex points on feet, 2-3 times daily
Dietary Supplementation:
Cleansing Trio, Essential Omegas, Juva Power, Agave Nectar (no processed sugars)

EPSTEIN-BARR VIRUS
(See also HYPOGLYCEMIA, FATIGUE, THYROID, ADRENAL GLAND IMBALANCE)

Also known as Chronic Fatigue Syndrome, the Epstein-Barr virus is a type of herpes virus that also causes mononucleosis.

Symptoms include indigestion, upper and lower gas, poor assimilation, poor electrolyte balance, allergic reaction to foods and other substances, emotional mood swings, fatigue, irritability, and a lack of motivation, discipline, and creativity.

Hypoglycemia is a precursor and can render the body susceptible to the Epstein-Barr virus. Treat the hypoglycemia, and the symptoms of the Epstein-Barr virus may begin to disappear.

Single Oils:
Thyme, clove, sandalwood, grapefruit, nutmeg, blue tansy, mountain savory, oregano, tea tree, rosemary
Blends:
ImmuPower, EndoFlex, Thieves, Longevity Di-Tone, Exodus II
EO Applications:
   INGESTION:
   CAPSULE, 00 size, 3 times daily
   TOPICAL:
   RAINDROP Technique, weekly with ImmuPower
   INHALATION:
   DIRECT, 4-5 times daily
Dietary Supplementation:
Super C Chewable, ImmuPro, Thyromin, ImmuneTune, Cleansing Trio, Berry Young Juice, JuvaTone, JuvaPower/Spice, ImmuGel, Power Meal, Mineral Essence, Royaldophilus, Detoxyme, Mega Cal

Mononucleosis
Infectious mononucleosis is a disease caused by the Epstein-Barr virus (EBV) which is a type of herpes virus. Symptoms usually last four weeks or more. The spleen enlarges and may even rupture in severe cases.

Single Oils:
Ravensara, hyssop, thyme, mountain savory, frankincense
Blends:
Thieves, R.C., Raven
   Mononucleosis blend:
   - 3 drops Thieves
   - 3 drops thyme
   - 3 drops mountain savory
   - 2 drops ravensara
EO Applications:
   INGESTION:
   CAPSULE, 00 size, 1 capsule twice daily
   TOPICAL:
   RAINDROP Technique twice a week
   VITA FLEX, massage 3-6 drops on bottom of feet twice daily
Dietary Supplements:
ImmuPro, Super C Chewable, Cleansing Trio

EXPECTORANT
(See MUCUS)

EYE DISORDERS
(See AGE-RELATED MACULAR DEGENERATION)

In 1997 Dr. Terry Friedmann, MD, eliminated his need for glasses after applying sandalwood and juniper on the areas around his eyes--above the eyebrows and on the cheeks (being careful never to get oil into eyes.) He also used the supplements of Chelex, VitaGreen, the Cleansing Trio, and JuvaTone for a complete colon and liver cleanse.

CAUTION: Never put any essential oils in the eyes or on eyelids.

Blocked Tear Ducts
Single Oils:
Lavender.
EO Applications:
1 drop lavender oil rubbed over the bridge of the nose has been reported to work in seconds.

Cataracts and Glaucoma
Cataracts are a clouding of the eye lens that often comes with aging. Glaucoma is a condition caused by an abnormal buildup of intraocular pressure in the eye.
Single Oils:
Clove, lavender
Clove oil is the most powerful known antioxidant and when taken internally it can slow or prevent both cataracts and glaucoma.
Blends:
Eye blend #1:
- 10 drops lemongrass
- 5 drops cypress
- 3 drops *Eucalyptus radiata*

Eye blend #2:
- 10 drops lemon
- 5 drops cypress
- 3 drops *Eucalyptus radiata*

EO Applications:
TOPICAL:
DILUTE 20-80, apply 2-4 drops in a wide circle around the eye, being careful not to get any oil in the eye or on the eyelid, 1-3 times daily. This may also help with puffiness. Also apply on temples and eye Vita Flex points on the feet and hands (the undersides of your two largest toes and your index and middle fingers.)
NOTE: If essential oils should ever accidentally get into the eyes, dilute with V-6 Advanced Oil Complex or other pure vegetable oil. NEVER rinse with water.
INGESTION:
CAPSULE, 0 size 2-3 times daily
Dietary Supplementation:
Alpha lipoic acid, Essential Omegas, Mineral Essence, Longevity Caps, AD&E, VitaGreen Selenium supports the eyes. Mineral Essence is a good source of all minerals, including selenium. AD&E is beneficial for all eye problems.
Topical Treatment:
NeuroGen

Blurred Vision
Single Oils:
Idaho Tansy, helichrysum, lavender, peppermint
Blends:
Aroma Life, PanAway
Dietary Supplementation:
Longevity Caps, Alpha lipoic acid, Mineral Essence, AD&E, Master Formula Vitamins, VitaGreen, Sulfurzyme, Super B, Essential Omegas, Super Cal, Power Meal, Mega Cal

Pink Eye
Blends:
Purification, 3 Wise Men, ImmuPower
EO Applications:
INHALATION:
DIFFUSER, at night while sleeping

FAINTING
(See SHOCK)
Single Oils:
Melissa, peppermint, sandalwood, cardamom, spearmint.
Blends:
Clarity, Brain Power, Trauma Life
EO Applications:
INHALATION:
DIRECT, 1-2 times as needed

FATIGUE
(See DIABETES, EPSTEIN-BARR VIRUS, HEART, THYROID, ADRENAL GLAND IMBALANCE)

Hormone imbalances may play a large role in fatigue as well as latent viral infections (Herpes virus and/or Epstein-Barr Virus). Also mineral deficiencies (especially magnesium) can play a large part in low energy.

Natural progesterone for women and DHEA for men can be instrumental in helping combat the fatigue that comes with age and declining hormone levels. Because pregnenolone is a precursor for all male and female hormones, both men and women can benefit from its supplementation.

Physical Fatigue
A lack of energy can be due to a host of factors, including poor thyroid function or adrenal imbalance. Other factors may also play a part, including diabetes, cancer and other conditions.

Single Oils:
Lemongrass, juniper, basil, lemon, peppermint, rosemary, nutmeg, black pepper, thyme, melissa, cypress
Blends:
Motivation, Valor, En-R-Gee, Hope, Clarity, Citrus Fresh, Awaken, Joy

VitaGreen is a plant-derived high-protein energy formula that athletes use to boost endurance. Longevity Caps increase energy and endurance.

Digestion and colon problems may cause fatigue. A colon and liver cleanse unburdens the digestive system and increases energy.

EO Applications:
INHALATION:
DIRECT, 2-5 times daily
DIFFUSION, 10 minutes 3 times daily
TOPICAL:
DILUTE 50-50, 2-4 drops on temples, in clavicle notch (over thyroid), and behind ears, 2-4 times daily as needed
Dietary Supplementation:
VitaGreen, Power Meal, Master Formula, Mineral Essence, WheyFit, Wolfberry Crisp bars, Berrygize bars, Longevity Caps, Super B, Thyromin

Mental Fatigue
Single Oils:
Black pepper, sage, peppermint, nutmeg, spearmint, pine
Blends:
En-R-Gee, Clarity, Live With Passion, Envision, Valor, Motivation
EO Applications:
TOPICAL:
DILUTE 50-50, 2-4 drops at base of throat, temples, back of neck, as needed
VITA FLEX, massage 1-3 drops on relevant Vita Flex points on feet

1-3 times daily
INHALATION:
DIRECT, 2-4 times daily
INGESTION:
SYRUP, 1-3 times daily

Dietary Supplementation:
Thyromin, Power Meal, VitaGreen, Master Formula Vitamins, Essential Omegas, Mineral Essence, Longevity Caps, Ultra Young, Berry Young Juice

Topical Treatments:
Morning Start Bath Gel, Peppermint/Cedarwood Bar Soap, Morning Start Bar Soap, Ortho Ease Massage oil

FERTILITY

Single Oils:
Clary sage, sage, anise seed, fennel, yarrow, geranium

Blends:
Dragon Time, Acceptance, Passion, Mister, Sensation

EO Applications:
TOPICAL:
NEAT or DILUTE 50-50, as desired, 2-4 drops on the reproductive Vita Flex points of hands and feet (inside of wrists, around the front of the ankles in line with the anklebone, on the lower sides of the anklebone, and along the Achilles tendon.) 1-3 times daily.

Dietary Supplementation:
PD 80/20, VitaGreen, Essential Manna
Use VitaGreen 3-8 capsules, 2-3 times daily, and Essential Manna

Topical Treatments:
Protec, Progessence, Prenolone
Women: Rub daily 1/2 tsp Prenolone or Progessence on lower back area and the lower bowel area near the pubic bone.
Men: Take 2-4 ProGen capsules daily to nourish the reproductive system. Also rub 4-6 drops Protec on the lower abdomen near the pubic bone and in the area between the scrotum and the rectum. (Alternatively, use 1 tablespoon of Protec in overnight rectal retention.)

FEVER
(See INFECTION)

Fevers are one of the most powerful healing responses orchestrated by the human body, and are especially valuable in fighting infectious diseases. However, if fever raises body temperature excessively (over 104º F) then neurological damage can occur.

Some essential oils are very cooling when applied to the skin and can help reduce fevers. Because of its menthol content, peppermint is used predominately for fever control.

Single Oils:
Peppermint, *Eucalyptus radiata*, rosemary, ledum, Idaho balsam fir

Blends:
ImmuPower, Melrose

EO Applications:
TOPICAL:
DILUTE 50-50, apply 2-3 drops to forehead, temples and back of neck.
INGESTION:
RICE MILK, sip slowly, 1-2 times as needed
CAPSULE, 00 size, 1-2 capsules, as needed
SYRUP, dissolve 1 tsp of the syrup/essential oil mixture in an 8 oz glass of cool water and sip slowly.
INHALATION:
DIRECT, 3-4 times as needed

Dietary Supplementation:
Super C Chewable, ImmuPro, ImmuneTune, Exodus, Essential Omegas, Longevity Caps,

Fresh Essence Plus
Topical Treatments:
Cinnamint Lip Balm

FIBRILLATION
(See HEART)

FIBROIDS
(See MENSTRUAL CONDITIONS)

Fibroids are fairly common benign tumors of the female pelvis that are composed of smooth muscle cells and fibrous connective tissue. Fibroids are not cancerous and neither develop into cancer nor increase a women's cancer risk in the uterus.

Fibroids can have a diameter as small as 1 mm or as large as 8 inches. They can develop in clusters or alone as a single knot or nodule.

Fibroids frequently occur in premenopausal women and are seldom seen in young women who have not begun menstruation. Fibroids usually stabilize or even regress in women who have been through menopause.

Single Oils:
Frankincense, cistus, lavender, Idaho tansy, oregano, pine, helichrysum

Blends:
Valor, EndoFlex, Cel-Lite Magic, Protec

EO Applications:
  INGESTION:
    CAPSULE, 0 size, 2 times daily
  TOPICAL:
    COMPRESS, warm on lower abdomen, daily

Dietary Supplementation:
Ultra Young, Thyromin, VitaGreen, AlkaLime, Essential Omegas, Power Meal, Prenolone, PD 80/20, and Essentialzyme

FIBROMYALGIA

Fibromyalgia is an autoimmune disorder of soft tissues. (By contrast, arthritis occurs in the joints.) Symptoms include general body pain, in some parts worse than others, usually brought on by short periods of exercise.

The pain is ubiquitous and continuous. It interrupts sleep patterns so that the fourth stage of sleep is never attained, and thus the body cannot rejuvenate and heal. Fibromyalgia is an acid condition in which the liver is toxic (see LIVER DISORDERS).

The best natural treatments for fibromyalgia are omega-3 fats such as flax seed, proteolytic enzymes such as bromelain and pancreatin, and MSM.

According to UCLA researcher, Ronald Lawrence, M.D. Ph.D., supplementation with MSM offers a breakthrough in the treatment of fibromyalgia.

Single Oils:
German chamomile, nutmeg, Idaho alsam fir

Blends:
PanAway, Relieve It, ImmuPower, Ortho Ease, Ortho Sport

Fibromyalgia blend #1:
- 8 drops Idaho balsam fir
- 6 drops white fir
- 4 drops wintergreen/birch
- 2 drops spruce

Fibromyalgia blend #2:
- 10 drops PanAway
- 8 drops wintergreen/birch
- 8 drops marjoram
- 6 drops spruce

EO Applications:
  TOPICAL:
    DILUTE 50-50, gently massage 2-4 drops on pain locations

COMPRESS, warm, on location, 3 times weekly
BODY MASSAGE, weekly Raindrop, adding Immune blend, weekly
INGESTION:
CAPSULE, 0 size, 2 times daily
Dietary Supplementation:
Sulfurzyme, Polzyme, Essential Omegas, Super C Chewable, VitaGreen, Coral Sea, Essentialzyme, ImmuneTune, Super Cal,
Topical Treatment:
Regenolone
Fibromyalgia Regiment:
1. Start cleansing by using Cleansing Trio.
2. Use 2 Tbsp. Sulfurzyme daily
3. Eat less acidic-ash foods and more alkaline-ash foods such as wheat sprouts or barley sprouts. The following is a list of alkalinizing supplements:
- VitaGreen: up to 4 times daily.
- Super C: 4-6 tablets daily.
- ImmuneTune: 2-6 times daily.
- Mineral Essence: 2-3 droppers, 2 times daily in water or cold apple juice will supply the trace minerals needed without increasing the acid condition.
- Super Cal or Mega Cal: 2-4 capsules daily, or as needed
- ImmuPower: Apply 4-6 drops along the spine and back along with Raindrop Technique (See chapter 5 on RAINDROP TECHNIQUE).

FLATULENCE (GAS)
(See DIGESTIVE PROBLEMS)

Flatulence (gas) can be caused by a lack of digestive enzymes and the consumption of indigestible starches that promote bifidobacteria production in the colon. Although increasing bifidobacteria production can lead to gas, it is highly beneficial to long term health, as the increase of beneficial flora crowds out disease-causing microorganisms such as Clostridium perfringens. Consumption of FOS (fructooligo-saccharides), an indigestible sugar, can create short term flatulence even as it drastically improves bifidobacteria production in the small and large intestine and increases mineral absorption.

Dietary Supplementation:
Royaldophilus, Carbozyme, Allerzyme, Essentialzyme Detoxzyme, Wolfberry Crisp, Cleansing Trio, Alkalime

FLU (Influenza)
(See INFLUENZA)

FOOD POISONING
Single Oils:
Tarragon, patchouly, rosemary
Blends:
Di-Tone, Exodus II, Thieves
EO Applications:
INGESTION:
CAPSULE, 00 size, 2 capsules, 2-3 times per day
Dietary Supplementation:
ComforTone, JuvaTone, AlkaLime, Polyzyme, Detoxzyme, Essentialzyme

FOOT PROBLEMS
Athlete's Foot
(see FUNGAL INFECTIONS)

Blisters on Feet
(see BLISTERS and BOILS)

Bunions
Bunions are caused from bursitis at the base of a toe. (See BURSITIS)

Blends:
Bunion Recipe:
- 6 drops *Eucalyptus radiata*
- 3 drops lemon
- 4 drops raven
- 1 drop wintergreen/birch

EO Applications:
TOPICAL:
NEAT or DILUTE 50-50, as needed. Apply 2-4 drops over bunion area 2-3 times daily

Corns
Single Oils:
Lemon, tangerine, grapefruit, oregano, myrrh

Blends:
Citrus Fresh

EO Applications:
TOPICAL:
NEAT, 1 drop directly on the corn 2-3 times daily

Sore Feet
Single Oils:
Peppermint, white fir, lavender, patchouly, myrrh, frankincense, sandalwood, vetiver

Blends:
Melrose, PanAway, Relieve It

EO Applications:
TOPICAL:
DILUTE 50-50, massage 6-9 drops onto each foot at night
COMPRESS, warm, for added effect and penetration
BATH SALTS, mix 10 drops essential oils in 1 Tbsp. Epsom salts and add to hot water in a basin large enough for footbath

Topical Treatment:
Ortho Sport or OrthoEase Massage Oils, Fresh Essence Plus mouthwash (used on the feet)

FRIGIDITY
(See SEXUAL DYSFUNCTIONS)

FUNGAL INFECTIONS

Fungi and yeast feed on decomposing or dead tissues. They exist everywhere: inside our stomachs, on our skin, and out on the lawn. When kept under control, the yeast and fungi populating our bodies are harmless and digest what our bodies cannot or do not use.

When we feed the naturally-occurring fungi in our bodies too many acid-ash foods, such as sugar, animal proteins, and dairy products, the fungal populations grow out of control. This condition is known as systemic candidiasis and is marked by fungi invading the blood, gastrointestinal tract, and tissues.

Fungal cultures such as candida excrete large amounts of poisons called mycotoxins as part of their life cycles. These poisons must be detoxified by the liver and immune systems. Eventually they can wreak enormous damage on the tissues and organs and are believed to be an aggravating factor in many degenerative diseases, such as cancer, arteriosclerosis, and diabetes.

Insufficient intake of minerals and trace minerals like magnesium, potassium, and zinc may also stimulate candida and fungal overgrowth in the body.

Symptoms of Systemic Fungal Infection:
- Fatigue/low energy
- Overweight
- Low resistance to illness
- Allergies
- Unbalanced blood sugar
- Headaches
- Irritability
- Mood swings
- Indigestion
- Colitis and ulcers
- Diarrhea/constipation

- Urinary tract infections
- Rectal or vaginal itch

Athlete's Foot
(See RINGWORM in this section).

Tinea pedis or athlete's foot is a fungal infection of the skin that infects the feet. (it is identical to ringworm which infects the skin in the rest of the body). This fungus thrives in the warm, moist environment to which many feet are subjected.

The best remedy is to keep feet cool and dry and avoid wearing tight-fitting shoes or heavy natural (ie. cotton) socks. Wear sandals, shoes, and socks woven from a light, breathable fabric.

It is especially important to control this fungus infection during showering or bathing, since the moist, warm environment favors the growth of the *Tinea* culture responsible for athlete's foot. Antifungal essential oils such as melaleuca and Melrose can be added to bath salts or Epsom salts and used in a the RainSpa shower head to create a mild, antifungal shower.

Single Oils:
Tea tree, niaouli (MQV), *Melaleuca ericifolia*, blue cypress, lemongrass (always dilute), Idaho balsam fir, lavender, peppermint, thyme, mountain savory

Blends:
Melrose, Thieves, Purification
Athlete's foot blend #1:
- 8 drops tea tree
- 2 drop lavender

Athlete's foot blend #2:
- 8 drops tea tree
- 4 drops peppermint
- 2 drops mountain savory

EO Applications:
TOPICAL:
NEAT or DILUTE 50-50 as needed. Apply 5-7 drops to affected areas between toes and around toenails
BATH SALTS, daily

Topical Treatments:
Thieves Antiseptic Spray, Ortho Ease Massage Oil. Fresh Essence Plus Mouthwash (used on the feet), Peppermint-Cedarwood Bar Soap, Rose Ointment

Candida Albicans (Intestinal)

Two of the most powerful weapons for fighting intestinal fungal infections such as candida are FOS (fructooligosaccharides) and *L. acidophilus* cultures.

FOS has been clinically documented in dozens of peer-reviewed studies for its ability to build up the healthy intestinal flora in the colon and combat the overgrowth of negative bacteria and fungi.

Acidophilus cultures have also been shown to combat fungus overgrowth in the gastrointestinal tract. Royaldophilus is an excellent source of *L. acidophilus* cultures, and Stevia Select is a superior source of plant-derived FOS.

Single Oils:
Tea tree, juniper, ravensara, thyme, cumin, peppermint, cistus, lavender, lemongrass, rosemary, geranium, palmarosa, rosewood

Blends:
Melrose, Raven, R.C., ImmuPower

EO Applications:
TOPICAL:
Dilute 50-50 or 20-80, as needed, massage 3-4 drops on thymus (at clavical notch, center of collarbone at base of throat) to stimulate the immune system. Also apply 3-6 drops on bottoms of the feet and on the chest. Also apply 5-10 drops on stomach. Do these applications 2 times daily.
VITA FLEX, massage 2-4 drops on relevant Vita Flex points of feet

2-4 times daily.
BATH SALTS, daily

INGESTION:
CAPSULE, 0 size, 2-3 times daily between meals
RICE MILK, 3 times daily between meals

Dietary Supplementation:
Royaldophilus, Stevia Select, Fiberzyme, Essentialzyme, ImmuPro, ImmuneTune, VitaGreen, Thyromin, Super C Chewable, AlkaLime, Exodus

Ringworm and Skin Candida

The ringworm fungus infects the skin causing scaly round itchy patches. It is infectious and can be spread from an animal or human host alike. Skin candida is a fungal infection that can erupt almost anywhere on the skin. It shows up in various places, such as behind the knees, inside the elbows, behind the ears, on temple area, and between the breasts.

Single Oils:
Tea tree, niaouli (MQV), *Melaleuca ericifolia*, blue cypress, lavender, rosemary, geranium, rosewood, myrrh

Blends:
Melrose, Raven, R.C., Ortho Ease

Ringworm blend:
- 3 drops tea tree
- 3 drops spearmint
- 1 drop peppermint
- 1 drop rosemary

Skin Candida blend:
- 2 drops Idaho tansy
- 10 drops tea tree
- 1 drop oregano
- 2 drops patchouly

EO Applications:
TOPICAL:
NEAT, massage 2-4 drops over affected area, then layer on Rose ointment, 2-4 times daily.

Combating Ringworm

Using antifungal essential oils while bathing or showering is especially important because fungal infections thrive in moist, warm environments. Essential oils like tea tree or Melrose can easily be added to bath salts or Epsom salts to combat fungal infections.

There are specially designed shower heads that can be filled with bath salts and essential oils. As the water passes over the mixture, it disperses the essential oils and salts into the shower spray, creating an antiseptic spa.

In severe cases, use 35 percent food-grade hydrogen peroxide to clean infected areas before applying essential oils. Saturate a gauze with essential oils and apply to affected area and wrap to hold in place.

Topical Treatment:
Thieves Antiseptic Spray, Ortho Sport or OrthoEase Massage Oils, Fresh Essence Plus (used topically), Rose Ointment

Thrush

Thrush is a fungal infection of the mouth and throat marked by creamy, curd-like patches in the oral cavity. Even though it appears in the mouth, thrush is usually a sign of systemic fungal overgrowth throughout the body. Thrush can usually be treated locally through the use of antifungal essential oils such as clove, cinnamon, rosemary CT cineol, peppermint, and rosewood.

Single Oils:
Cinnamon, clove, peppermint, rosemary cineol, geranium, rosewood, orange, lavender

Blends:
Thieves, Melrose, Purification, ImmuPower

> **Using Raindrop Technique to Purge Pathogenic Fungi**
>
> Pathogenic microorganisms have a tendency to hibernate along the spinal cord and in the lymphatic system. The body has the ability to hold them in a suspended state for long periods of time. When the immune system becomes compromised from stress, fatigue or other factors, they can be released and manifest illness and disease.
>
> Oregano, thyme, or hyssop along the spine using Raindrop Technique may help to drive the dormant fungi out of the spinal fluid.
>
> Additionally, lymphatic pump therapy will revitalize a sluggish lymphatic system to better combat pathogenic fungi. (see Chapter 6)

EO Applications:
ORAL:
GARGLE, 3-5 times daily
TOPICAL:
Dilute 50-50 or 20-80, as needed, massage 3-4 drops on thymus (at clavical notch, center of collarbone at base of throat) to stimulate the immune system. Also apply 3-6 drops on bottoms of the feet and on the chest. Also apply 5-10 drops on stomach. Do these applications 2 times daily
VITA FLEX, massage 2-4 drops on relevant Vita Flex points of feet, 2-4 times daily
INGESTION:
CAPSULE, 0 size, 2-3 times daily between meals
RICE MILK, 3 times daily between meals

NOTE: These applications are for adults, not infants. In cases of infants with thrush, consult a medical professional first.
Oral Hygiene:
Fresh Essence Plus Mouthwash, Thieves Lozenges

Vaginal Yeast Infection

Essential oils like tea tree have been documented to have highly antifungal activity. Positive results have been obtained on vaginal yeast infections using these oils in douches. Equally excellent results have been achieved by inserting a capsule of Royaldophilus into the vagina after douching.

Single Oils:
Lavender, tea tree, rosemary, Roman chamomile, geranium, rosewood, peppermint, spearmint, mountain savory, thyme, bay laurel
Blends:
Melrose, Purification, R.C., Di-Tone, Aroma Siez, Dragon Time, Mister
Vaginal yeast infection blend #1:
- 7 drops Purification
- 2 drops frankincense
- 5 drops mountain savory

Vaginal yeast infection blend #2:
- 12 drops tea tree
- 12 drops Purification
- 12 drops juniper

EO Applications:
RETENTION:
TAMPON, nightly for 5-10 days, as needed
INGESTION:
CAPSULE, 00 size, 3 times daily
Topical Treatment:
Fresh Essence Plus mouthwash

GALLBLADDER INFECTION

The gallbladder stores bile created by the liver and releases it through the biliary ducts into the duodenum to promote digestion. Bile is extremely important for fat digestion and the absorption of vitamins such as A, D, and E.

When bile flow is obstructed due to gallstones or inflamed due to infection, serious consequences can ensue, including poor digestion, jaundice, and severe abdominal pain.

Single Oils:

Lemon, ledum, carrot seed, celery, juniper, German chamomile

Blends:

JuvaFlex, Juva Cleanse, PanAway, Release

EO Applications:

   INGESTION:

      CAPSULE, 00 size, 1 capsule 3 times daily

   TOPICAL:

      NEAT, apply 6-10 drops over gallbladder area, 2-3 times daily
      COMPRESS, warm, 2-3 times daily
      VITA FLEX, massage 1-3 drops on liver Vita Flex points of the feet, 2-3 times daily

Dietary Supplementation:

Sulfurzyme, JuvaTone, Essentialzyme, Polyzyme

GALLSTONES

When bile contains excessive cholesterol, bilirubin, or bile salts, gallstones can form. Stones made from hardened cholesterol account for the vast majority of gallstones, while stones made from bilirubin, the brownish pigment in bile, constitute only about 20 percent of gallstones.

Gallstones can block both bile flow and the passage of pancreatic enzymes. This can result in inflammation in the gallbladder (cholecystitis) or pancreas (pancreatitis) and jaundice. In some cases, gallstones can be life-threatening, depending on where they are lodged.

Several Japanese studies show that limonene (a key constituent in orange, lemon, and tangerine oils) can effectively dissolve gallstone with no negative side effects.

Single Oils:

Lemon, orange, grapefruit, mandarin, tangerine, juniper, nutmeg, rosemary

Blends:

JuvaFlex, Juva Cleanse

Gallbladder blend:
- 2 drops ledum
- 1 drop Roman chamomile
- 1 drop lavender
- 1 drop rosemary
- 1 drop helichrysum
- 1 drop juniper

EO Applications:

   INGESTION:

      Capsule: 0 size, 2 times daily for 2 weeks

   TOPICAL:

      DILUTE 50-50, massage 6-10 drops over gallbladder twice daily
      COMPRESS, 2-3 times daily
      VITA FLEX, massage 1-3 drops on liver Vita Flex points of feet, 2-3 times daily

GANGRENE

Gangrene is the death or decay of living tissue caused by a lack of blood supply. A shortage of blood can result from a blood clot, arteriosclerosis, frostbite, diabetes, infection, or some other obstruction in the arterial blood supply. Gas gangrene (also known as acute or moist gangrene) occurs when tissues are infected with *Clostridium* bacteria. Unless the limb is amputated or treated with antibiotics, the gangrene can be fatal.

The part of the body affected with gangrene displays the following symptoms:

- Coldness
- Dark in color
- Looks rotten/decomposed
- Putrid smell

Other symptoms include:
- Fever
- Anemia

Dr. René Gattefossé suffered gas gangrene as a result of burns from a chemical explosion at the turn of the century. He successfully engineered his own recovery solely with the use of pure lavender oil.

NOTE: as with all serious medical conditions, consult your health care professional immediately if you suspect gangrene.

Single Oils:
Oregano, lavender, mountain savory, thyme, ravensara, cistus, blue cypress

Blends:
Exodus II, Thieves, ImmuPower, Melrose

EO Applications:
  TOPICAL:
  DILUTE 20-80, apply 2-4 drops on affected area, 3-5 times daily
  COMPRESS, warm, 3 times daily, every other day

Dietary Supplementation:
Exodus, PD 80/20, Essential Omegas, ImmuPro, ImmuneTune, Super C

Topical Treatment:
Regenolone, NeuroGen

GASTRITIS
(See DIGESTIVE PROBLEMS)

Gastritis occurs when the stomach's mucosal lining becomes inflamed and the cells become eroded. This can lead to bleeding ulcers and severe digestive disturbances. Gastritis may be caused by excess acid production in the stomach, alcohol consumption, stress, and fungal or bacterial infections.

Symptoms of gastritis:
- Weight loss
- Abdominal pain
- Cramping

Single Oils:
Tarragon, peppermint, fennel

Blends:
Di-Tone, Thieves

EO Applications:
  INGESTION:
  CAPSULE, 0 size, 2 times daily for 7 days
  TOPICAL:
  COMPRESS, warm, over stomach area, as needed

Dietary Supplementation:
Mineral Essence, Essentialzyme, Royaldophilus, Polyzyme

Supplementation regimen for gastritis
- Essentialzyme: 3-4 capsules, 3 times daily
- Polyzyme: 3-4 capsules, 3 times daily
- Royaldophilus: 2-4 capsules, 3 times daily
- Mineral Essence: 2-3 droppers, 3 times daily
- ComforTone and ICP: Begin after 2 weeks of using the products listed above.
- Alkalime: 1/2 tsp. each morning
- Mega Cal: 1 Tbsp. each morning in 8 oz. warm water

GINGIVITIS
(See ORAL CARE)

Essential oils are one of the best treatments against gum diseases such as gingivitis and pyorrhea. Clove oil, for example, is used as dental disinfectant; and the active principle in clove oil, eugenol, is one of the best-studied germ-killers available.

GLAUCOMA
(See EYE DISORDERS)

Common among people over 30 years of age,

glaucoma is an eye disease in which escalating pressure within the fluid of the eye eventually damages the optic nerve and causes blindness. Many people are unaware of that they have the disease until their peripheral vision is permanently lost.

Glaucoma usually develops in middle age or later, although glaucoma in newborns, children, and teenagers can occur.

GOUT
(See also KIDNEY DISORDERS)
(for pain, see JOINT STIFFNESS & PAIN)

Gout is a disease marked by abrupt, temporary bouts of joint pain and swelling that are most evident in the joint of the big toe. It can also affect the wrist, elbow, knee, ankle, hand, and foot. As the disease progresses, pain and swelling in the joints becomes more frequent and chronic, with deposits called tophi appearing over many joints, including the elbows and on ears.

Gout is characterized by accumulation of uric acid crystals in the joints caused by excess uric acid in the blood. Uric acid is a byproduct of the breakdown of protein that is normally excreted by the kidneys into the urine. To reduce uric acid concentrations, it is necessary to support the kidneys, adrenal, and immune functions. It is also necessary to detoxify by cleansing and drinking plenty of fluids.

Excess alcohol, allergy-producing foods, or strict diets can cause outbreaks of gout. Foods rich in purines, such as wine, anchovies, and animal liver, can also cause gout.

Single Oils:
Geranium, ledum, carrot seed, celery, juniper, Roman chamomile, lemon

Blends:
PanAway, JuvaFlex, Juva Cleanse
Gout blend:
- 10 drops geranium
- 8 drops juniper
- 5 drops rosemary
- 3 drops Roman chamomile
- 4 drops lemon
- 8 drops tea tree

EO Applications:
INGESTION:
CAPSULE, 0 size, 3 times daily for 10 days, then rest 4 days, repeat as needed
RICE MILK, 3 times daily
TOPICAL:
NEAT, gently massage 1-3 drops o affected joints 2-3 times daily

Dietary Supplementation:
Thyromin, Essential Manna, Mineral Essence, Super C, Super Cal, ArthroTune, VitaGreen, Sulfurzyme, Cleansing Trio, JuvaTone, JuvaPower/Spice

Supplementation regimen for gout:
- Mineral Essence: 3 droppers, 3 times daily
- ArthroTune: 3 capsules, 3 times daily
- JuvaTone: up to 10 tablets daily, reduce after 2 weeks.
- Super Cal: 2-4 capsules, 2 times daily
- Super C: 2-4 tablets, 2 times daily
- VitaGreen: 2-6 capsules, 2 times daily

Topical Treatment:
Ortho Ease Massage Oil, Ortho Sport Massage Oil

GRAVE'S DISEASE
(See THYROID)

GUM DISEASE
(See ORAL CARE)

HAIR AND SCALP PROBLEMS
Sulfur is the single most important mineral for maintaining the strength and integrity of the hair and hair follicle.

Single Oils:

Rosemary, lavender, clary sage, sage, basil, cedarwood, sandalwood, juniper, ylang ylang, sandalwood, lemon, cypress, rosewood
Rosemary adds body and conditions the hair.

Blends:

Blend for dry hair:
- 2 drops ylang ylang
- 8 drops rosewood
- 4 drops geranium

Blend for oily hair:
- 6 drops patchouly
- 2 drops lavender
- 6 drops lemon

Blend to help with split ends:
- 1 drop rosemary
- 3 drops sandalwood
- 1 drop ylang ylang

EO Applications:
TOPICAL:

DILUTE 20-80, massage 1 tsp into the scalp vigorously and thoroughly for 2-3 minutes; leave on scalp for 60-90 minutes. (An excellent time to do this would be during an exercise routine). Mix 2-4 drops of essential oils with 1-2 teaspoons of shampoo to wash hair after exercising.

A rinse to help restore the acid mantle of the hair:
- 1 drop rosemary
- 1 tsp. pure apple cider vinegar
- 8 oz. water.

Use as a final rinse on hair. Rub 1 or 2 drops on as hairdressing or on hairbrush to prevent static electricity.

NOTE: Quality shampoos containing essential oils do not lather up as much as other shampoos because they do not contain harmful, foaming agents.

Dietary Supplementation:
ParaFree, Thyromin, Super B, Master Formula, Longevity Caps, Sulfurzyme

Topical Treatment:
Lavender Volume Hair and Scalp Wash, Lemon Sage clarifying Hair and Scalp Wash, Rosewood Moisturizing Hair and Scalp Wash

Premature Graying

This condition is thought to be from a deficiency of biotin, an important B vitamin.

Sandalwood helps retard greying. Rosewood may lighten hair color.

Dandruff

Dandruff may be caused by allergies, parasites (fungal), and/or chemicals.

Melaleuca alternifolia (tea tree) has been shown to be effective in treating dandruff and other fungal infections.[23]

Single Oils:
tea tree, rosemary, cedarwood

Blends:
Citrus Fresh, Melrose

Dandruff blend:
- 5 drops lemon
- 1 drop rosemary or sage
- 1 drop lavender

EO Applications:
TOPICAL:

DILUTE 50-50, massage 1 tsp into the scalp vigorously and thoroughly for 2-3 minutes; leave on scalp for 60-90 minutes. (An excellent time to do this would be during an exercise routine). Mix 2-4 drops of essential oils with 1-2 teaspoons of shampoo to wash hair after exercising.

Topical treatment:
Lavender Volume Hair and Scalp Wash, Lemon-Sage Clarifying Hair and Scalp Wash

Hair Loss
(See ALOPECIA AREATA)

Hair loss is caused by hormonal imbalances (such as increase in testosterone), or inflammatory conditions (as in the case of alopecia areata).

Essential oils are excellent for cleansing, nourishing, and strengthening the hair follicle and shaft. Rosemary (cineol chemotype) encourages hair growth.

Single Oils:

Lavender, rosemary, cedarwood, sandalwood, clary sage

Blends:

Hair loss prevention blend #1:
- 3 drops rosemary
- 5 drops lavender
- 4 drops cypress
- 2 drops clary sage
- 2 drops juniper

Add 10 drops of the above blend to 1 tsp. of fractionated coconut oil and massage into the scalp where it is balding; then rub gently into the remainder of the scalp. This works best when done at night.

Hair loss prevention blend #2:
- 10 drops cedarwood
- 8 drops rosemary
- 10 drops sandalwood
- 10 drops lavender

Hair loss prevention blend #3:
- 6 drops rosemary cineol
- 8 drops ylang ylang
- 12 drops cedarwood
- 12 drops clary sage

EO Applications:
TOPICAL:

DILUTE 50-50, massage 1 tsp. into the scalp vigorously and thoroughly for 2-3 minutes; leave on scalp for 60-90 minutes. (An excellent time to do this would be during an exercise routine). Mix 2-4 drops of essential oils with 1-2 teaspoons of shampoo to wash hair after exercising

Dietary Supplementation:

Super B, Essential Omegas, Thyromin, Sulfurzyme.

Topical Treatment:

EndoBalance

HALITOSIS (Bad Breath)
(See also DIGESTION PROBLEMS and ORAL CARE) (See also CANDIDA in FUNGAL INFECTIONS)

Persistent bad breath or gum disease, may be a sign of poor digestion, candida/yeast infestation, or other health problems.

Single Oils:

Nutmeg, peppermint, spearmint, lemon, mandarin, cinnamon, tarragon

Blends:

Thieves

Bad breath blend:
- 4 drops spearmint
- 2 drops mandarin
- 2 drops cinnamon

Disinfectant mouthwash:
- 3 drops peppermint
- 2 drops lemon
- 2 drops clove
- 1 drop tea tree oil

Thoroughly stir the above essential oil blend into one bottle of Fresh Essence Plus Mouthwash or dilute blend in 2 tsp. agave nectar and 4 oz. of hot water. Gargle as needed.

EO Applications:
ORAL:

GARGLE, 2-4 times daily as needed
TONGUE, 2-4 times daily as needed

Oral Treatment:

Fresh Essence Plus Mouthwash, Dentarome

Ultra Toothpaste, Thieves Antiseptic Spray, Thieves Lozenges

HASHIMOTO'S THYROIDITIS
(See THYROID)

HEAD LICE

The most common remedy for lice (pediculosis) and their eggs (nits) is lindane (gamma benzene hexachloride) a highly toxic polychlorinated chemical that is structurally very similar to hazardous banned pesticides such as DDT and chlordane. It is so dangerous that Dr. Guy Sansfacon, head of the Quebec Poison Control Centre in Canada, has requested that lindane be banned.

Essential oils represent a safe and effective alternative. A 1996 study by researchers in Iceland showed the effectiveness against headlice of the essential oils of anise seed, cinnamon leaf, thyme, tea tree, peppermint, and nutmeg in shampoo and rinse solutions.[24]

Single Oils:
Eucalyptus radiata, lavender, peppermint, thyme, geranium, nutmeg, rosemary

Blends:
Head lice blend:
- 4 drops Eucalyptus radiata
- 2 drop lavender
- 2 drop geranium

EO Applications:
TOPICAL:
DILUTE 50-50, 1 tsp. applied to scalp. Massage into entire scalp, cover with disposable shower cap and leave for at least 1/2 hour. Then shampoo and rise well. Use the rinse below.

Head lice rinse:
- 2 drops Eucalyptus radiata
- 2 drops lavender
- 2 drops geranium
- 1/2 oz. vinegar
- 8 oz. water

Mix into a container with a watertight lid. Shake vigorously, then pour over hair making sure every strand is rinsed. This should be done leaning over bathtub or sink. This is not recommended if you are still in the bathtub as lice may cling to other body hairs. Dry naturally. Repeat daily until lice and eggs are gone.

Head lice rinse 2:
- 2 drops rosemary
- 2 drops clove
- 2 drops peppermint
- 1 Tbsp. fractionated coconut oil

Massage into scalp and let sit for 20 minutes. Remove with dry towel.

Head lice rinse 3

1 cup Fresh Essence Plus massaged into hair and scalp. Retain for 30 minutes before rinsing out.

Topical Treatment:
Ortho Ease, Ortho Sport

HEADACHES
(See also STRESS, HYPOGLYCEMIA)

Headaches are usually caused by hormone imbalances, circulatory problems, stress, sugar imbalance (hypoglycemia), structural (spinal) misalignments, and blood pressure concerns

Placebo-controlled double-blind crossover studies at the Christian-Albrechts University in Kiel, Germany, found that essential oils were just as effective in blocking pain from tension-type headaches as acetaminophen (ie., Tylenol).[25, 26]

Essential oils also promote circulation, reduce muscle spasms, and decrease inflammatory response.

Single Oils:
Peppermint, Idaho balsam fir, Roman chamomile, German chamomile, lavender, basil, spearmint, valerian, clove, rosemary, *Eucalyptus globulus*

> **Headache from Diffusing**
> (Clarity and Brain Power)
>
> People who get an instant headache from diffusing usually have a blockage related to heavy metals or synthetic chemicals from cosmetics and other topical chemicals.
> **Single Oils:** Helichrysum, rosemary
> **Blends:** Aroma Life, M-Grain, and Clarity.
>
> *Apply helichrysum, rosemary, Aroma Life, and M-Grain to the arteries in the neck or along upper parts of wrists or on other pulse points where arteries are closest to the surface of the skin.*
>
> *Continue to diffuse Clarity or the offending oil, for short periods of time, until headaches cease.*

Blends:

M-Grain, Brain Power, Clarity, Relieve It, PanAway, Thieves

Headache blend #1:
- 4 drops Idaho tansy
- 5 drops Roman chamomile
- 2 drops peppermint
- 2 drops lavender
- 1 drop basil
- 3 drops rosemary

Headache blend #2:
- 2 drops Idaho tansy
- 1 drop Roman chamomile
- 3 drops spearmint
- 7 drops lavender

EO Applications:
INHALATION:
DIFFUSION, 15 minutes 3-5 times daily
DIRECT, 3-8 times daily as needed
TOPICAL:
DILUTE 50-50, apply 1-3 drops on back of neck, behind ears, on temples, on forehead, and under nose. Be careful to keep away from eyes and eyelids.
ORAL:
TONGUE, place a drop on the tongue then push against the roof of the mouth

Dietary Supplementation:
VitaGreen, Essential Omegas, Power Meal, BodyGize, Essentialzyme

Topical Treatment:
Prenolone, Prenolone+, Progessence

Children's Headache
Single Oils:
German chamomile, grapefruit, peppermint, lavender, rosemary

Blends:
Peace & Calming, PanAway

Children's Headache blend:
- 1 drop German chamomile
- 10 drops grapefruit
- 5 drops peppermint
- 3 drops rosemary

EO Applications:
TOPICAL:
DILUTE 50-50, apply 2-4 drops on temples, forehead, and brainstem. Also massage on thumbs and big toes.

Hormone Imbalance Headache
(See MENSTRUAL CONDITIONS)

Migraines (Vascular-type Headache)
The vast majority of migraine headaches may be due to colon congestion or poor digestion. The Cleansing Trio is most important for cleansing the colon. Eye strain and decreased vision can accompany migraine headaches. AD&E contains large amounts of lutein, which is vital for healthy vision.

Single Oils:
Helichrysum, sandalwood, basil, rosemary,

peppermint, lavender, marjoram, melissa, German chamomile, *Eucalyptus radiata*

Blends:

M-Grain, Clarity

M-Grain is specially formulated for migraine headaches.

EO Applications:

TOPICAL:

NEAT, Apply 1-2 drops to temples, at base of neck, in center of forehead, and at nostril openings. Also massage on thumbs and big toes

INHALATION:

DIRECT, as needed

Dietary Supplementation:

AD&E, Polyzyme, Cleansing Trio, Essentialzyme

Sinus Headache

(See also SINUS INFECTION)

Single Oils:

Rosemary, tea tree, *Eucalyptus radiata*, lavender, lemon, geranium

Blends:

Melrose, R.C., Purification

Sinus headache blend:
- 5 drops *Melaleuca ericifolia*
- 9 drops rosemary
- 2 drops bergamot
- 7 drops lavender
- 3 drops lemon
- 4 drops geranium

EO Applications:

INHALATION:

DIFFUSION, 10 min. 2-5 times daily and at night

DIRECT, 2-5 times daily as needed

Dietary Supplementation:

Super C Chewable, AD&E, Essential Omegas, Master Formula Vitamins, ImmuPro

Tension Headache

(See also STRESS)

Single Oils:

Idaho balsam fir, peppermint, lavender, marjoram, lemongrass, rosemary, valerian, cardamom

Blends:

Valor, Aroma Siez, M-Grain

EO Applications:

TOPICAL:

DILUTE 50-50, apply 1-2 drops around the hairline, on the back of the neck, and across the forehead. Be careful not to use too much, as it will burn if any oil drips near eyes. If this should occur, dilute with a pure vegetable oil. Never with water.

HEARING IMPAIRMENT

Single Oils:

Helichrysum, juniper, geranium, peppermint, lavender, basil

Blends:

Melrose, ImmuPower, Purification

EO Applications:

TOPICAL:

NEAT, (1) apply 1 drop essential oil on a cotton ball, then place it carefully in the opening of the ear canal. Retain overnight. <u>Do NOT place oils directly in the ear canal</u>. NEAT, (2) massage 1-2 drops on each ear lobe, behind the ears, and down the jaw line (along the Eustachian tube).

Hearing Vita Flex Regimen:
- Apply 1-2 drops neat helichrysum to the area OUTSIDE the opening to the ear canal with fingertip or cotton swab. <u>Do NOT put oil inside the ear canal</u>
- After applying the helichrysum, hold ear lobes firmly and pull in circular motion 10 times to help stimulate absorption and circulation in the ear canal.

Tinnitus (ringing in the ears)
Single Oils:
Helichrysum, juniper, geranium, peppermint, lavender, basil

EO Applications:
TOPICAL:
NEAT, massage 1-2 drops on temples and forehead and back of neck. Additionally, apply 1 drop each on tips of toes and fingers, so that the oils get into the Vita Flex pathways. (A change in hearing can often be noticed within 15-20 minutes.)
VITA FLEX, Do the hearing Vita Flex regimen described above

HEART
(See CARDIOVASCULAR CONDITIONS and CONGESTIVE HEART FAILURE)

Many people do not understand how someone who is relatively healthy, with low cholesterol levels, suffers a heart attack with no explanation. The explanation is actually inflammation, the fundamental cause of heart disease.

Inflammation of the heart is caused when blood vessels leading to the heart are clogged and damaged. This releases a protein into the bloodstream called C-reactive protein. The level of this protein indicates the degree of inflammation in the linings of the arteries. Certain essential oils have been documented to be excellent for reducing inflammation. German chamomile contains azulene, a blue compound with highly anti-inflammatory properties. Peppermint is also highly anti-inflammatory. Other oils also have anti-inflammatory properties such as helichrysum, spruce, birch or wintergreen, and valerian. Clove, nutmeg and wintergreen are natural blood thinners and help reduce blood clotting.

Magnesium, the most important mineral for the heart, acts as a smooth muscle relaxant and supports the cardiovascular system. Magnesium will act as a natural calcium channel blocker for the heart, lowering blood pressure and dilating the heart blood vessels (according to Terry Friedmann, MD).

Heart Vita Flex
The foot Vita Flex point related to the heart is on the sole of the left foot, on the ring toe (second toe) and behind the knuckle. Massaging this point is as effective as massaging the hand and arm together.

The hand Vita Flex point related to the heart is in the palm of the left hand, one inch below the ring finger joint (at the lifeline). A secondary heart point is on the bottom of the left arm in line with the inside of the up-turned arm (approximately 2 inches up the arm from the funny bone), not on the muscle but up under the muscle. Have another person use thumbs and firmly press these two points alternately for 3 minutes, in a kind of pumping action. Work all 3 points when possible. Start with the foot first; then go to the hand and arm.

Angina
Single Oils:
Ginger, goldenrod, orange, melissa

Blends:
Aroma Life, Peace & Calming

EO Applications:
TOPICAL:
NEAT, massage 1-3 drops over heart area 1-3 times daily. Also apply to left chest, left shoulder and back of neck
VITA FLEX, massage 1 drop each of 2 or 3 of the recommended oils on heart Vita Flex points on foot, hand, and arm, as needed

Fibrillation

This is a specific form of heart arrhythmia that occurs when the upper heart chambers contract at a rate of over 300 pulsations per minute. The lower chambers cannot keep this pace, so efficiency is reduced and not enough blood is pumped. Palpitations, a feeling that the heart is beating irregularly, more strongly, or more rapidly than normal, are the most common symptoms.

Single Oils:

Goldenrod, ylang ylang, marjoram, valerian, lavender, rosemary, Idaho tansy

Blends:

Aroma Life, Peace & Calming, Joy

EO Applications:

TOPICAL:

NEAT, massage 1-3 drops over heart area 1-3 times daily. Also apply to left chest, left shoulder and back of neck

VITA FLEX, massage 1 drop each of 2 or 3 of the recommended oils on heart Vita Flex points on foot, hand, and arm, as needed

INHALATION:

DIRECT, as often as needed to bring calm

Dietary Supplementation:

HRT, CardiaCare, Mineral Essence, Super Cal, Wolfberry Crisp, BerryGize Bar, Sulfurzyme

Heart Attack (Myocardial Infarction)

A heart attack is a circulation blockage resulting in an interruption of blood supply to an area or the heart. Depending on the size of the area affected, it can be mild or severe.

NOTE: Contact your physical immediately if you suspect a heart attack.

Single Oils:

Goldenrod, thyme, lavender, Roman chamomile, helichrysum, Idaho tansy, clove nutmeg

Blends:

Longevity, Aroma Life, Peace & Calming, PanAway, Relieve It, Harmony, Valor

EO Applications:

TOPICAL:

NEAT, apply 1-2 drops to heart Vita Flex points on foot, hand, and arm as described under the 'Heart Vita Flex' section at the beginning of this heading. If there is not enough time to remove shoes to get at the feet, apply the 'pumping' action to left hand and arm points. Using 1-2 drops of Aroma Life on each point will increase effectiveness and may even revive an individual having a heart attack while waiting for medical attention.

Dietary Supplementation:

CardiaCare, HRT Tincture, Longevity Caps, CardiaCare, Mineral Essence, Essential Omegas, AD&E, Super Cal, Power Meal, Berry Berrygize Bars, Berry Young Juice, Sulfurzyme

Tachycardia

Another form of heart arrhythmia in which the heart rate suddenly increases to 160 beats per minute or faster.

Single Oils:

Marjoram, ylang ylang, lavender, goldenrod, Idaho tansy

Blends:

Aroma Life, Peace & Calming, Joy

EO Applications:

TOPICAL:

NEAT, massage 1-3 drops over heart area 1-3 times daily. Also apply to left chest, left shoulder and back of neck

VITA FLEX, massage 1 drop each of 2 or 3 of the recommended oils on heart Vita

Flex points on foot, hand, and arm, as needed
INHALATION:
DIRECT, as often as needed to bring calm
Dietary Supplementation:
CardiaCare, HRT Tincture, Sulfurzyme

Tonic-Stimulant
Single Oils:
Goldenrod, anise seed, mandarin, rosemary, peppermint, thyme, marjoram
Blends:
Aroma Life
EO Applications:
TOPICAL:
NEAT, massage 1-3 drops over heart area 1-3 times daily
VITA FLEX, massage 1 drop each of 2 or 3 of the recommended oils on heart Vita Flex points on foot, hand, and arm, as needed
INHALATION:
DIRECT, as often as needed to bring calm

HEARTBURN
(See Heartburn in DIGESTION PROBLEMS)

HEAVY METALS
(See also METAL TOXICITY, Aluminum)

We absorb heavy metals from air, water, food, skin care products, mercury fillings in teeth, etc. These chemicals lodge in the fatty tissues of the body, which, in turn, give off toxic gases that may cause allergic symptoms. Cleansing the body of these heavy metals is extremely important to have a healthy immune function, especially if one has amalgam fillings.

Drink at least 64 ounces of distilled water daily to flush toxins and chemicals out of the body.

Single Oils:
Helichrysum, cypress, frankincense, German chamomile, lemongrass, geranium
Blends:
Juva Cleanse
EO Applications:
TOPICAL:
DILUTE 50-50, apply 4-6 drops to under arms, kidney area and bottoms of feet, 1-3 times daily
RAINDROP Technique, 1-3 times monthly
INGESTION:
CAPSULE, 0 size, 1 capsule once a day
(See CIRCULATION PROBLEMS)
Dietary Supplementation:
JuvaTone, JuvaPower/Spice, VitaGreen, Super C, ImmuPro, ImmuneTune, ImmuGel, Longevity Caps, Chelex, K&B Tincture, HRT tincture, Rehemogen, AD&E, Essentialzyme
(See also CHEMICAL SENSITIVITY REACTION)

Vascular Cleansing
This regimen is to help cleanse the blood and tissues of heavy metal toxins. Certain essential oils and supplements can have a very beneficial effect in ridding the body of these toxins.

1. Chelex: Take 1 full dropper in 4 ounces of water 2 times daily to remove heavy metals. Cardamom essential oil and VitaGreen enhance this action.
2. Massage the body with Aroma Life and 1-2 drops of helichrysum, followed by Cel-Lite Magic Massage oil.
3. Vascular Cleansing blend:
   - 10 drops juniper
   - 10 drops cypress
   - 10 drops lemongrass
   - 1 Tbsp V6 Oil Complex

Rub 2-4 drops under arms, on arms, on skin above kidneys and on bottoms of feet 1-3 times daily.

4. To remove dental mercury from gum tissue, mix 3 drops helichrysum and 4 drops Thieves and put on a rolled gauze and place next to the gums. Only apply to one area at a time; for example, apply on lower left gum on the first night, the upper left the second night and so on.

NOTE: *For young or very sensitive gums, dilute with V-6 Oil Complex.*
(See CIRCULATION PROBLEMS)

HEMATOMA

A hematoma is a tumor-like mass of coagulated blood, caused by a break in the blood vessel or capillary wall. Essential oils, such as helichrysum or geranium, are excellent for balancing blood viscosity and dissolving clots. Clove oil and citrus rind oils, such as lemon and grapefruit, exert a blood-thinning effect that can help speed the dissolution of the clot.

Those who bruise easily are usually low in vitamin C, which may be caused by insufficient intake or poor absorption.

Single Oils:
Cypress, cistus, helichrysum, lemon, grapefruit, clove, nutmeg, wintergreen/birch

Blends:
Aroma Life, PanAway

Dietary Supplementation:
Super C Chewable, Mineral Essence

HEMORRHAGES

Some essential oils, when topically applied or used on pressure bandages, are excellent for slowing bleeding and initiating healing.

Single Oils:
Helichrysum, geranium, cistus, cypress, lavender, myrrh, hyssop

Blends:
Aroma Life, PanAway

EO Applications:
TOPICAL:
COMPRESS, cold, as needed
NEAT, 1-2 drops on location for small wounds

HEMORRHOIDS

Single Oils:
Cypress, cistus, helichrysum, myrrh, lemon, spikenard, basil, peppermint

Blends:
Aroma Siez, Aroma Life, PanAway
Hemorrhoid blend #1:
- 3 or 4 drops of basil
- 1 drop of wintergreen/birch
- 1 drop of cypress
- 1 drop of helichrysum

Hemorrhoid blend #2:
- 3 drops cypress
- 2 drops helichrysum
- 10 drops myrtle

EO Applications:
TOPICAL:
DILUTE 50-50, apply 3-5 drops on location. This may sting, but usually brings relief with one or two applications.
RETENTION:
RECTAL, once every other day for 6 days.

Dietary Supplementation:
Cel-Lite Magic, Royaldophilus, Essentialzyme, Polyzyme, VitaGreen, Super B, Longevity Caps
Cleanse using the Cleansing Trio

Topical Treatment:
Cel-Lite Magic

HEPATITIS

(See HEPATITIS in LIVER DISORDERS)

145

HERPES SIMPLEX
(See SEXUALLY TRANSMITTED DISEASES for Herpes Type II, COLD SORES for Herpes Type I, and CHICKEN POX for Herpes Zoster)

HICCUPS
Hiccups are usually caused by irritated nerves of the diaphragm, possibly caused from a full stomach or indigestion.
(See also DIGESTIVE PROBLEMS)

One technique for stopping hiccups that often works when others fail is to stimulate the Vita Flex point for hiccups by placing one drop of cypress and one drop of tarragon on the end of the index finger; then place that finger against the esophagus in the clavicle notch in the center, and curl inward and down, like you're curling down inside the throat, and release.

Cypress or tarragon either topically applied or taken as a dietary supplement may relax intestinal spasms, nervous digestion, and hiccups.

Single Oils:
Cypress, tarragon, peppermint

EO Applications:
TOPICAL:
DILUTE 50-50, apply 3-5 drops to chest and stomach areas.
INGESTION:
CAPSULE, 0 size, 1 capsule 2 times daily
RICE MILK, 2-4 times daily

HIVES
(See ITCHING in SKIN DISORDERS and LIVER DISORDERS)

Hives is a generalized itching or dermatitis that can be due allergies, damaged liver, chemicals, or other factors.

Single Oils:
Peppermint, patchouly, myrrh

EO Applications:
TOPICAL:
DILUTE 50-50, 2-4 drops on location as needed
COMPRESS, cold, as needed

Dietary Supplementation:
Super Cal, Coral Sea, Mega Cal, Mineral Essence, AD&E

Topical Treatment:
Tender Tush Ointment

HORMONE IMBALANCE
(See Hormone Imbalance under MENSTRUAL CONDITIONS)

HOT FLASHES
(See MENSTRUAL CONDITIONS)

HUNTINGTON'S CHOREA
(See NEUROLOGICAL DISEASES)

HYPERACTIVITY
Single Oils:
Lavender, cedarwood, vetiver, Roman chamomile, peppermint, valerian

EO Applications:
INHALATION:
DIRECT, 5 times daily for up to 30 days, then off 5 days, then repeat if necessary
TOPICAL:
NEAT, 2-4 drops on toes and balls of feet, as needed

HYPERPNOEA
Abnormally fast, labored breathing

Single Oil:
Ylang Ylang

EO Applications:
TOPICAL:
NEAT, 2-3 drops on solar plexus, base of throat and back of neck, as needed

HYPERTENSION
(See CARDIOVASCULAR CONDITIONS)

HYPOGLYCEMIA

Hypoglycemia may also be caused by low thyroid function (See THYROID).

Excessive consumption of sugar or honey will also cause reactive hypoglycemia, in which a rapid rise in blood sugar is followed by a steep drop to abnormally low levels.

In some cases, hypoglycemia may be a precursor to candida, allergies, chronic fatigue syndrome, depression, and chemical sensitivities.

Signs of hypoglycemia (low blood sugar) include:

- Fatigue, drowsiness, and sleepiness after meals.
- Headache or dizziness if periods between meals are too long.
- Craving for sweets.
- Allergic reaction to foods.
- Palpitations, tremors, sweats, rapid heart beat.
- Inattentiveness, mood swings, irritability, anxiety, nervousness, inability to cope with stress, and feelings of emotional depression.
- Lack of motivation, discipline, and creativity.
- Hunger that cannot be satisfied.

Often people with some of these symptoms are misdiagnosed as suffering either chronic fatigue or neurosis. Instead, they may be hypoglycemic.

To treat chronic hypoglycemia, it may be necessary to first treat the underlying candida or yeast overgrowth.
(See FUNGAL INFECTIONS).

Essential oils may reduce hypoglycemic symptoms by helping to normalize sugar cravings and supporting and stabilizing sugar metabolism in the body.

Single Oils:
Lavender, cinnamon, cumin, clove, thyme, coriander, lemon, dill

Blends:
Thieves, JuvaFlex, JuvaCleanse, Di-Tone, Exodus II

EO Applications:
  INGESTION:
    CAPSULE, 00 size, 1 times daily (coriander, dill and thyme work best through ingestion)
  INHALATION:
    DIRECT, 2-5 times daily as needed

Dietary Supplementation:
Power Meal, BodyGize, VitaGreen, Stevia, ThermaMist, ThermaBurn, Exodus, Mineral Essence, Essential Manna, Berry Young Juice

HYSTERECTOMY
(See Hysterectomy in MENSTRUAL CONDITIONS)

IMPOTENCE
(See also SEXUAL DYSFUNCTIONS)

Impotence (the inability to perform sexually) can be caused by physical limitations (an accident or injury) or psychological factors (inhibitions, trauma, stress, etc). In males, impotence is often linked to problems with the prostate or prostate surgery
(See also PROSTATE PROBLEMS)

If impotence is related to psychological trauma or unresolved emotional issues, it may be necessary to deal with these issues before any meaningful progress can be made.
(See also TRAUMA)

There is an extensive historical basis for the ability of fragrance to amplify desire and create a mood that can overcome frigidity or impotence. In fact, aromas such as rose and jasmine have been used since antiquity to attract the opposite sex and create a romantic atmosphere.

Modern research has shown that the fragrance of some essential oils can stimulate the emotional center of the brain. This may explain why essential oils have the potential to help people overcome impotence based on emotional factors or inhibitions.

Single Oils:
Ylang ylang, clary sage, sandalwood, myrrh, jasmine, frankincense, ginger, nutmeg, rose,

Blends:
Valor, Joy

Dietary Supplementation:
ProGen (for men)

INDIGESTION
(See DIGESTIVE PROBLEMS)

INFECTION (Bacterial and Viral)

Diffusing essential oils is one of the best ways to prevent the spread of airborne bacteria and viruses. Many essential oils, such as oregano, mountain savory, and rosemary, exert highly antimicrobial effects and can effectively eliminate many kinds of pathogens.

Viruses and bacteria have a tendency to hibernate along the spine. The body may hold a virus in a suspended state for long periods of time. When the immune system is compromised, these viruses may be released and then manifest into illness. Raindrop Technique along the spine helps reduce inflammation and kill the microorganism.

Oregano and thyme are generally used first for the Raindrop application. However, other oils may also be used and may be more desirable for some people. ImmuPower, R.C., and Purification all work well in the Raindrop application method.

Mountain savory, ravensara, and thyme applied during Raindrop Technique on the spine are beneficial for most infections, particularly chest-related.

(See also COLDS, LUNG-, SINUS-, and THROAT INFECTION)

Single Oils:
Mountain savory, rosemary lemongrass, spruce, clove, thyme, oregano, rosewood, sage, cistus, tea tree

Blends:
Purification, Melrose, R.C., Thieves, ImmuPower, Exodus II, 3 Wise Men

EO Applications:
TOPICAL:
DILUTE 20-80, 4-6 drops on location 2-3 times daily
RAINDROP Technique, 1-2 times weekly
INGESTION:
CAPSULE, 00 size, 1 capsule twice daily

Dietary Supplementation:
Super C Chewable, Exodus, Berry Young Juice, Longevity Caps, VitaGreen, ImmuPro, ImmuneTune, Rehemogen

INFERTILITY

Natural progesterone creams when used at the beginning of the cycle (immediately following the cessation of menstruation) can improve fertility. Some essential oils have hormone-like qualities that can support or improve fertility processes.

Single Oils:
Clary sage, anise seed, fennel, blue yarrow, geranium

To Kill Airborne Viruses and Bacteria

Periodically alternate diffusing ImmuPower and Thieves.

Topically apply 1 drop Melaleuca alternifolia and 1 drop rosemary to stem infection.

Single Oils: Tea Tree, cinnamon, clove, thyme, oregano, ravensara, or frankincense.

Blends: Thieves, Melrose, Purification

Blends:
Dragon Time, Mister, EndoFlex

EO Applications:
  INGESTION:
    CAPSULE, 0 size, 2 times daily
  TOPICAL:
    NEAT, for females, apply 2-4 drops to the lower back and lower abdomen areas, 2 times daily
    VITA FLEX, 1-3 drops applied to the reproductive Vita Flex points on hands and feet (These are the inside of wrists, inside and outside of the upper foot on either side of the anklebone, and along the achilles tendon) 2 times daily

Dietary Supplementation:
VitaGreen, Mineral Essence, Super Cal, Essential Manna, Ultra Young, Thyromin

Topical Treatment:
Progessence, Prenolone, Prenolone+, EndoBalance.

INFLAMMATION

Inflammation can be caused by a variety of conditions, including bacterial infection, poor diet, chemicals, hormonal imbalance, and physical injury.

Certain essential oils have been documented to be excellent for reducing inflammation. German chamomile contains azulene, a blue compound with highly anti-inflammatory properties. Peppermint is also highly anti-inflammatory. Other oils with anti-inflammatory properties include helichrysum, spruce, wintergreen/birch, and clove.

Some oils are better suited for certain types of inflammation. For example:

- Myrrh and helichrysum work well for inflammation due to tissue/capillary damage, and bruising.
- German chamomile and lavender are helpful with inflammation due to bacterial infection.
- Ravensara, hyssop, and thyme are appropriate for inflammation caused by viral infection.

Single Oils:
Wintergreen/birch, helichrysum, clove, nutmeg, lavender, ravensara, thyme, German chamomile, Roman chamomile, cypress, myrrh, hyssop, peppermint, spruce

Blends:
Purification, PanAway, Aroma Siez, Melrose, ImmuPro, Relieve It, Exodus II

Anti-inflammation blend #1:
- 10 drops fir
- 6 drops tea tree
- 4 drops German chamomile
- 2 drops peppermint
- 2 drops lemongrass

Anti-inflammation blend #2:
- 6 drops frankincense
- 6 drops fir
- 6 drops *Eucalyptus citriodora*
- 4 drops ravensara
- 3 drops wintergreen/birch
- 1 drop peppermint

EO Applications:
  TOPICAL:
    DILUTE 50-50, 2-4 drops on inflamed area, 2 times daily
    COMPRESS, cold, 1-3 times daily as needed
  INGESTION:
    CAPSULE, 0 size, 2 times daily

Topical Treatment:
Ortho Ease, Relaxation, Ortho Sport

INFLUENZA
(See COLDS)

Single Oils:
Idaho tansy, lemon, blue cypress, mountain

savory, oregano, *Eucalyptus radiata*, myrtle, peppermint

Blends:

ImmuPower, Di-Tone, Exodus II, Thieves, ParaFree, Essentialzyme, Polyzyme

EO Applications:

INGESTION:

RICE MILK, 2-4 times daily
CAPSULE, 00 size, 1 capsule 3 times daily

INHALATION:

DIRECT, 2-4 times daily

TOPICAL:

DILUTE 50-50, 2-4 drops on chest, stomach or lower back, as needed, 2 times daily
RAINDROP Technique, 1-2 times weekly
COMPRESS, warm, over lower abdomen, 1-2 times daily
BATH SALTS, (see below)

Influenza Recipe for bath:
- 2 drops Eucalyptus radiata
- 6 drops frankincense
- 3 drops helichrysum
- 6 drops spruce
- 15 drops ravensara
- 1 drop wintergreen or birch

Stir above essential oils thoroughly into 1/4 cup Epsom salt or baking soda, then add salt/oil mixture to hot bath water while tub is filling. Soak in hot bath until water cools.

Dietary Supplementation:

ParaFree, Essentialzyme, Polyzyme, ImmuPro, ImmuneTune, ImmuGel, Exodus, Essential Omegas

INSECT BITES

(See INSECT REPELLENT)

Because of their outstanding antiseptic and oil-soluble properties, essential oils are ideal for treating most kinds of insect bites. Essential oils such as lavender and peppermint reduce insect-bite-induced itching and infection.

Singles oils:

Lavender, eucalyptus globulus, citronella, tea tree, peppermint, rosemary

Blends:

Purification, Melrose, PanAway

Blend for stings and bites:
- 1 drop thyme
- 10 drops lavender
- 4 drops *Eucalyptus radiata*
- 3 drops Roman or German chamomile

EO Applications:

TOPICAL:

NEAT or DILUTE 50-50, apply 1-2 drops on bite location 2-4 times daily

Bee Stings

Single Oils:

Lavandin, Idaho tansy

Blends:

Purification, Melrose, PanAway

Bee Sting blend:
- 2 drops lavender
- 1 drop helichrysum
- 1 drop German chamomile
- 1 drop wintergreen/birch

Bee Sting Regimen:
- Flick or scrape stinger out with credit card or knife, taking care not to squeeze the venom sack.
- Apply 1-2 drops Purification, Melrose, lavender, or Idaho tansy on location. Repeat until the venom spread has stopped.
- Apply lavandin with or without one or more of the single oils listed, 2-3 times daily until redness abates. PanAway may be substituted for Purification.

Black Widow Spider Bite

Get victim to an emergency care facility immediately. Rub 1 drop lavender every 2-3 minutes over the bite until you reach the hospital.

Brown Recluse Spider Bite

The bite of this spider causes a painful redness and blistering which progresses to a gangrenous slough of the affected area. Seek immediate medical attention.

Blends:

Purification, Thieves
Spider Bite blend:
- 1 drop lavandin
- 1 drop helichrysum
- 1 drop Melrose

EO Applications:
  TOPICAL:
  NEAT, 1 drop of either of the two above blends every minute until you reach professional medical treatment.

Chiggers (Mites)
Single Oils:

Tea tree, lavender

Blends:

R.C., Purification

EO Applications:
  TOPICAL:
  NEAT, 2-6 drops, depending on size of affected area, 3-5 times daily

Ticks
Single Oils:

Thyme, oregano, peppermint

Blends:

R.C., Purification

EO Applications:
  TOPICAL:
  NEAT, apply 1 drop neat thyme or oregano to tick to loosen from skin. Apply 1 drop neat Purification on site to detoxify wound. Apply 1 drop neat peppermint every 5 minutes for 5 minutes to reduce pain and infection.

INSECT REPELLENT
Single Oils:

Peppermint, *Eucalyptus radiata,* lemon, lime, lavender, tea tree, cedarwood, geranium, Idaho tansy, rosemary, patchouly, citronella, lemongrass, thyme

Blends:

Purification, Thieves, Melrose
Insect Repellent blend:
- 6 drops peppermint
- 6 drops tea tree
- 9 drops *Eucalyptus radiata*

EO Applications:
  TOPICAL:
  DILUTE 20-80, apply to exposed skin as needed

Using Essential Oils As Insect Repellents

Mosquito-repellent: Lemon, peppermint, Eucalyptus radiata, lemongrass.

Moth repellent: Patchouly.

Horse-fly repellent: Idaho tansy floral water.

Aphids repellent: Mix 10 drops spearmint and 15 drops orange essential oils in 2 quarts salt water, shake well, and spray on plants.

Cockroach repellent: Mix 10 drops peppermint and 5 drops cypress in 1/2 cup salt water. Shake well and spray where roaches live.

Silverfish repellent: Eucalyptus radiata, citriadora

To repel insects, essential oils can be diffused or put on cotton balls or cedar chips (for use in closets or drawers).

INSOMNIA

After age 40, sleep quality and quantity deteriorates substantially as melatonin production in the brain declines. Supplemental melatonin has been researched to dramatically improve sleep/wake cycles and combat age-related insomnia.

Insomnia may also be caused by bowel or liver toxicity, poor heart function, negative memories and trauma, depression, mineral deficiencies, hormone imbalance, or underactive thyroid.

The fragrance of many essential oils can exert a powerful calming effect on the mind through their influence on the limbic region of the brain. Historically, lavender sachets or pillows were used.

Single Oils:
Valerian, lavender, cedarwood, lemon, German chamomile, Roman chamomile, mandarin, St. John's wort, Idaho balsam fir, rosemary, cypress

Blends:
Peace & Calming, Citrus Fresh, Harmony, Dream Catcher, Valor, Present Time, Gentle Baby, Citrus Fresh, 3 Wise Men

Insomnia blend #1:
- 12 drops orange
- 8 drops lavender
- 4 drops citrus hystrix
- 3 drops geranium
- 2 drops Roman chamomile

Insomnia blend #2:
- 15 drops lavender
- 15 drops Peace & Calming

EO Applications:
  INHALATION:
  DIFFUSION, 30-60 min. at bedtime. Or apply 1-3 drops on a cotton ball and place on or near your pillow.
  TOPICAL:
  NEAT, apply 1-3 drops to shoulders, stomach and on bottoms of feet.
  BATH SALTS, just before retiring at night

> **To Relax Before Sleep:**
>
> Rub Peace & Calming or Dream Catcher across the shoulders along with a little lavender or Roman chamomile if needed.
>
> Put 1 drop of Harmony on energy meridians to help balance the energy flow in the body. (1 drop on stomach, navel, thymus, throat, forehead, and crown of head).

Dietary Supplementation:
ImmuPro, Super Cal, Thyromin, HRT tincture, CardiaCare, PD80/20, PowerMeal
Take one 00 capsule of lavender oil 1 hour before bedtime.

Topical Treatment:
Progessence, Prenolone

Insomnia from Bowel Toxicity
(See also DIGESTIVE PROBLEMS)

Dietary Supplementation:
Essentialzyme, Comfortone, ICP

A fasting or cleansing program is important for combating insomnia caused by excess toxins accumulating in the liver and the gastrointestinal tract. Excessive toxins may also produce recurring migraine headaches, skin eruptions, discoloration, changes in pigmentation, acne, or bumpy skin.

Insomnia from Depression
(See also DEPRESSION)

Depression is a major cause of insomnia. St. John's wort has been proven highly effective in reducing depression. A lack of adequate mineral intake (ie., magnesium, zinc, copper, selenium, potassium) can also contribute to clinical depression.

Single Oils:
St. John's wort, melissa, frankincense, lemon

EO Applications:
   TOPICAL:
       NEAT, apply 1-3 drops to shoulders, stomach and on bottoms of feet.
Dietary Supplementation:
   Mineral Essence, Essential Manna, AD&E, Wolfberry Crisp, BerryGize Bar, Berry Young Juice, Master Formula Vitamins, Essential Omegas, Super B, Ultra Young

Insomnia from Thyroid Imbalance
(See also THYROID)

Hyperthyroidism (having an overactive thyroid) is caused by chlorine in the drinking water and can trigger insomnia.

Single Oils:
   Myrrh, myrtle
EO Applications:
   TOPICAL:
       NEAT, apply 1-3 drops to shoulders, stomach and on bottoms of feet.
Dietary Supplementation:
   Thyromin

IRRITABLE BOWEL SYNDROME
(See DIGESTIVE PROBLEMS)

Irritable bowel syndrome (IBS) is a common disorder of the intestines marked by the following symptoms:
- Cramps
- Gas and bloating
- Constipation
- Diarrhea and loose stools

IBS may be caused by a combination of stress and a high-fat diet. Fatty foods worsen symptoms by increasing the intensity of the contractions in the colon, thereby increasing symptoms. Chocolate and milk products, in particular, seem to have the most negative effect on IBS sufferers.

IBS is not the same as colitis, mucous colitis, spastic colon, and spastic bowel. Unlike colitis, IBS does not involve any inflammation and is actually called a "functional disorder" because it presents no obvious, outward signs of disease.

A number of medical studies have documented that peppermint oil (in enteric-coated capsules) is beneficial in treating irritable bowel syndrome and decreases pain.[27,28,29]

Single Oils:
   Peppermint, anise seed, fennel, tarragon
Blends:
   Di-Tone, Juva Cleanse
EO Applications:
   INGESTION:
       CAPSULE, 0 size, 2 times daily
       RICE MILK, 2-4 times daily
       SYRUP, 2-4 times daily
Dietary Supplementation:
   Royaldophilus, ICP, ComforTone, Stevia Select, Polyzyme, Essentialzyme, Lipozyme, Juva Power, Immugel

ITCHING
(See SKIN DISORDERS or FUNGAL INFECTIONS)

JAUNDICE
(See LIVER DISORDERS)

Jaundice refers to the yellowing of the skin that is a result of a stressed or damaged liver.

Single Oils:
   Ledum, amyris, carrot seed, German chamomile, thyme, geranium
Blends:
   JuvaFlex, JuvaCleanse, Release
EO Applications:
   INGESTION:
       CAPSULE, 0 size, once a day, using JuvaFlex, JuvaCleanse

TOPICAL:
   COMPRESS, warm, 2-3 times daily over the liver

Dietary Supplementation:
Cleansing Trio, JuvaTone, milk thistle, Rehemogen

JOINT STIFFNESS AND PAIN
(See also PAIN, ARTHRITIS and CONNECTIVE TISSUE)

Single Oils:
Spruce, Douglas fir, elemi, Idaho balsam fir, wintergreen/birch, German chamomile, cypress, peppermint, helichrysum, pine

Blends:
PanAway, Aroma Siez, Aroma Life, Relieve It

Joint Pain blend #1:
- 10 drops black pepper
- 2 drops rosemary
- 5 drops marjoram
- 5 drops lavender

Joint Pain blend #2:
- 8 drops spruce
- 8 drops sandalwood
- 7 drops fir
- 5 drops hyssop
- 4 drops lemongrass
- 5 drops helichrysum
- 4 drops wintergreen/birch
- 2 drops blue chamomile
- 3 drops vetiver
- 1 drop Idaho tansy

EO Applications:
   TOPICAL:
      DILUTE 50-50, massage 3-6 drops on location, repeat as needed to control pain
      VITA FLEX, apply to appropriate Vita Flex points on the feet. Repeat as needed

Dietary Supplementation:
Sulfurzyme, Power Meal, Ultra Young, ArthroTune, ArthroPlus

Topical Treatment:
Regenolone, Ortho Ease, Ortho Sport, Morning Start Bath Gel, Peppermint-Cedarwood Bar Soap, Melaleuca/Geranium Bar Soap

JUVENILE DWARFISM

Dwarfism is caused by insufficient production of growth hormone by the pituitary. The essential oil *Conyza canadensis* (Fleabane) was used by Daniel Pénoël, M.D., in his clinical practice for reversing retarded maturation. This essential oil is included in Ultra Young.

Singles:
Fleabane

Blends:
Brain Power
Brain Power stimulates the limbic system.

Dietary Supplementation:
Ultra Young, Ultra Young+, PD 80/20

Topical Treatment:
Prenolone+, EndoBalance

KIDNEY DISORDERS

The kidneys remove waste products from the blood, control blood pressure. The kidneys filter over 200 quarts of blood each day and remove over 2 quarts of waste products and water which flow into the bladder as urine through tubes called ureters.

Strong kidneys are essential for good health. Inefficient or damaged kidneys can result in wastes accumulating in the blood and causing serious damage.

High blood pressure can be a cause and a result of chronic kidney failure, since kidneys are central to blood regulation (see BLOOD PRESSURE, HIGH).

Symptoms of poor kidney function:
- Infrequent or inefficient urinations.
- Swelling, especially around the ankles.
- Labored breathing due to fluid accumulation in chest.

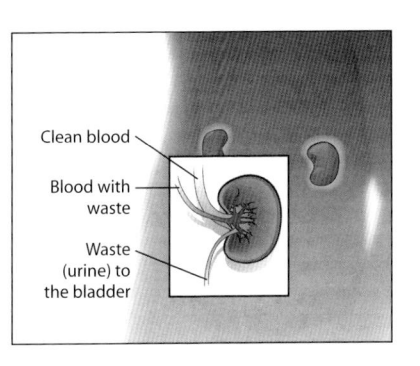

Clean blood
Blood with waste
Waste (urine) to the bladder

Diuretic (To Increase Urine Flow)
Single Oils:
Ledum, rosemary, juniper, fennel, anise seed, lemongrass, grapefruit, geranium, sage

Blends:
JuvaFlex, JuvaCleanse, EndoFlex, Di-Tone, Acceptance

Dietary Supplementation:
K & B Tincture, Cleansing Trio, and JuvaTone, JuvaPower/Spice

EO Applications:
  INGESTION:
  CAPSULE, 0 size, 3 times daily
  TOPICAL:
  DILUTE 50-50, massage 6-8 drops over kidney area on back, 1-2 times daily
  COMPRESS, warm, 1-2 times daily

Topical Treatment:
Cel-Lite Magic Massage Oil

Edema (Swelling)
(See EDEMA, WATER RETENTION)

Kidney Inflammation/Infection (Nephritis)
Kidney inflammation can be caused by structural defects, poor diet, or bacterial infection from *Escherichia coli, Staphylococcus aureus, Enterobacter,* and *Klebsiellabacteri.*

Abnormal proteins trapped in the glomeruli can also cause inflammation and damage to these tiny filtering units. This is called *glomerulonephritis*. This disease can be acute (flaring up in a few days), or chronic (taking months or years to develop). The mildest forms may not show any symptoms except through a urine test. At more advanced stages, urine appears smokey (as small amounts of blood are passed) and eventually red as more blood is excreted—the signs of impending kidney failure. As with all serious conditions, you should immediately consult a health care professional if you suspect a kidney infection of any kind.

Symptoms include:
- Feeling of discomfort in lower back
- Drowsiness
- Nauseous
- Smokey or red-colored urine

Damage to the glomeruli (tiny filtering units in the kidneys) caused by bacterial infections is called *pyelonephritis*. To reduce infection, drink a gallon of water mixed with 8 oz. of cranberry juice daily and use the following products:

Single Oils:
Myrrh, cypress, juniper, geranium, tangerine, marjoram

Blends:
Thieves, JuvaFlex, JuvaCleanse, Aroma Life, EndoFlex

A Simple Way To Strengthen the Kidneys

- Take 3 droppers K & B Tincture in 4 oz. distilled water, 3 times daily.
- Drink 8 oz. water with about 10 percent cranberry juice and the fresh juice of 1/2 lemon.
- Drink plenty of other liquids, preferably distilled water.

> **Case History**
>
> It was reported that a man had a heart bypass using a vein removed from his leg. The leg swelled up from fluid retention and could be moved around like jelly. The leg was first massaged from the foot up with 4 drops cypress mixed into Cel-Lite Magic Massage Oil. The massage was repeated with 4 drops each of fennel and geranium mixed into the same massage oil. After 20 minutes of massaging the swelling had dissipated.

EO Applications:
  INGESTION:
    CAPSULE, 00 size, 2 times daily for 10 days
    RICE MILK, 2-4 times daily
  TOPICAL:
    COMPRESS, cold, 1-2 times daily over kidney area
    VITA FLEX, massage 1-3 drops on kidney Vita Flex points on feet

Dietary Supplementation:
  K & B tincture

Kidney Compress regimen:
  Kidney Compress blend:
  - 5 drops juniper
  - 5 drops tangerine
  - 3 drops geranium
  - 1 drop helichrysum

  Mix the above oils with 1/2 tsp V6 Oil Complex or massage oil and massage 6-10 drops of the mixture on the back over the kidney area. Apply a COLD compress over the kidneys for one night.

  The following night do another COLD compress over the kidneys using 10 drops ImmuPower in 1/4 tsp. V6 Oil Complex. Each night, massage the kidney Vita Flex points on the feet. Repeat, if needed. Take 3 droppers of K & B three times daily.

Three Phase Kidney Support regimen:
  Phase I:
  Perform a colon and liver cleanse
  Phase II:
  Daily Regimen:
  - 4 servings of Power Meal and 6 capsules VitaGreen
  - 3 droppers Rehemogen 3 times daily
  - Apply 2-4 drops Aroma Life, JuvaFlex, or JuvaCleanse over the kidneys, on kidney Vita Flex points of the feet, and around the navel.
  - After 10 days, add ImmuneTune and Super C.

  Phase III:
  Drink a gallon of water mixed with 8 oz. of unsweetened cranberry juice daily.

Kidney Stones

A kidney stone is a solid piece of material that forms in the kidney from mineral or protein-breakdown products in the urine. Occasionally, larger stones can become trapped in a ureter, bladder, or urethra, which can block urine flow causing intense pain.

There are four types of kidney stones: Stones made from calcium (the most common type), stones made from magnesium and ammonia (a struvite stone), stones made from uric acid, and stones made from cystine (the most rare).

Some of the symptoms of kidney stones include:
- Persistent, penetrating pain in side
- A burning sensation during urination
- Blood in the urine
- Bad-smelling or cloudy urine
- Fainting

It is important to drink plenty of water *(at least 12 eight-ounce glasses daily)* to help pass or dissolve a kidney stone.

Single Oils:
Wintergreen/birch, geranium, juniper, helichrysum, fennel, lemongrass

Blends:
Kidney stone compress blend:
- 10 drops *Eucalyptus radiata*
- 10 drops geranium
- 10 drops juniper
- 1 Tbsp. V6 Oil Complex

EO Applications:
TOPICAL:
COMPRESS, warm, use 6-10 drops of above blend, over kidney area 1-2 times daily
VITA FLEX, massage 2-3 drops on kidney Vita Flex points of feet

INGESTION:
CAPSULE, 00 size, 2 times daily
RICE MILK, 2-4 times daily

Dietary Supplementation:
Cleansing Trio, Juvatone, K & B, Polyzyme, Essentialzyme, Detoxzyme, ComforTone
Other options for helping the body pass a stone:

Kidney Stone drink #1
- 5 drops rosemary
- 5 drops geranium
- 5 drops juniper
- 1 Tbsp. agave nectar
- juice from 1/2 lemon
- 8 oz. warm distilled water

Emulsify the three essential oils in the agave nectar, then add the lemon juice, stir briskly into 8 ounces of warm water and drink on empty stomach. Do this 2-3 times daily until stone passes.

Kidney Stone drink #2:
- 2 Tbsp. virgin olive oil
- 8 oz. organic apple juice

Mix the above in a sealed container, shake vigorously, then drink, 2-3 times daily until stone passes.

Detoxifing the Kidneys

The Chinese Wolfberry has been used in China for centuries as a kidney tonic and detoxifier. Essential oils can also assist in the detoxification due to their unique lipid-soluble properties.

Blends:
- Helichrysum with juniper or fennel.
- Helichrysum with Di-Tone, JuvaFlex or Juva Cleanse.

Place 1-3 drops in water and take as a dietary supplement three times a day. Apply as a compress over kidneys and bladder

Supplements: K & B tincture, Cleansing Trio, JuvaTone, VitaGreen, and Sulfurzyme.

Cleansing regimen to aid in passing a stone:
1. Start with colon cleanse using Cleansing Trio.
2. Support the liver by using JuvaTone 1 tablet 3 times daily during the first week; 2 tablets 3 times daily during succeeding weeks.
3. Take one dropper K & B in 8 oz pure water every 2 hours.
4. Drink as much extra water as you can comfortably consume to help flush kidneys.

Ureter Infection

The ureter is the duct from the kidney to the bladder.

Single Oils:
Lemon, myrtle

EO Applications:
INGESTION:
CAPSULE, 00 size, twice daily for 10 days
RICE MILK, 2-4 times daily

TOPICAL:
VITA FLEX, massage 1-3 drops on kidney Vita Flex points on feet

Dietary Supplementation:
Super C, AlkaLime

KNEE CARTILAGE INJURY
(See CONNECTIVE TISSUE)

LEUKEMIA
(See CANCER)

LEG ULCERS
(See SKIN DISORDERS)

LIVER DISORDERS

The liver is one of the most important organs in the body, playing a major role in detoxifying the body. When the liver is damaged, due to excess alcohol consumption, viral hepatitis, or poor diet, an excess of toxins can build up in the blood and tissues that can result in degenerative disease and death.

Symptoms of a stressed or diseased liver include:
- Jaundice (abnormal yellow color of the skin). This may be the only visible sign of liver disease.
- Nausea
- Loss of appetite
- Dark-colored urine
- Yellowish or grey-colored bowel movements
- Abdominal pain or ascites, a unusual swelling of the abdomen caused by an accumulation of fluid
- Itching, dermatitis, or hives
- Disturbed sleep caused by the build up of unfiltered toxins in blood
- General fatigue and loss of energy
- Lack of sex drive

Detoxification of Liver and Gall Bladder
Single Oils:
Ledum, *Citrus hystrix*, celery seed, helichrysum, mandarin, cardamom, geranium, carrot seed, German chamomile, Roman chamomile

Blends:
JuvaFlex, JuvaCleanse, Release, ImmuPower, Thieves, Di-Tone, EndoFlex

Liver blend:
- 2 drops German chamomile
- 3 drops helichrysum
- 10 drops orange
- 5 drops rosemary

Gall Bladder blend:
- 2 drops Roman chamomile
- 2 drops German chamomile

EO Applications:
INGESTION:
CAPSULE, 0 size, 2 times daily
RICE MILK, 2-4 times daily

TOPICAL:
COMPRESS, warm, over the liver 1-2 times daily
VITA FLEX, massage 1-3 drops on liver Vita Flex point of foot, 1-2 times daily
RAINDROP Technique, 1-2 times weekly

Dietary Supplementation:
JuvaTone, JuvaPower/Spice, Rehemogen, Sulfurzyme, Cleansing Trio, Power Meal, Chelex

Hepatitis

Viral hepatitis is a serious, life-threatening disease of the liver which results in scarring (cirrhosis) and eventual organ destruction and death. There are several different kinds of hepatitis: Hepatitis A (spread by contaminated food, water, or feces) and hepatitis B and C (spread by contaminated blood or semen).

A 2003 study conducted by Roger Lewis MD at the Young Life Research Clinic in Provo, Utah evaluated the efficacy of helichrysum, ledum, and celery seed in treating cases of advanced Hepatitis C. In one case of a male age 20 diagnosed with a Hepatitis C viral count of 13,200. After taking two capsules (approx. 750 mg each) of a blend of helichrysum, ledum, and celery seed (JuvaCleanse) per day for a month with no other intervention, patients showed that viral counts dropped to 2,580, an over 80 percent reduction.

Symptoms include jaundice, weakness, loss of appetite, nausea, brownish or tea colored urine, abdominal discomfort, fever and whitish bowel movements.

Single Oils:

Ledum, celery seed, ravensara, German chamomile, thyme, clove

Blends:

JuvaFlex, JuvaCleanse, Di-Tone, ImmuPower, Thieves, Release, Exodus II

EO Applications:

INGESTION:

CAPSULE, 0 size, 3 times daily
RICE MILK, 2-4 times daily

TOPICAL:

DILUTE 50-50, apply 1-3 drops on carotid arteries (on right and left side of throat just under jaw bone on either side), 2-5 times daily. (Carotid arteries are an excellent place to apply oils for fast absorption.)
COMPRESS, warm, over liver 1-2 times daily
VITA FLEX, massage 1-3 drops on liver Vita Flex point of foot, 1-3 times daily
RAINDROP Technique 2-3 times weekly

Dietary Supplementation:

Royaldophilus, JuvaPower/Spice, VitaGreen, JuvaTone, ImmuPro, ImmuneTune, Super C, ImmuGel, Rehemogen
NOTE: Avoid citrus juices.

How to Protect Your Liver

- Use supplements such as schizandra, milk thistle, and N-acetyl cysteine
- Avoid alcoholic beverages.
- Avoid unnecessary use of prescription drugs. Even some common over-the-counter pain relievers can have toxic effects on the liver in moderately high doses.
- Consume a diet high in selenium.
- Avoid mixing pharmaceutic drugs. Be especially cautious in mixing prescription drugs with alcohol.
- Avoid exposure to industrial chemicals whenever possible.
- Eat a healthy diet.
- The Chinese wolfberry (Ningxia variety) is widely used in China as a liver tonic and detoxifier.

Daily Hepatitis regimen:

- Begin with colon and liver cleanse using Cleaning Trio. After 3 days add JuvaTone, 1-2 tablets 3 times daily
- Super C Chewable: 6 tablets, 3 times daily.
- ImmuPro: Chew 8 tablets at night, 2-4 tablets morning and afternoon.
- VitaGreen: 2-6 capsules, 3 times daily, according to blood type
- Royaldophilus: 1-2 capsules at breakfast and bedtime
- Master Formula vitamins: 2-4 tablets, 3 times daily, according to blood type
- ImmuPro: 3 tablets, 4 times daily

LIVER CANCER

(See CANCER)

LIVER SPOTS (Senile Lentigenes)
(See also SKIN DISORDERS)
Single Oils:
Idaho tansy
EO Applications:
TOPICAL:
DILUTE 50-50, apply 2-4 drops over affected area 4 times daily for 2 weeks

LOU GEHRIG'S DISEASE (ALS)
(See NEUROLOGICAL DISORDERS)

LUMBAGO (LOWER BACK PAIN)
(See SPINE INJURIES AND PAIN)

LUNG INFECTIONS
Bronchitis

Bronchitis is characterized by inflammation of the bronchial tube tube lining accompanied by a heavy mucus discharge. Bronchitis can be caused by an infection or exposure to dust, chemicals, air pollution, or cigarette smoke.

When bronchitis occurs regularly over a long periods (i.e. 3 months out of the year for several years) it is known as chronic bronchitis. It can eventually lead to emphysema.

Symptoms:
- Persistent, hacking cough
- Mucus discharge from the lungs
- Difficulty breathing

Avoiding air pollution is an easy way to reduce bronchitis symptoms. In cases where bronchitis is caused by a bacteria or virus, the inhalation of high antimicrobial essential oils may help combat the infection. Heavy mucus may increase after eating foods containing processed sugar or flour.

Single Oils:
Rosemary, *Eucalyptus radiata*, ravensara, thyme, wintergreen/birch, spruce, pine, oregano, helichrysum, tea tree, spearmint, myrtle, Idaho balsam fir

Blends:
Exodus II, ImmuPower, Raven, R.C., Melrose, Thieves, Legacy, Purification, Brain Power

Bronchitis blend:
- 2 drops sage
- 4 drops myrrh
- 5 drops clove
- 6 drops ravensara
- 15 drops frankincense

NOTE: Essential oil blends work especially well in respiratory applications.

EO Applications:
TOPICAL:
DILUTE according to application code Appendix A). Apply 2-6 drops to neck and chest as needed.
COMPRESS, warm, on neck, chest and upper back areas 1-3 times daily
VITA FLEX, on lung points of feet, 2-4 times daily
ORAL:
GARGLE, hourly, or as needed
INHALATION:
DIRECT, 5-10 times daily as needed
DIFFUSION, 15 minutes, 3-10 times daily as needed. Alternate oils/blends each time.
Also diffuse at night during sleep
VAPOR, 2-4 times daily as needed
RETENTION:
RECTAL, using any of the recommended blends, combine 20 drops with 1 tablespoon olive oil. Insert into rectum with bulb syringe and retain throughout the night. Repeat nightly for 2-3 days.

Dietary Supplementation:
Super C, ImmuPro, ImmuGel, Immune-Tune, Exodus, Cleansing Trio, Fresh Essence +

Pneumonia
(See also THROAT INFECTION)
Single Oils:
Goldenrod, ledum, tea tree, rosemary, thyme, ravensara, *Eucalyptus globulus*, *Eucalyptus radiata*, mountain savory, clove, anise, fennel, wintergreen/birch, hyssop, spearmint, frankincense

Blends:
ImmuPower, Thieves, Raven, R.C., Aroma Siez, Sacred Mountain, Melrose, Inspiration, Exodus II
Pneumonia blend:
- 10 drops rosemary
- 8 drops ravensara
- 8 drops frankincense
- 2 drops oregano
- 2 drops peppermint

EO Applications:
TOPICAL:
DILUTE according to application code (Appendix A). Apply 2-6 drops to neck and chest as needed.
COMPRESS, warm, on neck, chest and VITA FLEX, on lung points of feet, 2-4 times daily

ORAL:
GARGLE, hourly, or as needed

INHALATION:
DIRECT, 5-10 times daily as needed
DIFFUSION, 15 minutes, 3-10 times daily as needed. Alternate oils/blends each time. Also diffuse at night during sleep
VAPOR, 2-4 times daily as needed

RETENTION:
RECTAL, using any of the recommend blends, combine 20 drops with 1 tablespoon olive oil. Insert into rectum with bulb syringe and retain throughout the night. Repeat nightly for 5-6 days.

For long-term chest congestion from welding, smoking, etc., use R.C. and myrtle in hot packs or compresses on chest and back.

The antibacterial and antiviral oils, which are very powerful prophylactic agents for protection against colds, flu, and chest infections, are basil, lavender, hyssop, frankincense, rosemary, bergamot, *Eucalyptus radiata,* tea tree, clove, oregano, cistus, thyme, and mountain savory.

Dietary Supplementation:
Super C, Longevity Caps, VitaGreen, ImmuPro, ImmuneTune, Rehemogen, Master Formula Vitamins, AD&E

Oral Care:
Thieves Lozenges, Fresh Essence Plus

Whooping Cough
This is a contagious disease affecting the respiratory system particularly in children. Lungs become infected, as the air passages become clogged with thick mucus. Over the course of several days, the condition worsens, resulting in long coughing bouts (up to 1 minute). The continual coughing makes breathing difficult and labored.

Single Oils:
Rosemary, lavender, lemongrass, thyme, myrtle, petitgrain, nutmeg, oregano, tea tree

Blends:
Thieves, Melrose, Purification, ImmuPower, Raven, R.C.

EO Applications:
TOPICAL:
DILUTE 20-80, apply 2-4 drops to neck and chest as needed.
COMPRESS, warm, on neck, chest and upper back areas 1-3 times daily
VITA FLEX, on lung points of feet, 2-3 times daily

INHALATION:
DIRECT, 5-10 times daily as needed

DIFFUSION, 15 minutes, 3-10 times daily as needed. Alternate oils/blends each time. Also diffuse at night during sleep.
VAPOR, 2-4 times daily as needed

Dietary Supplementation:
Super C, Longevity Caps, VitaGreen, ImmuPro, ImmuneTune, and Rehemogen.

NOTE: *Because whooping cough usually affects children, always dilute essential oils in V6 Oil Complex or other cold-pressed vegetable oil before topically applying. Start with low concentrations until response is observed. Diffuse intermittently and observe reaction.*

LUPUS

Lupus is an autoimmune disease that has several different varieties:

- *Lupus vulgaris* is characterized by lesions that form on skin. Brownish lesions may form on the face and become ulcerous and form scars.
- Discoid *Lupus erythematosus* is characterized by scaly red patches on the skin and oval or butterfly-shaped lesions on the face. It is milder than the systemic type.
- Systemic *Lupus erythematosus* is more serious than discoid lupus. It inflames the connective tissue in any part of the body, including the joints, muscles, skin, blood vessels, membranes surrounding the lungs and heart, and occasionally the kidneys and brain.

Because lupus is an autoimmune disease, it has been successfully treated using MSM, a form of organic sulfur.

Single Oils:
Cypress, lemongrass

Blends:
ImmuPower, Valor, EndoFlex, Joy, Acceptance, Present Time

Lupus blend:
- 30 drops cypress
- 30 drops lemongrass
- 30 drops EndoFlex

EO Applications:
TOPICAL:
BODY MASSAGE, once every other day
RAINDROP Technique, 1-2 times weekly

Lupus daily regimen:
1. BATH SALTS, using EndoFlex, add 30 drops to 1/2 cup Epsom salt or baking soda and add to hot bath. Soak for 30 minutes.
2. VITA FLEX: Massage EndoFlex on bottoms of the feet; follow two hours later with foot massage using Thieves.
3. TOPICAL: Massage 10-15 drops ImmuPower over liver and on feet 2-3 times daily.
4. SULFURZYME: 1-2 Tbsp powder or 5 capsules 1-2 times daily
5. SUPER CAL: 2-3 capsules, 2 times daily
6. IMMUNETUNE: 2-4 capsules 2 times daily
7. ESSENTIALZYME: 2-6 tablets, 2 times daily
8. VITAGREEN: 2-4 capsules, 2 times daily
9. ADRENAL SUPPORT (see ADRENAL GLAND IMBALANCES topic heading)

Dietary Supplementation:
Sulfurzyme, Super Cal, ImmuneTune, Essentialzyme, VitaGreen, Mega Cal

LYME DISEASE AND ROCKY MOUNTAIN SPOTTED FEVER

Viral infection caused by the bite of an infected tick. Lyme disease is caused by the microorganism *Borrelia burgdorferi*.

Singles:
   Thyme, oregano, clove, melissa, niaouli, blue cypress

Blends:
   PanAway, Melrose, Thieves, Exodus II, ImmuPower

EO Applications:
   INGESTION:
      CAPSULE, 00 size, 3 times daily

Dietary Supplementation:
   BodyGize, Power Meal, Polyzyme, ImmuPro, ImmuneTune, Wolfberry Crisp, BerryGize Bar, Berry Young Juice, Exodus, Thyromin
   Cleansing Trio and JuvaTone for a colon and liver cleanse.

(See also TICK BITES in INSECT BITES)
(See also RHEUMATOID ARTHRITIS)

LYMPHATIC SYSTEM

Essential oils have long been known to aid in stimulating and detoxifying the lymphatic system.

Single Oils:
   Ledum, sandalwood, helichrysum, myrtle, grapefruit, lemongrass, cypress, tangerine, orange, tangerine, rosemary

Blends:
   Di-Tone, JuvaFlex, JuvaCleanse, EndoFlex, Thieves, Acceptance, R.C., Aroma Life, En-R-Gee, Citrus Fresh

EO Applications:
   TOPICAL:
      DILUTE 50-50, massage 2-4 drops on sore lymph glands and under arms, 2-3 times daily
      RAINDROP Technique weekly or as needed
      COMPRESS, warm, over affected areas 1- 2 times daily

Massage oils on sore spots with sensitive lymph glands. Then apply Cel-Lite Magic and grapefruit or cypress oil, which helps detoxify chemicals stored in body fat.

Lymphatic Cleanse:
- 3 drops cypress
- 1 drop orange
- 2 drops grapefruit

Mix in 1/2 gallon distilled water. Grade B maple syrup may be added. Drink at least two 8 oz. glasses daily.

Dietary Supplementation:
   Super C, ImmuGel, Longevity Caps, VitaGreen
   Colon and liver cleanse: Cleansing Trio.

Topical Treatment:
   Cel-Lite Magic Massage Oil, Morning Start Bath Gel

LYMPHOMA
(See CANCER)

M.C.T. (Mixed Connective Tissue Disease)
(see LUPUS)

M.C.T. is an autoimmune disease similar to lupus in which the connective tissue in the body becomes inflamed and painful. This condition is usually due to poor assimilation of protein and mineral deficiencies.

Single Oils:
   Rosemary, nutmeg, clove, lemongrass, marjoram, peppermint, wintergreen/birch cypress

Blends:
   ImmuPower, Valor, Joy
   MCT blend (for aches and discomfort):
- 10 drops basil
- 8 drops wintergreen or birch
- 6 drops cypress
- 3 drops peppermint

EO Applications:
 TOPICAL:
  DILUTE 50-50, massage 4-8 drops on affected location 2-3 times daily
  VITA FLEX, massage 1-3 drops on liver Vita Flex points of the feet
  RAINDROP Technique, weekly or as needed.
  MCT/Lupus regimen:
  Rub 2-4 drops of ImmuPower over the liver and on liver Vita Flex Points on the bottom of the right foot 2-3 times daily. This has been reported to help lupus, which is similar to M.C.T.

Dietary Supplementation:
ImmuGel, Master Formula, Super C, Super B, VitaGreen, ImmuneTune, ArthroTune, Super Cal, Thyromin

MCT regimen:
1. Avoid acid-ash foods. Instead, use alkaline foods, such as barley or wheat sprouts.
2. VitaGreen: 2-6 capsules, 3 times daily.
3. Use Cleansing Trio to expel toxins. Avoid contact with or use of cigarettes, cleaning products, chemicals and chemical-using industries (auto garages, paint shops, etc.)
4. Build the body:
  - Super C: 1-3 tablets, 3 times daily.
  - Super Cal: 2-4 capsules, 2 times daily.
  - ImmuneTune: 2-4 capsules, 2 times daily.
  - Super B: 1 tablet, 4 times weekly.
  - Master Formula: 3-6 tablets, 2x daily.
  - ArthroTune: 2-3 capsules, 2 times daily.

MALARIA

Malaria is a serious disease contracted from several species of *Anopheles* mosquitoes. While malaria is largely confined to the continents of Asia and Africa, an increasing number of cases have arisen in North and South America. If not treated, malaria can be fatal.

Symptoms:
- Fever
- Chills
- Anemia

The best defense against malaria is to use insect repellents effective against *Anopheles* mosquitoes. Once a person has contracted the disease, oils such as lemon can help amplify immune response.

Single Oils:
Lemon, thyme, laurel

Topical/Oral Treatment:
Thieves Antiseptic Spray

EO Applications:
 INGESTION:
  Mix 3-6 drops lemon oil in 1 tsp agave syrup and 8 ox. water, shake, and sip regularly when outbreak is impending.

(See INSECT REPELLENT and INSECT BITES)

MALE HORMONE IMBALANCE

As men age, their DHEA and testosterone levels decline. Conversely, levels of dihydrotestosterone (DHT) increase, contributing to prostate enlargement and hair loss. Because pregnenolone is the master hormone from which all hormones are created, men can directly benefit from transdermal pregnenolone creams as a way of jump-starting sagging DHEA levels. Herbs such as saw palmetto and *Pygeum africanum* can prevent the conversion of testosterone into DHT, thereby reducing prostate enlargement and slowing hair loss.

Single Oils:
Rosemary, sage, fennel, ylang ylang, geranium, blue yarrow, clary sage

Blends:
Mister
EO Applications:
INGESTION:
CAPSULE, 0 size, once a day
Dietary Supplementation:
Progen, DHEA, saw palmetto, Cortistop (Men's)

MEASLES
Single Oils:
Lavender, Roman chamomile, tea tree, clove, thyme, German chamomile
Blends:
ImmuPower
Measles blend:
- 15 drops lavender
- 15 drops Roman chamomile
- 5 drops tea tree

EO Applications:
TOPICAL:
DILUTE 50-50, apply on spots, 3-5 x daily or as needed
BATH SALTS, soak at least 30 minutes in bath daily
Mix 6-9 drops of any of the above essential oils in 8 oz. water, shake well, and use to sponge down patient 1-2 times daily
Dietary Supplementation:
Super C, AD&E, Master Formula Vitamins, Essential Omegas

MEMORY
(See BRAIN DISORDERS)

MENSTRUAL CONDITIONS
Natural hormones such as natural progesterone and pregnenolone are the most effective treatment for menstrual difficulties and irregularities. The most effective method of administration is transdermal delivery in a cream. Just 20 mg applied to the skin twice a day is equivalent to 1000 mg taken internally.

As women reach menopause, progesterone production declines and a state of estrogen dominance often arises. The most commonly prescribed drugs are conjugated estrogens (from horse urine) or synthetic medroxyprogesterone. The molecules in these synthetic hormones are foreign to the human body and can dramatically increase the risk for ovarian and breast cancer with time.

Endometriosis
This occurs when the uterine lining develops on the outer wall of the uterus, ovaries, fallopian tubes, vagina, intestines, or on the abdominal wall. These fragments cannot escape like the normal uterine lining, which is shed during menstruation. Because of this, fibrous cysts often form around the misplaced uterine tissue. Symptoms can include abdominal or back pain during menstruation or pain that often increases after the period is over. Other symptoms may include heavy periods and pain during intercourse.
Single Oils:
Fennel, clary sage
Blends:
Melrose, Thieves
Dietary Supplementation:
ImmuPro, Super C Chewable, PD 80/20, Femalin, Protec
Topical Treatment:
Prenolone, Prenolone+, Progessence
Regimen:
- Colon and liver cleanse: Cleansing Trio.
- Hot compress of Melrose on the stomach.
- Apply Thieves to bottom of the feet.

Excessive Bleeding

Excessive Bleeding blend:
- 10 drops geranium
- 10 drops helichrysum
- 5 drops cistus

EO Applications:

TOPICAL:

DILUTE 50-50, apply 4-6 drops to forehead, crown of head, soles of feet, lower abdomen and lower back, 1-3 times daily

COMPRESS, warm, daily on lower back and abdomen

1/10 tsp. cayenne in 8 oz. warm water may help regulate bleeding during periods.

Hormone Imbalance

As women age, their levels of progesterone decline and contribute to osteoporosis, increased risk of breast and uterine cancers, mood swings, depression, and many other conditions. Estrogen levels can also decline and increase women's risk of heart disease. Replacing these declining levels using topically applied progesterone or pregnenolone creams may be the most effective way to replace and boost decline hormone levels. Pregnenolone may be especially effective, as it is the precursor hormone from which the body creates both progesterone and estrogens.

Single Oil:

Geranium, clary sage

Blends:

Mister, Dragon Time

Hormone Balancing blend #1:
- 10 drops basil
- 10 drops marjoram
- 8 drops hyssop
- 4 drops helichrysum
- 6 drops ylang ylang

Hormone Balancing blend #2:
- 5 drops bergamot
- 5 drops geranium

EO Applications:

TOPICAL:

DILUTE 50-50, apply 4-6 drops to forehead, crown of head, soles of feet, lower abdomen and lower back 1-3 times daily

VITA FLEX, massage 3-6 drops on reproductive Vita Flex points of feet

COMPRESS, warm, daily, on lower back or lower abdomen

Dietary Supplementation:

PD80/20

Topical Treatments:

Prenolone, Prenolone+, Progessence, Neurogen

BodyGize and WheyFit contain soy which helps balance hormones and activate (estrogen) receptors. Take BodyGize and WheyFit at least once a day.

Hysterectomy

(See Hormone Imbalance, above)

Single Oils:

Clary Sage

Dietary Supplementation:

FemiGen, PD 80/20.

Topical Treatment:

Progessence

Irregular Periods

Blends:

Period regulator blend #1:
- 5 drops peppermint
- 9 drops fleabane
- 16 drops clary sage
- 11 drops sage
- 5 drops jasmine absolute

Period regulator blend #2:
- 10 drops chamomile
- 10 drops fennel

EO Applications:
TOPICAL:
DILUTE 50-50, apply 4-6 drops to forehead, crown of head, soles of feet, lower abdomen, and lower back 1-3 times daily
VITA FLEX, massage 3-6 drops on reproductive Vita Flex points of feet, 2-3 times daily
COMPRESS, warm, daily, on lower back or lower abdomen

Menstrual Cramps
Single Oils:
Clary sage, rosemary, hops, sage, vitex, lavender, Roman chamomile, cypress, tarragon, vetiver, valerian

Blends:
Dragon Time, EndoFlex
Menstrual cramp relief blend:
- 10 drops Dragon Time
- 4 drops hops (*Humulus iupulus*)\

EO Applications:
TOPICAL:
COMPRESS, warm, over uterus area, 2-3 times weekly
VITA FLEX, massage 2-4 drops on reproductive Vita Flex points on feet (around ankles), also on lower back and stomach
INGESTION:
CAPSULE, 0 size, twice daily for 2 weeks prior to menses

Dietary Supplementation:
FemiGen, PD 80/20, Estro Tincture, VitaGreen, Master Formula HERS

Topical Treatment:
Prenolone, Prenolone+, EndoBalance
When migraine headaches accompany periods, a colon and liver cleanse may reduce symptoms.

Premenstrual Syndrome (PMS)

PMS is one of the most common hormone-related conditions in otherwise healthy women. Women can experience a wide range of symptoms for 10 to 14 days before menstruation, and even 2 to 3 days into menstruation. These symptoms include mood swings, fatigue, headaches, breast tenderness, abdominal bloating, anxiety, depression, confusion, memory loss, sugar cravings, cramps, low back pain, irritability, weight gain, acne, and oily skin and hair. Causes include hormonal, nutritional, psychological, and stress of the Western culture.

Single Oils:
Hops, clary sage, sage, anise seed, fennel, vitex, basil, ylang ylang, rose, neroli, bergamot

Blends:
Dragon Time, Mister, EndoFlex, Exodus II, Acceptance, Aroma Siez

EO Applications:
INHALATION:
DIRECT, 3-6 times daily
TOPICAL:
DILUTE 50-50, apply 4-6 drops to forehead, crown of head, soles of feet, lower abdomen and lower back 1-3 times daily
VITA FLEX, massage 2-4 drops on reproductive Vita Flex points of feet
COMPRESS, warm, daily, on lower back or lower abdomen
ORAL:
TONGUE, 1 drop of EndoFlex on the tongue and then hold the tongue against the roof of the mouth, 2-4 times daily

Dietary Supplementation:
Master Formula vitamins, VitaGreen, PD 80/20, Femalin, Berrygize Bars, Super B, Super Cal, Mineral Essence, AD&E, Estro Tincture, Ultra Young, ImmuneTune, Thyromin

Topical Treatment:
Prenolone, Prenolone Plus, Progessence

MENTAL FATIGUE
(See Mental Fatigue in FATIGUE heading)

METAL TOXICITY (Aluminum)
(See also HEAVY METALS)

Aluminum is a very toxic metal that can cause serious neurological damage in the human body—even in minute amounts. Aluminum has been implicated in Alzheimer's disease.

People unwittingly ingest aluminum from their cookware, beverage cans, and antacids. Even deodorants have aluminum compounds. The first step toward reducing aluminum toxicity in the body is to avoid these types of aluminum-based products.

Single Oils:
Clove, helichrysum, *Citrus hystrix*
Blends:
Juva Cleanse
EO Applications:
  INGESTION:
   CAPSULE, 00 size, 2 times daily
  TOPICAL:
   RAINDROP Technique, weekly
Dietary Supplementation:
Chelex, JuvaTone, Super Cal, ComforTone

MONONUCLEOSIS (Infectious)
(See EPSTEIN-BARR VIRUS)

MORNING SICKNESS
(See NAUSEA or MENSTRUAL CONDITIONS)

MOTION SICKNESS
(See NAUSEA)

MUCUS (Excess)
Many oils are natural expectorants, helping tissues discharge mucus, soft and hard plaque and toxins.

Single Oils:
Frankincense, ledum, lavender, rosemary, helichrysum, *Eucalyptus radiata*, cypress, lemon, marjoram, myrtle, peppermint
Blends:
Di-Tone, 3 Wise Men, Raven., R.C., Purification
Expectorant blend:
- 3 drops marjoram
- 3 drops ledum
- 1 drop lavender

EO Applications:
  INHALATION:
   DIRECT, 3-5 times daily
   DIFFUSION, 20 minutes 3 times daily
  INGESTION:
   CAPSULE, 0 size, 1 capsule twice a day
  TOPICAL:
   DILUTE 50-50, apply 2-4 drops on the T4 and T5 thoracic vertebrae (at the neck-to shoulder intersection), 3-5 times daily
   VITA FLEX, massage on relevant Vita Flex points on the feet 2-4 times daily

MULTIPLE SCLEROSIS (MS)
(See NEUROLOGICAL DISEASES)

MUMPS (Infectious Parotitis)
An acute, contagious, febrile disease marked by painful swelling and inflammation of the parotid glands and other salivary glands. The causative agent is a paromyxovirus, spread by direct contact, airborne droplets and urine.

Single Oils:
Thyme, melissa, myrrh, blue cypress, wintergreen/ birch.
Blends:
Raven, R.C., Thieves, Exodus II
EO Applications:
  TOPICAL:
   DILUTE 50-50, 2-4 drops behind the

ears
4 times daily
COMPRESS, warm, 1-3 times daily around throat and jaw
RAINDROP Technique 1-2 times weekly
INGESTION:
CAPSULE, 00 size, 1 capsule twice a day
Dietary Supplementation:
ImmuPro, Super C, Exodus

MUSCLES
Bruised Muscles
(see BRUISING)

To avoid excess blood clotting in a bruised muscle or tissue and increase circulation:
Single Oils:
Clove, German chamomile, helichrysum, wintergreen/birch, cypress, lavender, geranium, peppermint, vetiver, valerian
Blends:
Aroma Siez, Aroma Life, PanAway, Peace & Calming, Ortho Sport, Ortho Ease
E.O. Applications:
TOPICAL:
DILUTE 50-50, apply 2-4 drops to bruised area 3 times daily.
Sequence of application for bruise treatment: When a bruise displays black and blue discoloration and pain, start with helichrysum, wintergreen/ birch, Douglas fir, white fir, Idaho balsam fir, or oregano.

Once the pain and inflammation decrease, use cypress, then basil and Aroma Siez to enhance the muscle relaxation.

Follow with peppermint to stimulate the nerves and reduce inflammation. Finish with cold packs.
Dietary Supplementation:
ArthroTune, Super Cal, Mineral Essence, Essential Manna

General Rules

When selecting oils for injuries, think through the cause and type of injury and select oils for each segment. For instance, whiplash could encompass muscle damage, nerve damage, ligament damage, inflammation, bone injury, and possibly emotion. Select oils for each perceived problem and apply.

Cramps and Charley Horses
(See also Tight, Spasmed or Torn Muscles)

Magnesium and calcium deficiency may contribute to muscle cramps and charley horses.
Single Oils:
Rosemary, cypress, marjoram, lavender, elemi, German chamomile
Blends:
PanAway, Aroma Siez, Relieve It
E.O. Applications:
TOPICAL:
DILUTE 50-50, massage 2-4 drops on cramped muscle 3 times daily.
Dietary Supplementation:
Super Cal, Coral Sea, ArthroTune, Mineral Essence, Berry Young Juice, Essential Manna, Mega Cal, BLM
2-3 capsules of ArthroTune, taken each morning and night will help reduce night leg cramps.
Topical Treatment:
Ortho Sport, Ortho Ease

Inflammation Due to Injury

Tissue damage is usually accompanied by inflammation. Reduce inflammation by massaging with anti-inflammatory oils to minimize further tissue damage and speed healing.
Single Oils:
Peppermint, spearmint, German chamomile,

> **For Tired, Fatigued Muscles**
>
> Tired muscles may be lacking in minerals such as calcium and magnesium. Super Cal, Essential Manna, Berry Young Delights, and Mineral Essence are excellent sources of both trace and macro minerals and good for all muscle conditions. ArthroTune helps reduce stiffness from sitting for long periods.

myrrh, wintergreen/birch, marjoram, clove, Roman chamomile

Blends:

Aroma Siez, PanAway

Muscle Injury blend:
- 12 drops white fir
- 10 drops tea tree
- 8 drops lavender
- 6 drops marjoram
- 3 drops yarrow
- 3 drops spearmint
- 2 drops peppermint

EO Applications:
TOPICAL:
> DILUTE 50-50, massage 2-4 drops on inflamed muscle 3 times daily

Dietary Supplementation:
Arthro Plus, Super Cal, ArthroTune, Longevity Caps, Mineral Essence, Power Meal, Mega Cal Sulfurzyme, VitaGreen, Ultra Young, BLM

Inflammation Due to Infection
Single Oils:

Ravensara, hyssop, niaouli, blue cypress

EO Application
TOPICAL:
> DILUTE 50-50, massage 2-4 drops on inflamed muscle 3 times daily
> COMPRESS, cold, 1-3 times daily

Dietary Supplementation:
Arthro Plus, Super Cal, ArthroTune, Longevity Caps, Mineral Essence, Power Meal, Mega Cal Sulfurzyme, VitaGreen, Ultra Young, BLM

Sore Muscles
Single Oils:

Nutmeg, elemi, marjoram, black pepper, basil, spruce, Roman chamomile, wintergreen/birch, rosemary, peppermint

Blends:

Aroma Siez, Peace & Calming, M-Grain

Sore muscle blend #1:
- 4 drops rosemary
- 8 drops juniper
- 8 drops lavender
- 8 drops lemon
- 10 drops wintergreen/birch

Sore muscle blend #2:
- 9 drops cypress
- 8 drops rosemary
- 8 drops lavender
- 2 drops elemi
- 2 drops valerian

EO Applications:
TOPICAL:
> DILUTE 50-50, massage 4-6 drops into sore muscle 3 times daily.
> COMPRESS, warm, 1-3 times daily

Tight, Spasmed or Torn Muscles
Single Oils:

Elemi, wintergreen/birch, Idaho balsam fir, peppermint, basil, white fir, lemongrass, marjoram

Blends:

Aroma Siez, PanAway

Blend for tight muscles:
- 6 drops marjoram
- 4 drops cypress

- 4 drops wintergreen/birch
- 3 drops valerian
- 1 drop helichrysum

Blend for muscle spasms:
- 1-2 drops ravensara
- 4-5 drops Aroma Siez
- 1 drop black pepper

It is usually helpful to alternate cold and hot packs when applying the above essential oil blend to muscles that are in spasm.

Blend for torn muscle:
- 8 drops Idaho balsam fir
- 8 drops sandalwood
- 7 drops Douglas fir
- 5 drops hyssop
- 4 drop lemongrass
- 5 drops helichrysum
- 4 drops wintergreen/birch
- 2 drops vetiver
- 1 drops Idaho tansy

EO Applications:
TOPICAL:
DILUTE 50-50 in V-6 Mixing Oil, massage 2-6 drops on affected areas. Follow with Ortho Ease Massage Oil.

Muscle Weakness
Single Oils:
Ravensara, Douglas fir, lemongrass, juniper, nutmeg, white fir, Idaho balsam fir

Blends:
En-R-Gee

EO Applications:
TOPICAL:
DILUTE 50-50, massage 4-6 drops into weak muscle 3 times daily

Dietary Supplementation:
VitaGreen, AminoTech, WheyFit, Longevity Caps, Amino Tech, Power Meal

MUSCULAR DYSTROPHY
Single Oils:
Pine, lavender, marjoram, lemongrass, vetiver, Idaho balsam fir

Blends:
Aroma Siez, Relieve It

EO Applications:
TOPICAL:
DILUTE 50-50, massage 4-6 drops along spine 3 times daily

Dietary Supplementation:
Essentialzyme, Polyzyme, WheyFit, Power Meal, Essential Omegas, Sulfurzyme, VitaGreen, Mineral Essence, Thyromin, Ultra Young

Topical Treatment:
Ortho Ease, Ortho Sport

NAILS (Brittle or Weak)
Poor or weak nails, often containing ridges, indicate a sulfur deficiency.

Single Oils:
Frankincense, myrrh, lemon

Blends:
Citrus Fresh

EO Applications:
TOPICAL:
NEAT, 1-3 drops on nails and at base of nails, 3 times per week.

Dietary Supplementation:
Sulfurzyme, Super Cal, Mineral Essence, Mega Cal

Nail strengthening blend:
- 4 drops Wheat Germ Oil
- 4 drops frankincense
- 4 drops myrrh
- 4 drops lemon

Apply 1 drop of the above blend on each nail 2-3 times weekly.

NARCOLEPSY

A chronic ailment consisting of uncontrollable, recurrent attacks of drowsiness and sleep during daytime. May be aggravated by hypothalamus dysregulation or thyroid hormone deficiency.

(see also THYROID)

Single Oils:
Fleabane, rosemary, black pepper, cinnamon bark

Blends:
Brain Power

EO Applications:
  INHALATION:
    DIRECT, 4-8 times daily as needed
  TOPICAL:
    DILUTE 50-50, apply 1-2 drops on temples, behind ears, back of neck, on forehead, and under nostrils, as needed

Dietary Supplementation:
Mineral Essence, VitaGreen, Thyromin, BrainPower, Ultra Young.

NAUSEA

Patchouly oil contains compounds that are extremely effective in preventing vomiting due to their ability to reduce the gastrointestinal muscle contractions associated with vomiting.[30] Peppermint has also been found to be effective in many kinds of stomach upset, including nausea.

Single Oils:
Peppermint, patchouly, ginger, nutmeg, Idaho tansy

Blends:
Di-Tone

EO Applications:
  TOPICAL:
    DILUTE 50-50, massage 1-3 drops behind each ear (mastoids) and over navel 2-3 times hourly.
    COMPRESS, warm, over stomach, as needed
  INHALATION:
    DIRECT, 4-6 times hourly as needed
  ORAL:
    TONGUE, 1-4 times as needed

Morning Sickness

Single Oils:
Peppermint, spearmint

Blends:
Di-Tone

EO Applications:
  TOPICAL:
    DILUTE 50-50, massage 1-3 drops behind each ear (mastoids) and over navel 2-3 times hourly
    COMPRESS, warm, over stomach, as needed
  INHALATION:
    DIRECT, 4-6 times hourly as needed
  ORAL:
    TONGUE, 1-4 times as needed

Dietary Supplementation:
Polyzyme, Essentialzyme

Motion Sickness

Single Oils:
Patchouly, lavender, peppermint, ginger, spearmint

Blends:
Di-Tone, Valor, JuvaFlex, JuvaCleanse

EO Applications:
  TOPICAL:
    DILUTE 50-50, massage 1-3 drops behind each ear (mastoids) and over navel 2-3 times hourly
    COMPRESS, warm, over stomach, as needed
  INHALATION:
    DIRECT, 4-6 times hourly as needed

ORAL:
TONGUE, 1-4 times as needed
INGESTION:
RICE MILK, 1-2 times as needed

Motion Sickness Preventative:
- 4 drops peppermint
- 4 drops ginger
- 1 Tbsp. V6 Oil Complex

Rub 6-10 drops of the above blend on chest and stomach 1 hour before traveling.

Dietary Supplementation:
Polyzyme, Detoxzyme, Essentialzyme

NERVE DISORDERS

Nerve disorders usually involve peripheral or surface nerves and include neuritis, neuropathy, neuralgia, Bell's palsy, and carpal tunnel syndrome. In contrast, neurological disorders are usually associated with deep neurological disturbances in the brain, and these conditions include Lou Gehrig's disease, MS, and cerebral palsy. (See NEUROLOGICAL DISEASES)

Single Oils:

Peppermint, lavender, cedarwood, German chamomile, Roman chamomile, sage, rosemary, spruce, tangerine, sandalwood

Blends:

Valor, Peace & Calming, Citrus Fresh
General blend for nerve disorders:
- 2 drops peppermint
- 10 drops juniper
- 1 drop geranium
- 8 drops marjoram
- 4 drops helichrysum

EO Applications:
TOPICAL:
NEAT or DILUTE 50-50 as required, apply 2-4 drops to affected area 3-5x daily

Dietary Supplementation:
Super Cal, VitaGreen, Sulfurzyme, Power Meal, Super C, Super B, Mega Cal

Super Cal and Mega Cal provide calcium necessary to maintain nerve signal transmissions along neurological pathways.

Sulfur deficiency is very prevalent in nerve problems. Sulfur requires calcium and vitamin C for the body to metabolize. Super B and Sulfurzyme work well together to help repair nerve damage and the myelin sheath.

Bell's Palsy

A type of neuritis, marked by paralysis on one side of the face and inability to open or close the eyelid.

Single Oils:

Peppermint, helichrysum, juniper

Blends:

Aroma Siez, PanAway, Relieve It

EO Applications:
TOPICAL:
NEAT, massage 1-3 drops on the facial nerve, which is in front and behind the ear and any areas of pain 3-5 times daily until symptoms end.

Dietary Supplementation:
Ultra Young

Carpal Tunnel Syndrome

Nerves pass through a tunnel formed by wrist bones (known as carpals) and a tough membrane on the underside of the wrist that binds the bones together. The tunnel is rigid, so if the tissues within it swell for some reason, they press and pinch the nerves creating a painful condition known as carpal tunnel syndrome. This condition is primarily sports-related or due to activities that involve strenuous or repeated use of wrists. A similar but less common condition can occur in the ankle (tarsal tunnel syndrome), or elbow.

Single Oils:

Peppermint, basil, wintergreen or birch, cypress, marjoram, helichrysum, lemongrass

Blends:
PanAway, Relieve It
  Carpal tunnel blend:
- 5 drops wintergreen or birch
- 3 drops cypress
- 1 drop peppermint
- 2 drops marjoram
- 3 drops lemongrass

EO Applications:
TOPICAL:
NEAT or DILUTE 50-50 as required, apply 2-4 drops to affected area 3-5 times daily
COMPRESS, cold, on location 2-3 times daily

Dietary Supplementation:
Super C, Super Cal, Mega Cal, BLM, Mineral Essence, Essential Manna

Topical Treatments:
Regenolone, NeuroGen, Ortho Ease, Ortho Sport

Neuralgia

Neuralgia is pain from a damaged nerve. It can occur in the face, spine, or elsewhere. This reoccuring pain can be traced along a nerve pathway. Carpal tunnel syndrome is a specific type of neuralgia. The primary symptom is temporary sharp pain in the peripheral nerve(s).

Single Oils:
Marjoram, helichrysum, peppermint, juniper, nutmeg

Blends:
PanAway, Relieve It, Juva Flex, Peace & Calming

EO Applications:
TOPICAL:
NEAT or DILUTE 50-50 as required, apply 2-4 drops to affected area 3-5 times daily
COMPRESS, cold, on location 2-3 times daily

INHALATION:
DIRECT, Peace & Calming, 2-4 times daily

Dietary Supplementation:
Ultra Young, Sulfurzyme, Super B, Chelex, PD 80-20, JuvaTone, JuvaPower/Spice

Topical Treatment:
Regenolone, NeuroGen, Ortho Ease, Ortho Sport

Neuritis

Neuritis is a painful inflammation of the peripheral nerves.

It is usually caused by prolonged exposure to cold temperature, heavy-metal poisoning, diabetes, vitamin deficiencies (beriberi and pellagra), and infectious diseases such as typhoid fever and malaria.

Symptoms:
- Pain
- Burning
- Numbness or tingling
- Muscle weakness or paralysis

Single Oils:
Peppermint, lavender, juniper, oregano, thyme, blue yarrow, clove

Blends:
Valor, Aroma Siez, Peace & Calming

EO Applications:
TOPICAL:
NEAT or DILUTE 50-50 as required, apply 2-4 drops to affected area 3-5 times daily
COMPRESS, cold, on location 2-3 times daily

INHALATION:
DIRECT, Peace & Calming, 2-4 times daily

Dietary Supplementation:
Ultra Young, Sulfurzyme, Super B, Chelex, PD 80-20, JuvaTone, JuvaPower/Spice

Topical Treatment:
Regenolone, NeuroGen, Ortho Ease, Ortho Sport

Neuropathy

Neuropathy refers to actual damage to the peripheral nerves, usually from an auto-immune condition.

Damage to these peripheral nerves (other than spinal or those in the brain), generally starts as tingling in hands and feet and slowly spreads along limbs to the trunk.

Numbness, sensitive skin, neuralgic pain, weakening of muscle power can all develop in varying degrees. Most common causes include complications from diabetes (diabetic neuropathy), alcoholism, vitamin B12 deficiency, tumors, too many pain killers, exposure and absorption of chemicals, metallics, pesticides, and many other causes.

B vitamins and minerals such as magnesium, calcium, potassium, and organic sulfur are important in repairing nerve damage and quenching pain from inflamed nerves.

Fleabane may boost production of pregnenolone and human growth hormone. Pregnenolone aids in repairing damage to the myelin sheath.[31] Juniper also may help in supporting nerve repair.

If paralysis is a problem, a regeneration of up to 60 percent may be possible. If, however, the nerve damage is too severe, treatment may not help. If the damage starts to reverse, there will be pain. Apply a few drops of PanAway neat on location.

Symptoms:
- Tingling or numbness
- Gangrene

Single Oils:
Peppermint, fleabane, juniper, blue yarrow, goldenrod, helichrysum, lemongrass

Blends:
Aroma Siez, PanAway, Peace & Calming
Neuropathy blend #1:
- 10 drops juniper
- 10 drops geranium
- 10 drops helichrysum

Neuropathy blend #2:
- 15 drops geranium
- 10 drops helichrysum
- 6 drops cypress
- 10 drops juniper
- 5 drops peppermint

EO Applications:
  TOPICAL:
    NEAT or DILUTE 50-50 as required, apply 2-4 drops to affected area 3-5 times daily
    COMPRESS, cold, on location 2-3 times daily
  INHALATION:
    DIRECT, Peace & Calming, 2-4 times daily

Dietary Supplementation:
Super B, Longevity Capsules, Mineral Essence, Essential Omegas, Super Cal, Mega Cal, Super C, VitaGreen, Sulfurzyme, Essential Manna, BodyGize, Ultra Young, Master Formula Vitamins

Topical Treatment:
Regenolone, NeuroGen, Peppermint-Cedarwood Bar Soap

NERVOUS FATIGUE

Nervous fatigue can cause motor skill problems.

Single Oils:
St. John's wort, blue yarrow, juniper, goldenrod, helichrysum, thyme, peppermint

Blends:
Brain Power, Clarity, Peace & Calming, Humility, Hope, Trauma Life

EO Applications:
INHALATION:
DIRECT, 4-8 times daily as needed
TOPICAL:
DILUTE 50-50, apply 1-2 drops on temples, behind ears, back of neck, on forehead, and under nostrils, as needed.

NERVOUS SYSTEM (Autonomic)

The autonomic nervous system controls involuntary activities such as heartbeat, breathing, digestion, glandular activity, and contraction and dilation of blood vessels.

The autonomic nervous system is composed of two parts that balance and complement each other: the parasympathetic and sympathetic nervous systems.

The sympathetic nervous system has stimulatory effects and is responsible for secreting stress hormones such as adrenaline and noradrenaline.

The parasympathetic nervous system has relaxing effects and is responsible for secreting acetylcholine which slows the heart and speeds digestion.

To Stimulate Parasympathetic Nervous System
Single Oils:
Lavender, patchouly, rose, marjoram
Blends:
Valor, ImmuPower, Peace & Calming
EO Applications:
INHALATION:
DIRECT, 1-2 times daily, as needed
INGESTION:
CAPSULE, 0 size, 1 capsule 2 times daily
TOPICAL:
RAINDROP Technique, biweekly

To Stimulate Sympathetic Nervous System
Single Oils:
Peppermint, fennel, grapefruit, ginger, *Eucalyptus radiata*, black pepper
Blends:
Clarity, Brain Power
EO Applications:
INHALATION:
DIRECT, 1-2 times daily, as needed
INGESTION:
CAPSULE, 0 size, 1 capsule twice daily
TOPICAL:
RAINDROP Technique, biweekly
Dietary Supplementation:
Power Meal, Super Cal, Sulfurzyme, Ultra Young, Mineral Essence, Mega Cal

NEURITIS, NEUROPATHY, NEURALGIA
(See NERVE DISORDERS)

NEUROLOGICAL DISEASES
ALS (Lou Gehrig's Disease)

Lou Gehrig's Disease is another name for Amyotrophic Lateral Sclerosis (ALS), a degenerative nerve disorder. ALS affects the nerve fibers in the spinal cord which control voluntary movement. Muscles require continuous stimulation by their associated nerves to maintain their tone. Removal or deadening of these nerves results in muscular atrophy. The lack of control forces the muscles to spasm, resulting in twitching and cramps. The sensory pathways are unaffected so feeling is never lost in the afflicted muscles.

Juniper promotes nerve function. Frankincense may help clear the emotions of fear and anger, which is common with people who have these neurological diseases. When these diseases are contracted, people often become suicidal.

Hope, Joy, Gathering, and Forgiveness will help work through the psychological and emotional aspects of the disease.

Single Oils:

Frankincense, helichrysum, oregano, sage, juniper, rosemary, clove, cardamom, vitex.

Blends:

Acceptance, Joy, Gathering, Brain Power, Clarity, Forgiveness

ALS blend:
- 1 drop rosemary
- 1 drop helichrysum
- 1 drop ylang ylang
- 1 drop clove

EO Applications:

INHALATION:

DIRECT, 3-4 times daily

DIFFUSION, 30 minutes, 2-3 times daily

TOPICAL:

DILUTE 50-50, 1-3 drops on brain reflex points on forehead, temples and mastoids (just behind ears). Use a direct pressure application, massaging 6-10 drops of diluted oil from the base of the skull down the neck and down the spine. Put a few drops of the oil on a loofah brush and rub along the spine vigorously. (Always use a natural bristle brush, since the oils may dissolve plastic bristles.)

RAINDROP Technique, 3 times monthly, but use a cold compress instead of a warm one

NOTE: *Never use hot packs for neurological problems. Always use cold packs to reduce pain and inflammation. In other words, reduce the temperature of the damaged site.*

Dietary Supplementation:

Sulfurzyme, JuvaTone, JuvaPower/Spice, Ultra Young, VitaGreen, Power Meal, Chelex, Chelex, Super Cal, Super C, Super B Sulfur deficiency is very prevalent in neurological diseases. Sulfur requires calcium and Vitamin C for the body to metabolize. Super B and Sulfurzyme work well together to help repair nerve damage and the myelin sheath.

Huntington's Chorea

Huntington's Chorea is a degenerative nerve disease that generally becomes manifest in middle age. It is marked by uncontrollable body movements, which are followed—and occasionally preceded—by mental deterioration. (Not to be confused with Sydenham's chorea (often called St. Vitus Dance, chorea minor, or juvenile chorea) which affects children, especially females, usually appearing between between the ages of 7 and 14. The jerking symptoms eventually disappear.)

Single Oils:

Peppermint, juniper, basil

Blends:

Aroma Siez

Nerve blend:
- 5 drops peppermint
- 10 drops juniper
- 3 drops basil
- 5 drops Aroma Siez

EO Applications:

INHALATION:

DIRECT, 3-4 times daily

DIFFUSION, 30 minutes, 2-3 times daily

TOPICAL:

DILUTE 50-50, 1-3 drops on brain reflex points on forehead, temples and mastoids (just behind ears). Use a direct pressure application, massaging 6-10 drops of diluted oil from the base of the skull down the neck and down the spine. Put a few drops of the oil on a loofah brush and rub along the spine vigorously. (Always use a natural bristle brush, since the oils

may dissolve plastic bristles.)
RAINDROP Technique, 3 times monthly, but use a cold compress instead of a warm one.

NOTE: *Never use hot packs for neurological problems. Always use cold packs to reduce pain and inflammation. In other words, reduce the temperature of the affected area.*

Dietary Supplementation:
Sulfurzyme, JuvaTone, JuvaPower/Spice, Ultra Young, VitaGreen, Power Meal, Rehemogen, Chelex, Super Cal, Super C, Super B, Mega Cal

Multiple Sclerosis (MS)
Multiple Sclerosis is a progressive, disabling disease of the nervous system (brain and spinal cord) in which inflammation occurs in the central nervous system. Eventually, the myelin sheaths protecting the nerves are destroyed, resulting in a slowing or blocking of nerve transmission.

MS is an autoimmune disease, in which the body's own immune system attacks the nerves. Some researchers believe that MS is triggered by a virus, while others make a case that it has a strong genetic or environmental component.

Symptoms:
- Muscle weakness in extremities
- Deteriorating coordination and balance
- Numbness or prickling sensations
- Poor attention or memory
- Speech impediments
- Incontinence
- Tremors
- Dizziness
- Hearing loss

Single Oils:
Juniper, basil eugenol, helichrysum, geranium, peppermint, thyme, oregano, wintergreen/ birch, cypress, marjoram, rosemary

Blends:
Valor, Aroma Siez, Acceptance, Awaken

MS Recipe:
- 10 drops helichrysum
- 10 drops peppermint
- 10 drops rosemary
- 5 drops basil

EO Applications:
INHALATION:
DIRECT, 3-4 times daily
DIFFUSION, 30 minutes, 2-3 times daily

TOPICAL:
DILUTE 50-50, 1-3 drops on brain reflex points on forehead, temples and mastoids (just behind ears). Use a direct pressure application, massaging 6-10 drops of diluted oil from the base of the skull down the neck and down the spine. Put a few drops of the oil on a loofah brush and rub

---

> **Maintaining MS Status Quo**
>
> One of the simplest ways to keep MS symptoms from becoming more severe is to keep the body cool and avoiding any locations or physical activities which heat the body (including hot showers or exercise). Cold baths and relaxed swimming are two of the best activities for relieving symptoms.
>
> Applying heat is the worst thing to do for MS. If an MS patient is experiencing increasingly severe symptoms, lower their body temperature (by up to 3 degrees F) by laying them on a table, covering them with a sheet, ice, shower curtain, and blankets (in that order). Work the feet with oils and watch for benefits.

along the spine vigorously. (Always use a natural bristle brush, since the oils may dissolve plastic bristles.)
RAINDROP Technique, 3 times monthly, but use a cold compress instead of a warm one.

NOTE: *Never use hot packs for neurological problems. Always use cold packs to reduce pain and inflammation. In other words, reduce the temperature of the affected area.*

MS Regimen (to be performed daily):
1. Layer neat applications of 4-6 drops of helichrysum, juniper, geranium and peppermint, Raindrop-style, along the spine. Lightly massage oils in the direction of the MS paralysis. For example, if it is in the lower part of the spine, massage down; if it is in the upper part of the spine, massage up. Follow the application with 30 minutes of cold packs (change cold packs as needed).
2. Apply 4-6 drops Valor on the spine. If the MS affects the legs, rub down the spine; if it affects the neck, rub up the spine.
3. Apply 2-3 drops each of cypress and juniper to the back of the neck then cover with 2-3 drops of Aroma Siez.

To to give additional emotional support to the person with MS symptoms, use Acceptance and Awaken. Be patient. Overcoming MS is a long-term endeavor.

Dietary Supplementation:
Sulfurzyme, JuvaTone, JuvaPower/Spice, Ultra Young, VitaGreen, Power Meal, Rehemogen, Chelex, Super Cal, Mega Cal, Super C, Super B

Parkinson's Disease

Parkinson's Disease involves the deterioration of specific nerve centers in the brain and affects more men than women by a ratio of 3:2. The main symptom is tremors, an involuntary shaking of hands, head, or both. Other symptoms include rigidity, slowed movement, and loss of balance. In many cases these are accompanied by a continuous rubbing together of thumb and forefinger, stooped posture, mask-like face, trouble swallowing, depression, and difficulty performing simple tasks. These symptoms may all be seen at different stages of the disease. The tremors are most severe when the affected part of the body is not in use. There is no pain or other sensation, other than a decreased ability to move. Symptoms appear slowly, in no particular order and may end before they interfere with normal activities. Restoring dopamine levels in the brain can reduce symptoms of Parkinson's. Ultra Young contains a vegetable source of dopamine. Sulfurzyme provides a source of organic sulfur, a vital nutrient for nerve and myelin sheath formation.

Vitex has been shown to reduce the symptoms of Parkinson's disease by 89 percent in animal studies.[32]

Single Oils:
Juniper, peppermint, vitex

Blends:
Peace & Calming, Valor, Juva Cleanse

EO Applications:
INHALATION:
DIRECT, 3-4 times daily
DIFFUSION, 30 minutes, 2-3 times daily

TOPICAL:
DILUTE 50-50, 1-3 drops on brain reflex points on forehead, temples and mastoids (just behind ears). Use a direct pressure application, massaging 6-10 drops of diluted oil from the base of the skull down the neck and down the spine. Put a few drops of the oil on a loofah brush and

rub along the spine vigorously. (Always use a natural bristle brush, since the oils may dissolve plastic bristles.)
RAINDROP Technique, 3 times monthly, but use a cold compress instead of a warm one

NOTE: *Never use hot packs for neurological problems. Always use cold packs to reduce pain and inflammation. In other words, reduce the temperature of the affected area.*

Dietary Supplementation:
Sulfurzyme, Ultra Young, Super B, Juva Power, PD80/20, BLM
Juniper promotes nerve function.

NIGHT SWEATS
(See MENSTRUAL CONDITIONS)
Single Oils:
Sage, clary sage, blue yarrow.
Blends:
Mister, EndoFlex, Dragon Time
EO Applications:
TOPICAL:
DILUTE 50-50, apply 3-5 drops over lower abdomen and back of neck before retiring
VITA FLEX, apply 2-3 drops to heart, to brain and to liver Vita Flex points on feet
Dietary Supplementation:
Estro, Prenolone, Prenolone, Ultra Young, Thyromin.
Topical Treatment:
Dragon Time Bath Gel or Massage Oil

NOSE
Nosebleeds
Nosebleeds usually are not serious. However, if bleeding does not stop in a short time or is excessive or frequent, consult your doctor.

Single Oils:
Helichrysum, geranium, lavender, cypress
Blends:
Nosebleed blend:
- 2 drops helichrysum
- 2 drops lavender
- 2 drops cypress

EO Applications:
TOPICAL:
NEAT, apply 2-4 drops to the bridge and sides of nose and back of neck. Repeat as needed.
Nosebleed regimen:
Put 1 drop helichrysum, lavender, or cypress on a tissue paper and wrap the paper around a chip of ice about the size of a thumb nail, push it up under the top lip in the center to the base of the nose. Hold from the outside with lip pressure. This usually will stop bleeding in a very short time.

Dry Nose
Single Oils:
Lavender, lemon, peppermint
Dry nose blend:
- 2 drops lavender
- 1 drop myrrh

EO Applications:
INHALATION:
DIRECT, 3-5 times daily as needed
DIFFUSION, 20 minutes 3 times daily and before retiring
TOPICAL:
DILUTE 50-50, apply 1-2 drops to nostril walls with cotton swab twice daily
Nasal Irrigation Regimen:
Rosemary and Melaleuca ericifolia oils can be used in a saline solution for very effective nasal irrigation that clears and decongests sinuses. As recommended by Daniel Pénoël,

MD, the saline solution is prepared as follows:
- 12 drops rosemary cineol
- 4 drops tea tree
- 8 tablespoons very fine salt

The essential oils are mixed thoroughly in the fine salt and stored in a sealed container. For each nasal irrigation session, 1 teaspoon of this salt mixture is dissolved into 1 1/2 cups distilled water.

This oils/salt/water solution is then placed in the tank of an oral irrigator to irrigate the nasal cavities, which is done while bending over a sink. This application has brought surprisingly positive results in treating latent sinusitus and other nasal congestion problems.

Dietary Supplementation:
AD&E.

Loss of Smell
(Due to Chronic Nasal Catarrh)
Single Oils:
Basil, peppermint, rosemary, goldenrod, frankincense
EO Applications:
  INHALATION:
    DIRECT, 3-5 times daily, or as needed
Dietary Supplementation:
ImmuneTune, Exodus, Power Meal

Polyps (Nasal)
Single Oils:
Citronella
Blends:
Purification
EO Applications:
  TOPICAL:
    DILUTE 50-50, carefully apply 1 drop on location inside the nostrils with a cotton swab 1-3 times daily

OBESITY
(see DEPRESSION)

Hormone treatments using natural progesterone (for women) and testosterone (for men) may be one of the most powerful treatments for obesity. In women, progesterone levels drop dramatically after menopause and this can result in substantial weight gain, particularly around the hips and thighs. Using transdermal creams to replace declining progesterone can result in substantial declines in body fat.

Diffusing or directly inhaling essential oils can have an immediate positive impact on moods and appetites. Olfaction is the only sense that can have direct effect on the limbic region of the brain. Studies at the University of Vienna have shown that some essential oils and their primary constituents can stimulate blood flow and activity in the emotional centers of the brain.[33]

Fragrance influences the satiety center in the brain in such a manner that frequent inhalation of pleasing aromas can significantly reduce appetite. Dr. Alan Hirsch, in his landmark studies, showed dramatic weight loss in research subjects using aromas from peppermint oil and vanilla absolute to curb food cravings.[34]

Single Oils:
Peppermint, jasmine absolute, ylang ylang vanilla absolute
Blends:
Joy, Citrus Fresh, Juva Cleanse
EO Applications:
  INHALATION:
    DIRECT, 5-20 times daily or as often as needed
Dietary Supplementation:
BodyGize, Power Meal, ThermaBurn, Juva Power, Berrygize Bars, Amino Tech, WheyFit, BeFit
  Topical Treatments:
Progessence, Prenolone, Prenolone+

ORAL CARE (Teeth and Gums)
(see HALITOSIS)

Poor oral hygiene has not only been linked to bad breath (halitosis) but also cardiovascular disease. Some of the same bacteria that populate the mouth have now been implicated in arteriosclerosis.

Essential oils make excellent oral antiseptics, analgesics and anti-inflammatories. Clove essential oil has been used in mainstream dentistry for decades to numb the gums and help prevent infections. Similarly menthol (found in peppermint oil), methyl salycilate (found in wintergreen oil), thymol (found in thyme essential oil) and eucalyptol (found in eucalyptus and rosemary essential oils) are approved OTC drug products for combating gingivitis and periodontal disease.

Dental Visits

Prior to visiting the dentist, rub one drop each of helichrysum, clove and PanAway on gums and jaw. Clove may interfere with bonding of crowns so keep it off the teeth if this procedure is planned.

Dental Pain and Infection Control
Single Oils:

Wintergreen/birch, helichrysum, tea tree, *Eucalyptus radiata*, clove, thyme, oregano

Blends:

PanAway, Thieves, R.C.

EO Applications:
  TOPICAL:

  DILUTE 50-50, apply 1-2 drops on gums and around teeth. Repeat as needed. Just before a tooth extraction, rub 1-2 drops of helichrysum, Thieves and R.C. around the gum area. Rubbing R.C. on gums may also help to bring back feeling after numbness from anesthesia.

Oral Treatments:

Fresh Essence Plus Mouthwash, Dentarome Ultra Toothpaste, Thieves Lozenges, Thieves Antiseptic Spray

Gingivitis & Periodontitis

Periodontal diseases are infections of the gum and bone that hold the teeth in place. Gingivitis affects the upper areas of the gum, where it bonds to the visible enamel, while periodontitis is a more internal infection affecting the gum at the root level of the tooth. In advanced stages, these diseases can lead to painful chewing problems and even tooth loss. Oils such as peppermint, wintergreen, clove, thyme, and eucalyptus can kill bacteria and effectively combat a variety of gum infections.

Single Oils:

Mountain savory, clove, tea tree, oregano, peppermint, wintergreen/birch, thyme

Blends:

Exodus II, Thieves

EO Applications:
  ORAL:

  GARGLE, up to 10 times daily as needed

Dietary Supplementation:

Super C, Super C Chewable, Dentarome, Dentarome Plus, Fresh Essence Plus Mouthwash, Thieves lozenges

Super C Chewable: Take 1-3 tablets at regular intervals throughout the day.

Oral Treatments:

Fresh Essence Plus Mouthwash, Dentarome Ultra Toothpaste, Thieves Lozenges, Thieves Antiseptic Spray

Bleeding Gums
Single Oils:

Cinnamon, peppermint, mountain savory, wintergreen/birch, myrrh

Blends:
Thieves, Melrose, PanAway
Blend for combatting gum bleeding:
- 2 drops myrrh
- 2 drops thyme
- 1 drop Thieves
- 1 drop Exodus II

EO Applications:
ORAL:
GARGLE, 3-10 times daily, as needed
TOPICAL:
DILUTE 50-50, apply 1-2 drops on gums 2-3 times daily

Dietary Supplementation:
ImmuGel

Oral Hygiene Regimen:
1. Gargle three times daily with Fresh Essence Plus Mouthwash.
2. Brush teeth and gums two times daily with Dentarome Ultra toothpaste.
3. For infection or inflammation, place ImmuGel on a piece of gauze. Roll like a piece of rope place along the gum, and hold in mouth for at least 30 minutes. This works particularly well for leukemia patients because their gums tend to inflame, swell, and become infected.

Mouth Ulcers
Single Oils:
Myrrh, oregano, tea tree
Blends:
Thieves, Exodus II
EO Applications:
ORAL:
GARGLE, 3-10 times daily, as needed
TOPICAL:
DILUTE 50-50, apply 1-2 drops on gums2 times daily

Oral Hygiene:
Dentarome Ultra Toothpaste, Fresh Essence+ Mouthwash, Thieves lozenges, Thieves Antiseptic Spray, Immugel
Gargle with Fresh Essence+ Mouthwash or Thieves Antiseptic Spray. Add 1-2 drops of Thieves, clove, and Exodus II to strengthen therapeutic action.
If infection is due to leukemia, saturate a rolled piece of gauze with ImmuGel and 1-3 drops Thieves. Place gauze between gums and inner cheek skin and change gauze pads morning and evening. Massage abscessed area with 1-2 drops Thieves.

Teeth Grinding
Single Oils:
Lavender, valerian
Blends:
Peace & Calming
EO Applications:
INHALATION:
DIRECT, 1-3 times daily and before retiring
DIFFUSION, 30 minutes twice a day and before retiring
TOPICAL:
NEAT, massage 1-3 drops each of lavender and valerian on bottoms of feet each night before retiring

Dietary Supplementation:
Mineral Essence

Toothache and Teething Pain
Single Oils:
Clove, wintergreen/birch, German chamomile, tea tree, Idaho tansy
Blends:
Thieves, Exodus
EO Applications:
TOPICAL:
DILUTE 50-50, apply on affected tooth and gum area as needed

ORAL:

GARGLE, 4-6 times daily or as needed

Dietary Supplements:

ImmuGel, MegaCal, Coral Sea, AD&E

Oral Hygiene:

Thieves Antiseptic Spray, Dentarome Ultra, Fresh Essence Plus Mouthwash.

NOTE: All essential oils should be diluted 20-80 before being used orally on small children.

OSTEOPOROSIS (Bone Deterioration)

Osteoporosis is primarily caused by four main factors:

- Progesterone Deficiency
- Lack of Magnesium and boron in diet
- Lack of Vitamin D in diet
- Lack of dietary calcium

Natural progesterone is the single most effective way to increase bone density in women over age 40. Clinical studies by John Lee, MD, showed dramatic increases in bone density using just 20 mg of daily topically-applied progesterone

Calcium, magnesium, and boron are a few of the most important minerals for bone health and are usually lacking or deficient in most modern diets. Magnesium is especially important to bone strength, but most Americans consume only a fraction of the daily 400 mg daily value needed for bone health. Calcium and magnesium may not be adequately metabolized when consumed because of poor intestinal flora and excess phytates in the diet (a problem with vegetarians). Phytates occur in many nuts, grains, and seeds including rice. Enzymes like phytase are essential for increasing calcium absorption by liberating calcium from insoluble phytates complex.

Lack of vitamin D (cholecalciferol) has become epidemic among older people and has contributed to a lack of absorption of calcium in the diet.

Single Oils:

Wintergreen/birch, elemi, spruce, balsam fir, pine, cypress, peppermint, marjoram, rosemary, basil

Blends:

Aroma Siez, Purification, Melrose, Sacred Mountain, Relieve It, PanAway

EO Applications:

TOPICAL:

DILUTE 50-50, massage 6-10 drops on spine (or area affected) 2-3 times daily

Dietary Supplementation:

Polyzyme, Essentialzyme, Super Cal, Mega Cal, BLM, Coral Sea, AlkaLine, AD&E, Mineral Essence, WheyFit, Sulfurzyme, Thyromin, Ultra Young

Topical Treatments:

Prenolone, Prenolone+, Progessence Super Cal, AlkaLime, and Mineral Essence are all excellent sources of calcium and magnesium which is essential for strong bones. Super Cal not only includes calcium, but also magnesium and boron which are both vital for maintaining bone composition. Mineral Essence is an excellent source magnesium and other trace minerals. Especially avoid consuming carbonated drinks which can leach calcium out of the body due to their phosphoric acid content. Ultra Young helps stimulate growth hormone production which can result in much stronger bones.

Studies show that the majority of women that do resistance training 3-4 times a week do not develop osteoporosis.

Topical Treatments:

Prenolone, Prenolone+, EndoBalance

OVARIAN AND UTERINE CYSTS

(See CANCER, MENSTRUAL CONDITIONS)

Single Oils:
Frankincense, geranium, tea tree, oregano, clary age, cypress

Blends:
Melrose, DragonTime, Mister
Female Cyst blend #1:
- 9 drops frankincense
- 5 drops basil

Female Cyst blend #2:
- 8 drops frankincense
- 8 drops geranium
- 8 drops cypress

EO Applications:
  RETENTION:
  TAMPON, nightly for 4 nights.
  NOTE: if irritation occurs, discontinue use for 3 days before resuming use.

  TOPICAL:
  COMPRESS, warm, on location, as needed
  VITA FLEX, massage 1-3 drops on the reproductive Vita Flex points, located around the anklebone, on either side of the foot. Work from the ankle bone down to the arch of the foot.

Dietary Supplementation:
Master Formula Hers, PD80/20, FemiGen, Protec

Topical Treatments:
Prenolone, Prenolone+, Progessence

PAIN

One of the most effective essential oils for blocking pain is peppermint. A recent study by in 1994 showed that peppermint oil is extremely effective in blocking calcium channels and substance P, important factors in the transmission of pain signals.[35] Other essential oils also have unique pain-relieving properties, including helichrysum, Idaho balsam fir, and Douglas fir.

> **How MSM Works to Control Pain**
>
> When fluid pressure inside cells is higher than outside, pain is experienced. The MSM found in Sulfurzyme equalizes fluid pressure inside cells by affecting the protein envelope of the cell so that water transfers freely in and out.

MSM, a source of organic sulfur, has also been proven to be extremely effective for killing pain, especially tissue and joint pain. The subject of a best-selling book by Dr. Ronald Lawrence and Dr. Stanley Jacobs, MSM is defining the treatment of pain, especially associated with arthritis and fibromyalgia. Sulfurzyme is an excellent source of MSM.

Natural pregnenolone can also blunt pain. (See ARTHRITIS or HEADACHES)

Bone-Related Pain
Single Oils:
Wintergreen/birch, cypress, fir, spruce, pine, peppermint, helichrysum

Blends:
PanAway, Relieve It

EO Applications:
  TOPICAL:
  DILUTE 50-50, 2-4 drops on location as needed
  VITA FLEX, apply to relevant points on feet, repeat as needed

Dietary Supplementation:
Sulfurzyme, Super Cal, Mega Cal, BLM

Topical Treatment:
Ortho Ease, Regenolone, Neurogen

Chronic Pain
To pinpoint the most effective essential oil for quenching pain, it may be necessary to try each

of the essential oils in these categories in order to find the one that is most effective for your particular pain situation.

Single Oils:
Peppermint, helichrysum, spruce, ginger, wintergreen/birch, clove, elemi, oregano, Douglas fir, Idaho balsam fir, rosemary

Blends:
Relieve It, PanAway, Aroma Siez, Release, Sacred Mountain

EO Applications:
  TOPICAL:
    DILUTE 50-50, 2-4 drops on location as needed
    COMPRESS, warm, on location as needed
  INGESTION:
    CAPSULE, 0 size, 2 times per day

Dietary Supplementation:
Sulfurzyme, Super Cal, ArthroTune, Mega Cal, BLM

Topical Treatment:
Regenolone, Neurogen, Ortho Ease, Morning Start Bath Gel, Ortho Sport, Morning Start, Peppermint-Cedarwood Bar Soap.

Inflammation Pain
(see INFLAMMATION)

Joint Pain:
(See JOINT STIFFNESS and ARTHRITIS)

Muscle-related Pain
Single Oils:
Peppermint, rosemary, marjoram, nutmeg

Blends:
PanAway, Aroma Siez, Relieve It.

EO Applications:
  TOPICAL:
    DILUTE 50-50, 2-4 drops on location as needed
    VITA FLEX, apply to relevant points on feet, repeat as needed

Dietary Supplementation:
Sulfurzyme, WheyFit, Mineral Essence, Berrygize Bars, Super Cal

Topical Treatment:
Ortho Ease, Ortho Sport, Neurogen

Trauma-related Pain
Single Oils:
Sandalwood, geranium
Massage around hairline of the head and tips of the toes.

Blends:
Trauma Life, Valor, Release
Trauma pain relief blend:
- 12 drops Idaho balsam fir
- 10 drops tea tree
- 8 drops lavender
- 6 drops marjoram
- 3 drops spearmint
- 2 drops peppermint

EO Applications:
  TOPICAL:
    DILUTE 50-50, 2-4 drops on location, 2-4 times daily. Also massage around hairline and on the tops of the toes.
    COMPRESS, warm, on location as needed

Dietary Supplementation:
Sulfurzyme, Super Cal, Mega Cal

Topical Treatment:
Ortho Ease, Ortho Sport.

Warm compresses help the oils penetrate faster and deeper when applied on location.

PANCREATITIS

Pancreatitis is an inflammation of the pancreas that can be either acute or chronic. Acute pancreatitis can be caused by a sudden blockage in the main pancreatic duct, which results in enzymes becoming backed-up and literally digesting the pancreas unless remedied. Chronic pancreatitis occurs more gradually, with attacks recurring over weeks or months.

Symptoms:
- Abdominal pain
- muscle aches
- vomiting
- abdominal swelling
- sudden hypertension
- jaundice
- rapid weight loss
- fever.

In the case of acute pancreatitis, a total fast for at least 4-5 days is one of the safest and most effective methods of treatment. In the case of infection, fasting should be combined with immune stimulation by using Exodus combined with Vitamin C and B-complex vitamins.

Single Oils:

Geranium, vetiver, peppermint, mountain savory, oregano

Blends:

Exodus II, ImmuPower, Thieves

EO Applications:

RETENTION:
RECTAL, 3 times per week
TOPICAL:
RAINDROP Technique, once a week
INGESTION:
CAPSULE, 0 size, 1 capsule 3 times per week

Dietary Supplementation:

Exodus, ImmuGel, VitaGreen, Super B, Super C, Essentialzyme

PARASYMPATHETIC NERVOUS SYSTEM
(See NERVOUS SYSTEM-AUTONOMIC)

PARASITES, Intestinal
(See FOOD POISONING)

Many types of parasites use up nutrients, while giving off toxins. This can leave the body depleted, nutritionally deficient, and susceptible to infectious disease.

Occasionally parasites can lie dormant in the body and then become active due to ingestion of a particular food or drink. This can result in the appearance and disappearance of symptoms even though parasites are always present.

The parasite, *Cryptosporidium parrum,* may be present in many municipal or tap waters. To remove, water must be distilled or filtered using a .3 micron filter.

Symptoms:
- Fatigue
- Weakness
- Diarrhea
- Gas and bloating
- Cramping
- Nausea
- Irregular bowel movements.

The first step to controlling parasites is beginning a fasting and/or cleansing program. A colon cleanse is particularly important.

Single Oils:

Tarragon, anise seed, Idaho tansy, basil, peppermint, ginger, lemongrass, nutmeg, fennel, juniper, rosewood, tea tree, rosemary

Blends:

Di-Tone, JuvaFlex, JuvaCleanse

Blend for parasite retention enema:
- 10 drops ginger
- 10 drops Di-Tone
- 1 Tbsp. V6 Oil Complex

EO Applications:

INGESTION:
CAPSULE, 00 size, 3 times per week
RICE MILK, 1-3 times daily

TOPICAL:
COMPRESS, warm, over intestinal area, 2 times weekly
VITA FLEX, daily massage up to 6 drops to the instep area on both feet (small intestine and colon Vita Flex points)
RETENTION:
RECTAL, use above blend nightly for 7 nights, then rest for 7 nights. Repeat this cycle 3 times to eliminate all stages of parasite development. Alternatively, substitute 2 tbsp liquid ParaFree for the retention blend and retain overnight every other day for a week.

Dietary Supplementation:
Polyzyme, Essentialzyme, ComforTone, ICP, ParaFree, Fresh Essence Plus

Oral Treatments:
Fresh Essence Plus Mouthwash, Thieves Lozenges Dentarome Ultra Toothpaste

PERIODONTAL DISEASE
(See ORAL CARE)

PERSPIRATION (EXCESSIVE)
Excessive perspiration may indicate adrenal and thyroid problems or diabetes. Sage helps regulate sweating.

Single Oils:
Geranium, rosewood, sage, nutmeg

Blends:
Purification, EndoFlex, En-R-Gee

EO Applications:
TOPICAL:
DILUTE 20-80, apply 2-4 drops under arms daily
INGESTION:
CAPSULE, 0 size, 1 capsule twice a day

PH BALANCE
(See ACIDOSIS)

PHLEBITIS - THROMBOSIS
(See CARDIOVASCULAR CONDITIONS)

Phlebitis refers to inflammation of a blood vein. Symptoms include pain and tenderness along the course of the vein, discoloration of the skin, inflammatory swelling, joint pain, and acute edema below the inflamed site.

Natural progesterone is an effective anti-inflammatory.

Single Oils:
Helichrysum, clove, cistus, orange, goldenrod, Idaho tansy, lavender

EO Applications:
INGESTION:
CAPSULE, 0 size, 1 capsule daily
TOPICAL:
DILUTE 50-50, apply 5-7 drops on location or over the heart, 3 times daily
RAINDROP Technique, weekly

Dietary Supplementation:
Essential Omegas, Polyzyme, Essentialzyme, Super Cal, Coral Sea, Power Meal, Mega Cal
Rehemogen: (3 droppers in water, 3 times daily)

Topical Treatment:
Progessence, Prenolone+

PINKEYE
(See EYE DISORDERS)

PLAQUE
(See CARDIOVASCULAR CONDITIONS)

PLEURISY
Inflammation of the pleura, or outer membranes covering the lungs and the thoracic cavity.

Single Oils:
Ravensara, mountain savory, thyme

Blends:
Raven, R.C., ImmuPower, Exodus II

EO Applications:
TOPICAL:
DILUTE 20-80, massage 5-7 drops on neck and chest 2-3 times daily
COMPRESS, warm, on neck, chest and upper back areas, daily
VITA FLEX, 1-3 drops on lung Vita Flex points of feet daily
RAINDROP Technique, 1-2 times weekly

Dietary Supplementation:
Exodus, ImmuPro, ImmuneTune, Super C, Ultra Young, Mineral Essence, Sulfurzyme

PNEUMONIA
(See LUNG INFECTIONS)

POLIO
Polio (Poliomylitis) is an acute infectious disease usually manifested in epidemics and caused by a virus. It creates an inflammation of the gray matter of the spinal cord. It is characterized by fever, sore throat, headache, and vomiting, sometimes stiffness of the neck and back. If it develops into the major illness, it can involve paralysis and atrophy of groups of muscles ending in contraction and permanent deformity.

Single Oils:
Frankincense, melissa, wintergreen/birch, tea tree, sandalwood, ravansara, blue cypress

Blends:
Polio blend:
- 2 drops lemon
- 10 drops ylang ylang
- 7 drops frankincense
- 10 drops wintergreen or birch
- 7 drops myrtle
- 8 drops cypress
- 15 drops myrrh
- 10 drops tarragon
- 6 drops sage

EO Applications:
INGESTION:
CAPSULE, 0 size, 2 times daily

Dietary Supplementation:
ImmuPro

PREGNANCY
(See also BREASTFEEDING, Postpartum Depression in DEPRESSION, and Diaper Rash and Stretch Marks in SKIN DISORDERS)

Essential oils can be invaluable companions during pregnancy. Oils like lavender and myrrh may help reduce stretch marks and improve the elasticity of the skin. Geranium and Gentle Baby blend have similar effects and can be massaged on the perineum (tissue between vagina and rectum) to lower the risk of tearing or the need for an episiotomy (an incision in the perineum) during birth.

Single Oils:
Lavender, myrrh, geranium, ylang ylang, helichrysum

Blends:
Gentle Baby, Joy, Envision, Valor
Blend for use during labor:
- 4 drops helichrysum
- 2 drops fennel
- 2 drops peppermint
- 5 drops ylang ylang
- 2 drops clary sage

EO Applications:
TOPICAL:
DILUTE 50-50, massage 2-4 drops on reproductive Vita Flex points on sides of ankles. Apply ONLY after labor has started. Also massage 4-6 drops on lower stomach and lower back.

INHALATION:
DIFFUSION, diffuse Gentle Baby, Joy or Valor to reduce stress before and after the birth. (Expectant fathers will also find this helps to reduce anxiety while waiting for delivery.)

PROSTATE PROBLEMS

Natural progesterone is one of the best natural remedies for prostate inflammation (BPH) that can obstruct urinary flow and lead to impotence. Transdermal creams are the most effective means of hormone delivery.

Scientists are tracing the higher incidence of hormone-dependent cancers including cancer of the breast, prostate and testes to exposure to endocrine disrupters in the environment.[36] Petrochemical contamination from DDT, PCB, pesticides, the phylate DBP, and synthetic steroids in meat, are all implicated in interfering with hormone receptors, rendering them unable to function properly, eventually leading to cancer.

For prostate problems, peppermint acts as an anti-inflammatory to the prostate. Saw palmetto, Pygeum africanum, and pumpkin seed oil also reduce prostate swelling.[37]

Single Oils:

Oregano, frankincense, myrrh, orange, Idaho balsam fir, cumin, thyme, blue cypress

Blends:

Mister, EndoFlex, Dragon Time, Australian Blue

EO Applications:

TOPICAL:

DILUTE 20-80, apply 2-4 drops between the rectum and scrotum twice daily. Mister works especially well here

VITA FLEX, massage 4-6 drops on Vita Flex reproductive points on the feet 2 times daily

RETENTION:

RECTAL, nightly for 7 days; rest 7 days, then repeat

Dietary Supplementation:

ProGen, Longevity Caps, Protec, ImmuPro, Master Formula HIS, Wolfberry Crisp

Zinc helps reduce prostate swelling. ImmuPro, ProGen, and Master Formula HIS are excellent sources of zinc.

Topical Treatments:

Prenolone, Prenolone +, Progessence

Benign Prostate Hyperplasia (BPH)

Almost all males over age 50 have some degree of prostate hyperplasia, a condition which worsens with age. BPH can severely restrict urine flow and result in frequent, small urinations.

Three herbs which are extremely effective for treating this condition are saw palmetto, pumpkin seed oil, and *Pygeum africanum*. The mineral zinc is also important for normal prostate function and prostate health. The hormone-like activity of some essential oils can support a nutritional regimen to reduce BPH swelling.

Single Oils:

Ledum, frankincense, myrrh, orange, Idaho balsam fir, cumin, tsuga, blue cypress

Blends:

Mister, EndoFlex, Dragon time, Australian Blue

EO Applications:

TOPICAL:

DILUTE 50-50, 1-3 drops between the rectum and scrotum 1-3 times daily

VITA FLEX, 1-3 drops on reproductive Vita Flex points on feet, 2 times daily

INGESTION:

CAPSULE, 00 size, 1 capsule 3 times daily

RICE MILK, 2-4 times daily

RETENTION,

RECTAL, 3 times per week, at night

BPH Specific Regimen:

The following regimen reduced PSA (prostate specific antigen) counts 70 percent in 2 months: PSA counts typically rise when BPH occurs.

BPH blend:
- 10 drops frankincense
- 5 drops myrrh
- 3 drops sage

Use the above blend for the following three applications simultaneously:
1. Mix the above amounts of essential oils with 1 tablespoon olive oil and use 3 times weekly as overnight rectal retention enema.
2. Massage 1-3 drops neat on Vita Flex reproductive points on both feet daily
3. Dilute above blend 50-50 with V6 Oil Complex and apply 2-4 drops topically between the rectum and the scrotum daily.

Dietary Supplementation:
ProGen, Master Formula vitamins, Longevity Caps, Protec, ImmuPro, Mineral Essence

Topical Treatments:
Prenolone, Prenolone +, Progessence

Other:
1 oz. Protec with 1-2 drops tsuga essential oil in a rectal retention enema. Retain overnight, 3 times weekly

Prostate Cancer
(See Prostate Cancer in CANCER)

Prostatitis
Prostatitis is an inflammation of the prostate that can present symptoms similar to benign prostate hyperplasia: frequent urinations, restricted flow, etc.

Single Oils:
Rosemary, myrtle, thyme, tsuga, peppermint

Blends:
Mister, Dragon Time, Aroma Siez, Di-Tone

EO Applications:
 INGESTION:
  CAPSULE, 0 size, twice daily
 RETENTION:
  RECTAL, 3 times per week, at night
 TOPICAL:
  DILUTE 20-80, apply 1-3 drops to the area between the rectum and the scrotum daily
  VITA FLEX, massage 4-6 drops on reproductive foot Vita Flex points daily

Dietary Supplementation:
ProGen, Master Formula HIS, Longevity Caps, Protec, ImmuPro, Mineral Essence

Topical Treatment:
Prenolone, Prenolone+, Progessence

PSORIASIS
(See SKIN DISORDERS)

PYORRHEA
(See ORAL CARE)

Essential oils are one of the best treatments against gum diseases such as gingivitis and pyorrhea. Clove oil, for example, is used as a dental disinfectant; and the active principle in clove oil, eugenol, is one of the best-studied germ-killers available.

RADIATION DAMAGE
Many cancer treatments use radiation therapy that can severely damage both the skin and vital organs. Using antioxidant essential oils topically, as well as proper nutrients internally, is helpful in minimizing radiation damage.

Single Oils:
Tea tree, neroli

Blends:
Melrose

EO Applications:
 TOPICAL:
  NEAT or DILUTE 50-50, massage 2-4 drops on affected area 1-2 times daily

Dietary Supplementation:
Essential Omegas, AD&E, Super C, Power Meal, ImmuPro, ImmuneTune, Berry Young Juice, Essential Manna

RESTLESS LEG SYNDROME
(See also ATTENTION DEFICIT SYNDROME)

Single Oils:
Oregano, basil, marjoram, lavender, cypress, Roman chamomile, peppermint

Blends:
Peace & Calming, Aroma Siez

EO Applications:
INHALATION:
DIRECT, 6-8 times daily as needed
DIFFUSION, 20 minutes, 4 times daily
TOPICAL:
RAINDROP Technique, weekly

Dietary Supplementation:
Mineral Essence, Thyromin, VitaGreen, Mega Cal

RHEUMATIC FEVER

Rheumatic fever results from a *Streptococcus* infection that primarily strikes children (usually before age 14). It can lead to inflammation that damages the heart muscle and valve.

Rheumatic fever is caused by the same genus of bacteria that causes strep throat and scarlet fever. Diffusing essential oils can help reduce the likelihood of contracting the disease. Essential oils such as mountain savory, rosemary, tea tree, thyme, and oregano, have powerful antimicrobial effects.

In cases where a person is already infected, the use of essential oils in the Raindrop Technique may be appropriate.

Single Oils:
Mountain savory, peppermint, thyme, rosemary, tea tree, black pepper, oregano

Blends:
Thieves, Exodus II, ImmuPower

EO Applications:
INHALATION:
DIFFUSION, 1 hour, 3 times daily

TOPICAL:
DILUTE 50-50, massage 3-5 drops on bottoms of feet and on carotid artery spots under ear lobes
RAINDROP Technique, once weekly

Dietary Supplementation:
Exodus, ImmuPro, ImmuneTune, Super C, Sulfurzyme, AD&E, Berry Young Juice, HRT

RINGWORM
(See Ringworm or Athlete's Foot in FUNGAL INFECTIONS)

SALMONELLA
(See FOOD POISONING and INFECTION)

SCABIES
(See also LICE in SKIN DISORDERS)

Scabies are caused by eight-legged insects known as itch mites—tiny parasites the burrow into the skin, usually in the fingers and genital areas. The most common variety, *Sarcoptes scabiei,* can quickly infest other people. Although it only lives six weeks, it continually lays eggs once it digs into the skin.

The most common remedy for scabies and lice is lindane (gamma benzene hexachloride) a highly toxic polychlorinated chemical that is structurally very similar to hazardous banned pesticides such as DDT and chlordane. It is so dangerous that Dr. Guy Sansfacon, head of the Quebec Poison Control Centre in Canada, has requested that lindane be banned.

Natural plant-derived essential oils have the same activity as commercial pesticides but are far safer. Essential oils have been studied for their ability to not only repel insects, but also kill them and their eggs as well. Because many oils are nontoxic to humans, they make excellent treatments to combat scabies infestations.

Single Oils:
Citronella, peppermint, palmarosa, lavandin, *Eucalyptus globulus,* black pepper, ginger

Blends:
Di-Tone, Purification, Peace & Calming

EO Applications:
TOPICAL:
NEAT, or Dilute 50-50 if needed, apply 2-4 drops on location, 3 times daily
DILUTE 20-80, massage thoroughly 1 tsp. into scalp at night before retiring.
To treat hair or scalp, add 2-4 drops of essential oil to 1 tsp. of shampoo.

Topical Treatment:
Lavender Hair and Scalp Wash, Lemon-Mint Hair and Scalp Wash

SCAR TISSUE

Some essential oils may be valuable for reducing or minimizing the formation of scar tissue:

Single Oils:
Helichrysum, lavender, cypress, elemi, blue yarrow, rose, cistus, myrrh, sandalwood

Blends:
3 Wise Men, Inspiration
Scar prevention blend:
- 4 drops helichrysum
- 6 drops lavender
- 8 drops myrrh
- 2 drops sandalwood

EO Applications:
TOPICAL:
NEAT, gently apply 2-6 drops over wound or cut daily until healed

Dietary Supplementation:
AD&E, Essential Omegas, Super C, Sulfurzyme, Power Meal, Essential Manna

Topical Application:
Tender Tush Ointment

SCIATICA
(See SPINE INJURIES and PAIN)

SCHIZOPHRENIA

A neurological disease that involves identity confusion. Onset is typically between the late teens and early 30's. Abnormal neurological findings may show a broad range of dysfunction including slow reaction time, poor coordination, abnormalities in eye tracking, and impaired sensory gating. Typically schizophrenia involves dysfunction in one or more areas such as interpersonal relations, work, education, or self-care. Some cases are believed to be caused by viral infection.

Single Oils:
Peppermint, cardamom, cedarwood, vetiver, melissa, frankincense, rosemary

Blends:
Brain Power, Clarity, Valor, M-Grain

EO Applications:
INHALATION:
DIRECT, 4-6 times daily
TOPICAL:
RAINDROP Technique, once weekly

Dietary Supplementation:
Mineral Essence, Super Cal, Essential Omegas, Ultra Young, Wolfberry Crisp, Berry Young Juice

SCLERODERMA

Also known as systemic sclerosis, scleroderma is a non-infectious, chronic, autoimmune disease of the connective tissue. Caused by an over-production of collagen, the disease can involve either the skin or internal organs and can be life-threatening. Scleroderma is far more common among women than men.

Single Oils:
Frankincense, Roman chamomile, lavender, patchouly, sandalwood, myrrh

Blends:
Melrose
Scleroderma blend #1:
- 3 drops Roman chamomile
- 3 drops lavender
- 3 drops patchouly

Scleroderma blend #2:
- 4 drops sandalwood
- 4 drops myrrh

EO Applications:
  TOPICAL:
  DILUTE 50-50, massage 4-6 drops on location 3 times daily. Alternate between blend #1 and blend #2 (above) each day

Dietary Supplementation:
PD 80/20, Cleansing Trio, Essential Omegas, JuvaTone, JuvaPower/Spice, Thyromin, Mineral Essence, Power Meal, Sulfurzyme, Detoxyme

Topical Treatment:
Prenolone

SCOLIOSIS

(See SPINE INJURIES and Chapter 5: Raindrop Technique)

Scoliosis is an abnormal lateral or side-to-side curvature or twist in the spine. It is different from hyperkyphosis (hunchback) or hyperlordosis (swayback) which involve excessive front-to-back accentuation of existing spine curvatures.

While a few cases of scoliosis can be attributed to congenital deformities (such as MS, cerebral palsy, Down's syndrome, or Marfan's syndrome), the vast majority of scoliosis types are of unknown origin.

Some medical professionals believe that scoliosis may be caused by persistent muscle spasms that pull the vertebrae of the spine out of alignment. Others feel - and there is a growing body of research documenting this hypothesis - that it begins with hard-to-detect inflammation along the spine caused by latent viruses. (See citations in Chapter 5.)

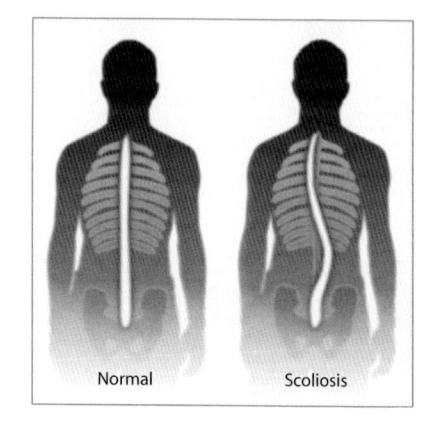

Symptoms:
- When bending forward, the left side of the back is higher or lower than the right side (the patient must be viewed from the rear).
- One hip may appear to be higher or more prominent than the other.
- Uneven shoulders or scapulas (shoulder blades).
- When the arms are hanging loosely, the distance between the left arm and left side is different than the distance between the right arm and right side.

The Raindrop Technique is proving to be one of the most effective therapies for straightening spines misaligned due to scoliosis.

Single Oils:
Oregano, thyme, basil, wintergreen/birch, cypress, marjoram, peppermint.

Blends:
Aroma Siez, PanAway, Valor

EO Applications:
  TOPICAL:
  RAINDROP Technique, 3-5 times monthly

DILUTE 50-50, as a supplement to RAINDROP Technique, apply 3-6 drops along spine daily or as needed

Dietary Supplementation:
Mineral Essence, Super Cal, Essential Manna, Power Meal, Sulfurzyme

Topical Treatments:
Ortho Ease, Ortho Sport

SCURVY

A condition due to deficiency of vitamin C in the diet and marked by weakness, anemia, spongy gums, bleeding of the gums and nose, and a hardening of the muscles of the calves and legs.

Supplements:
Super C, Super C Chewable, Berry Young Juice, Power Meal

SEIZURES

Most seizures can be treated by removing all forms of sugar, artificial colors, and flavors from diet. Avoid using personal care products with ammonium-based compounds, such as quaterniums and polyquaterniums.
(See BRAIN DISORDERS or EPILEPSY)

Single Oils:
Frankincense, sandalwood, melissa, jasmine, basil

Blends:
Valor, Aroma Siez, Exodus II

EO Applications:
   TOPICAL:
   DILUTE 50-50, massage 10 drops into scalp 3 times daily to help reduce risk of seizure. Supplement with inhalation therapy below

   INHALATION:
   DIRECT, 3-5 times daily

Seizure regimen (do all the following):
- Massage 4-6 drops Valor on bottoms of feet daily
- Diffuse Peace & Calming for 30 minutes 3-4 times daily
- Massage 4-6 drops Joy over heart daily
- Do a Raindrop Technique on spine weekly

Dietary Supplements:
Stevia Select, Agave Nectar, Mineral Essence, AD&E, Master Formula Vitamins, Vita-Green, Super B, Longevity Caps, Power Meal, Sulfurzyme

SEXUAL DYSFUNCTION
(See IMPOTENCE)

Lack of Libido
Single Oils:
FOR WOMEN: Geranium, ylang ylang, clary sage, nutmeg, rose, black pepper
(These oils can be inhaled or taken orally as dietary supplements. Jasmine absolute can also be used in inhalation therapy or topical use, but must never be ingested.)
FOR MEN: Myrrh, black pepper, pine, ylang ylang, ginger, nutmeg, rose

- Ylang Ylang helps balance sexual emotion and sex drive problems. Its aromatic influence elevates sexual energy and enhances relationships.
- Clary sage can help with lack of sexual desire particularly with women by regulating and balancing hormones.
- Nutmeg supports the nervous system to overcome frigidity.

Blends:
Joy, Live with Passion, Sensation, Mister, Dragon Time, Valor

Dietary Supplementation:
Ultra Young, Sensation Moisture Cream, VitaGreen, FemiGen, ProGen, FemiGen, Sulfurzyme

Sulfurzyme provides MSM (sulfur), which can harmonize libido.

Topical Treatment:
Progessence, Prenolone, Prenolone+, NeuroGen

Excessive Sexual Desire
Single Oils:
Marjoram, lavender, St. John's wort
Blends:
Peace & Calming, Acceptance, Surrender
EO Applications:
  INHALATION:
    DIRECT, 3-5 times daily
  TOPICAL:
    DILUTE 50-50, massage 4-6 drops on neck, shoulders and lower abdomen, 1-3 times daily
Dietary Supplementation:
Mineral Essence, Super B, PD80/20, Mega Cal

Frigidity
Single Oils:
Jasmine absolute, ylang ylang, rose
Blends:
Joy, Valor, Chivalry
EO Applications:
  INHALATION:
    DIRECT, 3-5 times daily
  TOPICAL:
    DILUTE 50-50, massage 4-6 drops on neck, shoulders and lower abdomen, 1-3 x daily
Topical Treatment:
Progessence, Prenolone, Prenolone+, NeuroGen

SEXUALLY TRANSMITTED DISEASES
(See INFECTIONS)

Herpes Simplex Type II

The Herpes Simplex Virus Type 2, is transmitted by sexual contact and results in sores or lesions. Four to seven days after contact with an infected partner, tingling, burning, or persistent itching usually heralds an outbreak. One or two days later, small pimple-like bumps appear over reddened skin. The itching and tingling continue, and the pimples turn into painful blisters, which burst, bleeding with a yellowish pus. Five to seven days after the first tingling, scabs form, and healing begins.

Antiviral essential oils have generally been very effective in treating herpes lesions and reducing their onset. Oils such as tea tree, melissa, and rosemary have been successfully used for this purpose by Daniel Pénoël, M.D. in his clinical practice. A study at the University of Buenos Aires found that sandalwood essential oil inhibited the replication of Herpes Simplex viruses-1 and -2.[38]

Those with herpes should avoid diets high in the amino acid L-arginine, substituting instead L-lysine. Lysine retards the growth of the virus. Foods such as amaranth are very high in lysine. (Amaranth is used in Essential Manna).

Single Oils:
Melissa, ravensara, tea tree, sandalwood, blue cypress, oregano, thyme, cumin, rosemary
Blends:
Melrose, Thieves, Exodus II, ImmuPower, Purification

Herpes blend #1 (topical):
- 1 drop lavender
- 1 drop tea tree oil

Herpes blend #2 (vaginal):
- 2 drops sage
- 2 drops melissa
- 4 drops ravensara
- 2 drops lavender

EO Applications:
 TOPICAL:
  NEAT, apply Herpes blend #1 (above) on lesion as soon as it appears. Apply 1-2 drops of neat oil 2-3 times daily, alternating between the above herpes blend and Melrose each day.
  RAINDROP Technique, 1-2 treatments
 RETENTION:
  TAMPON, for vaginal treatment of herpes, use Herpes blend #2 (above), diluted 20-80 in tampon/ pad application nightly. If tampon/pad stings after 5 minutes, remove and change dilution rate to 10-90.

Dietary Supplementation:
Exodus, ImmuPro, ImmuneTune, Power Meal, Sulfurzyme, Essential Manna, Super C Chewable, Super B, VitaGreen, Master Formula Vitamins, Cleansing Trio.
Avoid using Ultra Young since this supplement is high in L-arginine.

Topical Treatment:
Thieves Antiseptic Spray, ImmuGel

Genital Warts

Genital warts are a form of viral infection caused by the human papillomavirus (HPV), of which there are more than 60 different types.

One type of HPV virus is among the most common sexually transmitted diseases. Up to 24 million Americans may be currently infected with HPV, usually spread through sexual contact. HPV lives only in genital tissue. HPV can later lead to cervical cancer in women.

Single Oils:
Melissa, oregano, thyme, Idaho tansy, tea tree, *Melaleuca ericifolia,* lavender

Blends:
Melrose, Thieves, ImmuPower

EO Applications:
 TOPICAL:
  NEAT or DILUTE 50-50, 1-3 drops 2 times daily for 10 days
 RETENTION:
  TAMPON, nightly

Topical Treatment:
Thieves Antiseptic Spray, ImmuGel, Fresh Essence Plus

Gonorrhea and Syphilis

NOTE: Seek immediate professional medical attention if you suspect you may have either of these diseases.

Single Oils:
Oregano, melissa, thyme, mountain savory, cinnamon

Blends:
Thieves, Exodus II

EO Applications:
 INGESTION:
  CAPSULE, 00 size, 1 capsule 2 times daily for 15 days

Dietary Supplementation:
Exodus, ImmuPro, Essential Manna

Topical Treatment:
Thieves Antiseptic Spray, ImmuGel

SHINGLES (Herpes Zoster)
(See CHICKEN POX)

SHOCK

Shock can be described as a state of profound depression of the vital processes associated with reduced blood volume and pressure. The blood rushes to the vital organs after trauma.

It may be caused by the sudden stimulation of the nerves and convulsive contraction of the muscles caused by the discharge of electricity. Other causes include sudden trauma, terror, surprise, horror, or disgust.

Symptoms or signs:
- Irregular breathing

- Low blood pressure
- Dilated pupils
- Cold and sweaty skin
- Weak and rapid pulse
- Dry mouth

Any injury that results in the sudden loss of substantial amounts of fluids can trigger shock.

Shock can also be caused by allergic reactions (anaphylactic shock), infections in the blood (septic shock), or emotional trauma (neurogenic shock).

Shock should be treated by covering the victim with a blanket and elevating the victim's feet unless there is a head or upper torso injury. Inhaling essential oils can also help—especially in cases of emotional shock.

Single Oils:
Cardamom, helichrysum, peppermint, tea tree, frankincense, basil, rosemary, sandalwood

Blends:
Clarity, Legacy, Trauma Life, 3 Wise Men, Valor, Harmony, Present Time, Thieves

EO Applications:
   INHALATION:
   DIRECT, 1-2 drops, as needed
   TOPICAL:
   DILUTE 50-50, rub 1-2 drops on temples, back of neck, and under nose.

NOTE: When applying essential oil to the temples be careful not to get the oil too close to the eyes.

SINUS INFECTIONS
(See also COLDS and THROAT INFECTIONS)

Nasopharyngitis
Inflammation of the mucous membranes of the back of the nasal cavity where it connects to the throat and the eustachian tubes.

Single Oils:
Eucalyptus radiata, thyme, ravensara

Blends:
Raven, R.C., Thieves, Exodus II

EO Applications:
   TOPICAL:
   DILUTE 50-50, apply just under jawbone on right and left sides, 4-8 times daily
   INHALATION:
   DIRECT, 4-8 times daily
   ORAL:
   GARGLE, 2-5 times daily

Dietary Supplementation:
Super C, Super C Chewable, ImmuPro, ImmuGel, Dentarome Ultra, Fresh Essence Plus Mouthwash, Thieves lozenges, Exodus

Rhinitis
Inflammation of the mucous membranes of the sinus

Single Oils:
Basil, *Eucalyptus radiata*, ravensara, tea tree, Melaleuca ericifolia, peppermint

Blends:
R.C., Melrose, Raven

EO Applications:
   INHALATION:
   DIRECT, 4-8 times daily
   TOPICAL:
   NEAT, apply 2-4 drops on forehead and bridge of nose, being careful not to get oils in or near eyes or eyelids. 3-6 times daily.

Dietary Supplementation:
AD&E, ImmuGel, Dentarome Ultra, Fresh Essence Plus Mouthwash, Thieves lozenges, ImmuPro, Super C, Super C Chewable, Exodus

Nasal Irrigation Regimen:
Rosemary and tea tree oils can be used in a

saline solution for very effective nasal irrigation that clears and decongests sinuses. As recommended by Daniel Pénoël, MD, the saline solution is prepared as follows:
- 12 drops rosemary
- 4 drops Melaleuca ericifolia
- 8 tablespoons very fine salt (salt flower)

The essential oils are mixed thoroughly in the fine salt and kept in a sealable container. For each nasal irrigation session, 1 teaspoon of this salt mixture is dissolved into 1 1/2 cups distilled water. This oils/salt/water solution is then placed in the tank of an oral irrigator to irrigate the nasal cavities, which is done while bending over a sink. This application has brought surprisingly positive results in treating latent sinusitus and other nasal congestion problems.[39]

Sinus Congestion
Single Oils:
Sandalwood, goldenrod, ledum, Idaho balsam fir, ravensara, thyme, *Eucalyptus radiata*, Melaleuca ericifolia, tea tree, peppermint, fennel, rosemary

Blends:
Di-Tone, Raven, R.C., Thieves, Exodus II

EO Applications:
  INHALATION:
    DIRECT, 3-8 times daily, or as needed
    VAPOR, 2-5 times daily, as needed
  INGESTION:
    SYRUP, 3-6 times daily
  ORAL:
    GARGLE, 3-6 times daily
  TOPICAL:
    DILUTE 50-50, massage 1-3 drops on each of the following areas: forehead, nose, cheeks, lower throat, chest and upper back, 1-3 times daily
    VITA FLEX, massage 1-3 drops on Vita Flex points on the feet, 2-4 times daily
    RAINDROP Technique, 1-2 times weekly
    BATH SALTS, daily
    Use Nasal Irrigation Regimen: (see Rhinitis)

Dietary Supplementation:
Super C, Super C Chewable, Exodus, AD&E, ImmuGel, Dentarome Ultra, Fresh Essence Plus Mouthwash, Thieves lozenges, ImmuPro

Sinusitis
Essential oils, such as *Eucalyptus radiata* and ravensara strengthen the respiratory system, open the pulmonary tract, and fight respiratory infection.

Single Oils:
Clove, ravensara, myrtle, Melaleuca ericifolia, *Eucalyptus radiata*, *Eucalyptus globulus*, thyme, rosemary, lemon, cypress, lemongrass

Blends:
R.C., Raven, Thieves, Purification, ImmuPower

Sinus blend #1:
- 3 drops *Melaleuca ericifolia*
- 3 drops Raven

Sinus blend #2:
- 10 drops peppermint
- 5 drops *Eucalyptus radiata*
- 2-3 drops tea tree

EO Applications:
  INHALATION:
    DIRECT, 3-5 times daily
  TOPICAL:
    DILUTE 50-50, apply 1-2 drops to a cotton swab, and swab inside of nostrils 3 times daily. The sinusitis blend is ideal for this method.
  ORAL:
    GARGLE, 2-5 times daily
    Use Nasal Irrigation Regimen: (see Rhinitis)

SKIN DISORDERS

(See also BLISTERS and BOILS, LIVER DISORDERS and MENSTRUAL CONDITIONS)

Our skin is our armor and the largest absorbent organ of the body. Protecting the skin environment is essential. Many chemical molecules are too large to be absorbed and lay on the surface of the skin, causing irritation, resulting in rashes, itching, blemishes, flaky and dry skin, dandruff, and allergies. Essential oils are soluble through lipids in the skin and are easily absorbed.

Many skin conditions may be related to dysfunctions of the liver. It may be necessary to cleanse, stimulate, and condition the liver and colon for 30 to 90 days before the skin begins to improve.

Abscesses/Boils:

Skin abscesses are small pockets of pus that collect under the skin. They are usually caused by a bacterial or fungal infection.

A number of essential oils may reduce inflammation and combat infection, helping to bring abscesses/boils to a head, so they can close and heal.

Single Oils:

Tea tree, frankincense, helichrysum, peppermint, lavender, lemon, German chamomile, *Eucalyptus radiata,* rosemary, thyme, mountain savory, palmarosa, patchouly, rosewood, juniper, ravensara, oregano

Blends:

Melrose, Purification, Exodus II, ImmuPower, Thieves, Sacred Mountain

EO Applications:

TOPICAL:

DILUTE 50-50, apply on location 3-6 times daily

Dietary Supplementation:

JuvaTone, Essential Omegas, Cleansing Trio, AD&E

Acne

(See Clogged Pores in this section)

Acne results from an excess accumulation of dirt and sebum around the hair follicle and the pores of the skin. This accumulation may be due to an over-production of sebum, an oily substance that is secreted by the sebaceous glands in the hair follicles. As the pores and hair follicles become congested, bacteria begins to feed on the sebum. This leads to inflammation and infection around the hair follicle and the formation of a pimple or a puss-filled blackhead.

One of the most common forms of acne, *Acne vulgaris,* occurs primarily in adolescents due to hormone imbalances which stimulate the creation of sebum.

Acne in adults can be also be caused by hormone balances, as well as use of chlorinated compounds, endocrine system imbalances, or poor dietary practices. Heavy or greasy makeup can also contribute to acne.

Tips for Clearing Up Acne

- Eliminate dairy products, fried foods, chemical additives, and sugar from diet.
- Avoid use of makeup or chlorinated water.
- Avoid contact with plastics which may exude estrogenic chemicals.
- Topically apply essential oils such as tea tree to problem areas. Tea tree was shown to be equal to benzoyl peroxide in the treatment of acne, according research published in the Medical Journal of Australia.[40]
- Begin a cleansing program with the Cleansing Trio and Sulfurzyme.

Stress may also play a role. According to research conducted by Dr. Toyoda in Japan, acne and other skin problems are a direct result of physical and emotional stress.[41]

Essential oils are outstanding for treating acne because of their ability to dissolve sebum, kill bacteria, and preserve the acid mantle of the skin. Because essential oils may be slightly drying to the skin when applied undiluted, it may be necessary to dilute them with V6 Oil Complex or grapeseed oil to keep the skin hydrated.

Single Oils:
Tea tree, geranium, vetiver, blue cypress, lavender, patchouly, German or Roman chamomile, rosewood, cedarwood, *Eucalyptus radiata,* orange, clove

Blends:
Melrose, Thieves, Gentle Baby, Purification, JuvaFlex, JuvaCleanse

EO Applications:
TOPICAL:
NEAT or DILUTE 50-50 as required. Gently massage 3-5 drops into oily areas 1-3 times daily. Alternate oils daily for maximum effect

Dietary Supplementation:
Essential Omegas, Power Meal, Mineral Essence, Exodus, Super C, Super C Chewable, Stevia, VitaGreen, Cleansing Trio, Wolfberry Crisp

To resolve acne caused by hormonal imbalance: Estro Tincture, Ultra Young, Progessence Cream

Topical Treatment:
Mint Satin Scrub, Juniper Satin Scrub, Progessence Cream, Ortho Ease, Melaleuca-Geranium Bar Soap, Lemon-Sandalwood Bar Soap.

Burns
(See BURNS)

Chapped, Dry, or Cracked Skin
Single Oils:
Roman chamomile, neroli, rose, cedarwood, palmarosa, sandalwood, lavender, spikenard, myrrh, rosewood

Blends:
Chapped skin blend:
- 1 drop rosewood
- 1 drop patchouly
- 1 drop geranium

Dry skin blend:
- 1 drop rose
- 1 drop Roman chamomile
- 1 drop sandalwood

EO Applications:
TOPICAL:
DILUTE 20-80 in a quality, unperfumed lotion base or other high grade emolient, skin oil, apply on location as often as needed

Topical Treatment:
Tender Tush Ointment, Sandalwood Moisturizing Cream, Satin Body Lotion, Rose Ointment

Lip Treatment:
Cinnamint Lip Balm

Combine 3-5 drops of essential oils with 1 tsp of Sensation and Genesis Body lotion to create a very effective lotion for rehydrating the skin of chapped hands and maintaining the natural pH balance of the skin.

Alternate oils of rose, Roman chamomile, or sandalwood with body lotion.

Bath and shower gels, such as Dragon Time, Evening Peace, Morning Start, and Sensation, are formulated to help balance the acid mantle of the skin. The AromaSilk Bar Soaps are rich in moisturizers.

Drink at least 8 glasses per day of purified water

> **Essential oils that help the skin**
>
> **To rejuvenate and heal skin:**
> - Rosewood
>
> **To prevent and retard wrinkles:**
> - Lavender, spikenard, and myrrh
>
> **To regenerate the skin:**
> - Geranium, helichrysum, and spikenard
>
> **To restore skin elasticity**
> - Rosewood, lavender
> - Ylang ylang with lavender
>
> **To combat premature aging of the skin:**
>
> Mix the following recipe into 1 tablespoon of high grade, unperfumed skin lotion and apply on location twice daily.
> - 6 drops rosewood
> - 4 drops geranium
> - 3 drops lavender
> - 2 drops frankincense

Clogged Pores
Single Oils:

Lemon, orange, tea tree, geranium

Blends:

Purification

EO Applications:

TOPICAL:

NEAT, apply 2-4 drops to affected area and gently remove with cotton ball

Topical Treatment:

AromaSilk, Bar Soaps especially Melaleuca-Rosewood, and Sandalwood Toner. Juniper or Mint Facial Scrub are gentle exfoliators designed to clarify skin and reduce acne. (If their texture is too abrasive for your skin, mix them with Orange Blossom Facial Wash. This is excellent for those with severe or mild acne.)

Spread scrub over face and let dry for perhaps 5 minutes to draw out impurities, pulling and toning the skin at the same time. Put a hot towel over face for greater penetration. Wash off with warm water by gently patting skin with warm face cloth. If you do not have time to let the mask dry, gently massage in a circular motion for 30 seconds, then rinse. Afterwards, apply Sandalwood Moisture Cream or AromaSilk Satin Body Lotion. This also works well underneath foundation makeup.

Diaper Rash
Single Oils:

Lavender, helichrysum, German chamomile cypress

Blends:

Gentle Baby

EO Applications:

TOPICAL:

DILUTE 50-50, apply on location 2-4 times daily

Topical Treatment:

Tender Tush Ointment, Lavaderm Cooling Mist, Lavender-Rosewood Bar Soap

Eczema / Dermatitis
(See Psoriasis in this section)

Eczema and dermatitis are both inflammations of the skin and are most often due to allergies, but also can be a sign of liver disease (See LIVER DISORDERS).

Dermatitis usually results from external factors, such as sunburn or contact with poison ivy, metals (wristwatch, earrings, jewelry, etc.). Eczema usually results from internal factors, such as irritant chemicals, soaps and shampoos, allergy to wheat (gluten), etc. In both dermatitis and eczema, skin becomes red, flaky and itchy. Small blisters may form and if broken by scratching, can become infected.

Single Oils:
   Lavender, juniper, ledum, *Citrus hystrix*, celery seed, cistus, Roman and German chamomile, geranium, rosewood, thyme
Blends:
   JuvaFlex, JuvaCleanse, Purification, Melrose, Gentle Baby
EO Applications:
   TOPICAL:
      DILUTE 50-50, apply as needed on location
Dietary Supplementation:
   Cleansing Trio, JuvaTone, Rehemogen, Rose Ointment, Juva Power, Detoxyme

Freckles
Single Oils:
   Idaho tansy.
EO Applications:
   TOPICAL:
      DILUTE, 4-6 drops in 1/2 teaspoon of high grade, unperfumed skin lotion. Spread lightly over freckle areas. Use 2-3 times weekly

Fungal Skin Infection
(See FUNGAL INFECTIONS)
Single Oils:
   Oregano, lemongrass, tea tree, naiouli, *Melaleuca ericifolia*
Blends:
   Melrose
   Antifungal skin blend:
   - 10 drops patchouly
   - 4 drops lavender
   - 2 drops German chamomile
   - 5 drops lemon
EO Applications:
   TOPICAL:
      DILUTE 50-50, apply on location, 3-5 times daily

Lemongrass and Skin Care

Lemongrass helps clears acne and balances oily skin conditions. Lemongrass is the predominant ingredient in Morning Start Bath and Shower Gel, which can be used to balance the pH of the skin, decongest the lymphatics and stimulate circulation.

Dietary Supplementation:
   Royaldophilus, Cleansing Trio, Mineral Essence, AD&E, Essential Omegas
Topical Treatment:
   Sandalwood Moisturizer Cream, Rose Ointment

Itching
Itching can be due to dry skin, impaired liver function, allergies, or over-exposure to chemicals or sunlight.
Single Oils:
   Peppermint, oregano, lavender, German chamomile, helichrysum, patchouly, nutmeg
Blends:
   Aroma Siez
EO Applications:
   TOPICAL:
      DILUTE 50-50, Apply 2-6 drops on location as needed
Dietary Supplementation:
   Juva Flex, Essential Omegas, JuvaTone, ComforTone
Topical Treatment:
   Tender Tush Ointment

Melanoma
(See CANCER)

Moles

To remove moles: Apply 1-2 drops of oregano neat, directly on the mole, 2-3 times daily.

Poison Oak - Poison Ivy
Single Oils:
Peppermint, *Eucalyptus dives*, German chamomile, lemongrass, lemon, Idaho tansy, tea tree, rosemary, basil

Blends:
Thieves, Purification, Sensation, Melrose, Gentle Baby, R.C., JuvaFlex, JuvaCleanse, Release

EO Applications:
 TOPICAL:
  DILUTE 50-50, apply 4-6 drops to affected areas twice daily
  COMPRESS, Cold, apply on affected area, twice daily

Dietary Supplementation:
Master Formula vitamins

Topical Treatment:
Rose Ointment, Stevia, Satin Body Lotion, Morning Start Bath and Shower Gel, Thieves Antiseptic Spray

Psoriasis

Psoriasis is a non-infectious skin disorder that is marked by skin lesions that can occur in limited areas (such as the scalp) or that can cover up to 80-90 percent of the body.

The overly rapid growth of skin cells is the primary cause of the lesions associated with psoriasis. In some cases, skin cells grow four times faster than normal, resulting in the formation of silvery layers that flake off.

Symptoms:
- Occurs on elbows, chest, knees, and scalp.
- Slightly elevated reddish lesions covered with silver-white scales.
- The disease can be limited to one small patch or can cover the entire body.
- Rashes subside after exposure to sunlight.
- Rashes recur over a period of years.

Single Oils:
Roman chamomile, tea tree, patchouly, helichrysum, rose, German chamomile, lavender

Blends:
Melrose, JuvaFlex, JuvaCleanse
Psoriasis blend:
- 2 drops patchouly
- 2 drops Roman chamomile
- 2 drops lavender
- 2 drops Melrose

EO Applications:
 TOPICAL:
  NEAT, apply 2-4 drops to affected area twice daily. 6-10 drops can be added to 1 tsp of regular skin lotion and applied daily or as needed
  COMPRESS, warm, 3 times weekly
 INGESTION:
  CAPSULE, 0 size, 1 per day

Dietary Supplementation:
Essential Omegas, Cleansing Trio, AlkaLime, JuvaTone, JuvaPower, Sulfurzyme

Topical Treatment:
Tender Tush Ointment, Rose Ointment

Sagging Skin
Single Oils: joke
Lavender, helichrysum, patchouly, cypress

Topical Treatment:
Cel-Lite Magic, Boswellia Wrinkle Cream
Skin firming blend (morning):
- 10 drops tangerine
- 10 drops cypress

Skin firming blend (night):
- 8 drops geranium
- 5 drops cypress

- 5 drops helichrysum
- 1 drop peppermint

EO Applications:
   TOPICAL:
      NEAT or DILUTE 50-50, massage 4-6 drops on affected area twice daily. Use morning blend before dressing in the morning; evening blend before bed at night. Strength training with weights can help tighten sagging skin.

Skin Ulcers
Single Oils:
   Rosewood, clove, helichrysum, Roman chamomile, patchouly, myrrh, lavender

Blends:
   Melrose, Purification, Relieve It, 3 Wise Men, Gentle Baby

EO Applications:
   TOPICAL:
      NEAT or DILUTE 50-50, massage 4-6 drops on affected areas 2 times daily

Dietary Supplementation:
   Super C, Exodus, Cleansing Trio

Topical Treatment:
   Tender Tush Ointment, AromaSilk Satin Body Lotion, Boswellia Wrinkle Cream

Stretch Marks
Stretch marks are most commonly associated with pregnancy, but can also occur during growth spurts and periods of weight gain.

Single Oils:
   Lavender, frankincense, elemi, spikenard, geranium, myrrh

Blends:
   Gentle Baby

EO Applications:
   TOPICAL:
      NEAT or DILUTE 50-50, apply on affected areas 2 times daily

Dietary Supplementation:
   Sulfurzyme, Essential Omegas

Topical Treatment:
   Tender Tush Ointment, Rose Ointment

Vitiligo
A skin disorder marked by patches of skin devoid of skin pigmentation.

Single Oils:
   Vetiver, sandalwood, myrrh

Blends:
   Purification, Melrose

EO Applications:
   TOPICAL:
      NEAT, apply 2-4 drops on location, 2 times daily

Wrinkled or Rough Skin
Single Oils:
   Frankincense, helichrysum, cypress, rose, lavender, ylang ylang, patchouly, sage, geranium, clary sage, rosewood, sandalwood, jasmine, neroli, palmarosa, spikenard

Blends:
   Gentle Baby, Sensation
   Wrinkle-reducing blend:
- 5 drops sandalwood
- 5 drops helichrysum
- 5 drops geranium
- 5 drops lavender
- 5 drops frankincense

EO Applications:
   TOPICAL:
      DILUTE 50-50 in high grade, unperfumed body lotion (AromaSilk Satin Body Lotion) or an emollient vegetable oil and apply on location as needed.
      NOTE: Be careful not to get lotion or oils near the eyes.

Dietary Supplementation:
   Ultra Young, Berry Young Juice, Master Formula vitamins, Thyromin, Stevia

Topical Treatment:
   AromaSilk Satin Body Lotion, Rose Ointment, Lavender, Valor and Lemon-Sandalwood Bar Soaps, NeuroGen, Boswellia Wrinkle Cream, Sandalwood Moisture Cream

   Boswellia wrinkle cream is excellent for dry or prematurely aging skin.

   Rose Ointment was developed to feed and rehydrate the skin and to supply nutrients necessary to slow down the aging process. Moreover, it contains no synthetic chemicals which can cause skin irritation.

SLEEP DISORDERS
(See also APNEA, INSOMNIA, or LIVER DISORDERS)

   Melatonin is the most powerful natural remedy for restoring both quality and quantity of sleep. It improves the length of the time the body sustains deep, Stage 4 sleep, when the immune system and growth hormone production reaches its maximum. ImmuPro not only contains melatonin, but mineral and polysaccharide complexes to restore natural sleep rhythm and eliminate insomnia.

Single Oils:
   Lavender, valerian, goldenrod, marjoram, Roman chamomile, orange

Blends:
   Peace & Calming, Surrender, Inspiration, Hope, Humility

EO Applications:
   INGESTION:
      CAPSULE, 0 size, 1 per day
   INHALATION:
      DIRECT, 1-3 times before bed
      Diffuser: 30 minutes before bed
   TOPICAL:
      BATH SALTS, daily, just before bedtime

Dietary Supplementation:
   ImmuPro, Essential Omegas, Essentialzyme

SMOKING CESSATION
(See also ADDICTIONS)

Single Oils:
   Cinnamon, clove, nutmeg

Blends:
   Harmony, JuvaFlex, JuvaCleanse, Peace & Calming, Thieves, Exodus II

EO Applications:
   INHALATION:
      DIRECT, whenever the urge for a cigarette arises
      DIFFUSION, 30 minutes, 3 times a day as needed

Dietary Supplementation:
   Cleansing Trio, Rehemogen, JuvaTone, Stevia Select, Stevia

   Cleanse colon and liver with Cleansing Trio and JuvaTone.

   JuvaTone, JuvaPower/Spice detoxifies the liver and reduces the cravings for nicotine and caffeine, Take 3 tablets of JuvaTone 3 times daily, and two tablespoons JuvaPower/Spice daily.

   Rehemogen cleanses and detoxifies the blood and works synergistically with JuvaTone and JuvaFlex in rebuilding the liver.

   Stevia may also decrease cravings for sugar, tobacco and alcohol.

SNAKE BITES

Single Oils:
   Clove

Topical Treatment:
   Thieves Antiseptic Spray

EO Applications:
   NOTE: Get medical attention immediately.

TOPICAL:
DILUTE 50-50, Apply 2-3 drops on location every 15 minutes until professional medical help is available

SNORING
Rub 4-6 drops thyme diluted 50-50 on the soles of both feet at bedtime.

SORE THROAT
(See COLDS OR THROAT INFECTION)

SPASTIC COLON
(See DIGESTION PROBLEMS)

SPINA BIFIDA
Spina bifida (SB) is a defect in which the spinal cord of the fetus fails to close during the first month of pregnancy. This results in varying degrees of permanent nerve damage, paralysis in lower limbs, and incomplete brain development.

SB has three different variations:
- The most severe form is Myelomeningocele. The spinal cord and its protective sheath (known as the meninges) protrude from an opening in the spine.
- The next most severe form is Meningocele. Only the meninges protrude from the opening in the spine
- The mildest form is Occulta. It is characterized by malformed vertebrae. Symptoms of this disease range from bowel and bladder dysfunctions to excess build up in the brain of cerebrospinal fluid.

The easiest way to prevent SB is with folic acid supplementation (at least 400 mcg daily), (found in Super B) by all women of child-bearing age.

To Prevent:
Dietary Supplementation:
Master Formula vitamins, Super B, Super C

To Reduce Symptoms:
Single Oils:
Mountain savory, helichrysum, thyme, tea tree
Blends:
Melrose, Thieves, Exodus II
EO Applications:
TOPICAL:
RAINDROP, weekly
COMPRESS, warm, 2 times weekly
Dietary Supplementation:
ImmuGel, Essential Omegas, Super B, uper C

SPINE INJURIES AND PAIN
According to numerous chiropractors, the Raindrop Technique using therapeutic-grade essential oils is revolutionizing the treatment of many types of back pain, spine inflammation, and vertebral misalignments. (See chapter 5: RAINDROP TECHNIQUE)

All of the essential oils described in this chapter can be used effectively in a Raindrop Application as well as in traditional massage therapy.

The following essential oils, blends, and supplements and are used for supporting the structural integrity of the spine and reducing discomfort:

Single Oils:
Wintergreen/birch, Douglas fir, spruce, peppermint, marjoram, basil
Blends:
Valor, Aroma Siez, Thieves, ImmuPower, PanAway
EO Applications:
TOPICAL:
DILUTE 50-50, 6-10 drops on location twice a day or as needed
COMPRESS, warm,1-2 times daily (if not inflamed)

RAINDROP Technique, 3 times a month for one month
Dietary Supplements:
Super C, Mineral Essence, Super Cal, WheyFit, Longevity Caps, ArthroTune, MegaCal, BLM

Backache
Single Oils:
Lavender, German chamomile, basil, peppermint, geranium, elemi
Blends:
Backache blend:
- 5 drops clary sage
- 5 drops lavender
- 5 drops chamomile

EO Applications:
  TOPICAL:
  NEAT, apply 2-4 drops to aching area 1-3 times daily as needed
  COMPRESS: warm, if there is no inflammation; cold, if there is inflammation, 1-2 times daily
  RAINDROP, weekly for 3 weeks
Topical Treatment:
Regenolone, Ortho Sport, Ortho Ease, Peppermint-Cedarwood Bar Soap, Morning Start Bar Soap, Valor Bar Soap, Morning Start Bath Gel
(See MUSCLES)

Calcification of Spine
Single Oils:
Geranium, rosemary, *Eucalyptus radiata*, ravensara, oregano, vetiver, elemi
Blends:
R.C.
EO Applications:
  TOPICAL:
  RAINDROP Technique, 3 times a month

Dietary Supplementation:
ArthroTune, Sulfurzyme, Super Cal, BLM, MegaCal
Topical Treatment:
Regenolone, Ortho Ease Massage Oil

Herniated Disk / Disk Deterioration
For this situation, it is best to consult a specialist.

For temporary relief until medical attention can be given:
Single Oils:
Helichrysum, basil, thyme, melissa, Idaho balsam fir, spruce, vetiver, valerian
Blends:
Relieve It, PanAway, Aroma Siez
EO Applications:
  TOPICAL:
  DILUTE 50-50, apply on location for pain relief
  COMPRESS: Cold, on location as needed
  RAINDROP, weekly (after medical attention). Stimulate vertebrae with the "pointer technique" (see grey box)
Dietary Supplementation:
Sulfurzyme, ArthroTune, Super Cal, BLM, MegaCal
Topical Treatments:
Regenolone, Neurogen, Ortho Sport, Ortho Ease

Lumbago (Lower back pain)
Chronic lower back pain can have many causes, including a damaged or pinched nerve (neuralgia) or a congested colon.
Single Oils:
Marjoram, nutmeg, basil, wintergreen/birch, helichrysum, German chamomile, elemi, peppermint

Blends:
Di-Tone, Relieve It, PanAway

EO Applications:
TOPICAL:
DILUTE 50-50, 6-10 drops on location twice a day or as needed, Also apply to navel
VITA FLEX, massage 2-3 drops on stomach and intestine Vita Flex points on the feet
COMPRESS, warm, 1-2 times daily (if not inflamed)
RAINDROP Technique, 3 times a month

Dietary Supplementation:
Cleansing Trio, Royaldophilus, MegaCal, Mineral Essence

Topical Treatments:
Regenolone, Neurogen, Ortho Sport and Ortho Ease Massage Oils, Raindrop Technique

Neck Pain and Stiffness
Single Oils:
Basil, marjoram, helichrysum, wintergreen/birch, Douglas fir, Idaho balsam fir, nutmeg, elemi, peppermint

Blends:
Neck stiffness blend:
- 5 drops basil
- 5 drops marjoram
- 3 drops lavender

Neck pain blend:
- 2 drops helichrysum
- 10 drops wintergreen/birch
- 8 drops cypress
- 15 drops basil
- 4 drops peppermint

EO Applications:
TOPICAL:
DILUTE 50-50, apply 4-6 drops to neck area and massage 1-3 times daily, as needed

---

Pointer Technique for Nerve Damage

The "pointer technique" may also be used on the foot Vita Flex points.

If there is nerve damage, apply about 6 drops of peppermint along the spine, starting at the hips and ending at the neck, using Raindrop Technique. Starting at the bottom of the spine, use a small-nosed pointer (about the size of a pencil but with a round end).

Stimulate each vertebra between each rib on the vertebra knuckles all the way up on each side of the spine. Use medium pressure and a rocking motion for 1-10 seconds at each location. Then follow the same procedure once more up the center of the spine directly on each vertebra.

How to Make Your Own High-Powered Massage Oil

Add these formulas to 4 oz. of vegetable or massage oil to create a custom muscle-toning formula.

Massage Oil #1:
- 10 drops wintergreen or birch
- 10 drops balsam fir
- 10 drops marjoram
- 8 drops elemi
- 8 drops vetiver
- 5 drops helichrysum
- 5 drops cypress
- 5 drops peppermint

Massage Oil #2:
- 20 drops wintergreen or birch
- 15 drops marjoram
- 10 drops juniper
- 10 drops cypress
- 6 drops spruce

> Chiropractors have found that by applying Valor on the bottom of the feet, spinal manipulations take 60 percent less time and work, and the results last 75 percent longer.

COMPRESS: warm, on neck area, daily
or as needed (if no inflammation)

Dietary supplementation:

Mineral Essence, AD&E, MegaCal, BLM

Sciatica

Sciatica is characterized by pain in the buttocks and down the back of the thigh. The pain worsens during coughing, sneezing, or extension or flexion of the back. The pain is caused by pressure on the sciatic nerve as it leaves the spine in the lower pelvic region, due to spinal misalignment, nerve inflammation or both. The sciatic nerve is the largest in the body, with branches throughout the legs and feet, and sciatica pain can be intense and immobilizing.

Acute sciatica has a sudden onset and is usually triggered by a misaligned vertebra pressing against the sciatic nerve due to accident, injury, pregnancy, or inflammation.

Symptoms:
- Lower back pain
- Swelling or stiffness in a leg
- Loss of sensation in a leg
- Muscle wasting in a leg

Sulfurzyme and Super B work well together to help rebuild nerve damage and the myelin sheath.

Single Oils:

Helichrysum, peppermint, nutmeg, thyme, spruce, wintergreen/birch, basil, rosemary, clove, tarragon

Blends:

Aroma Siez, PanAway, Relieve It, Aroma Life

EO Applications:
  TOPICAL:
    DILUTE 50-50, 6-10 drops on location twice a day or as needed
    COMPRESS, warm, 1-2 times daily (if not inflamed)
    VITA FLEX, 2-3 drops on Vita Flex points on feet, 2-4 times daily
    RAINDROP Technique, 3 times a month
  INGESTION:
    CAPSULE, 0 size, 2 times daily

Dietary Supplementation:

ArthroTune, Sulfurzyme, Super B

Topical Treatments:

Regenolone, Neurogen, Ortho Sport, Ortho Ease

SPRAIN

(See also CONNECTIVE TISSUE)

Single Oils:

Wintergreen/birch, Idaho balsam fir, lemongrass, basil, pine, spruce, cypress, peppermint

Blends:

PanAway, Relieve It, Aroma Siez

EO Applications:
  TOPICAL:
    DILUTE 50-50, apply 4-6 drops on location 3-5 times daily
    COMPRESS, cold, on location, 2 times daily

Dietary Supplementation:

Sulfurzyme, Mineral Essence, MegaCal

Topical Treatment:

Regenolone, Prenolone, Ortho Sport

STOMACHACHE

(See DIGESTIVE DISORDERS)

STRESS
Single Oils:
Lavender, chamomile, blue tansy, marjoram, rose, sandalwood, frankincense, cedarwood
Blends:
Humility, Harmony, Valor, Joy
EO Applications:
  INHALATION:
    DIRECT, as needed
    DIFFUSION, 30 minutes 1-3 times daily
  INGESTION:
    CAPSULE, 0 size, 2 times a day
  TOPICAL:
    DILUTE 50-50, apply on temples, neck, and shoulders twice daily, or as needed
    BATH SALTS, daily
Dietary Supplementation:
Super B, Ultra Young, Super C, VitaGreen, Thyromin, Master Formula Vitamins, MegaCal
Topical Treatment:
Ortho Ease, Ortho Sport

STRETCH MARKS
(See SKIN DISORDERS)

STROKE
(See BRAIN DISORDERS)

SUNBURN
(See BURNS)

SYMPATHETIC NERVOUS SYSTEM
(See NERVOUS SYSTEM-AUTONOMIC)

TACHYCARDIA
(See HEART, CARDIOVASCULAR CONDITIONS)

TENDONITIS
(See CONNECTIVE TISSUE)

TEETHING PAIN
(See ORAL CARE)

TEETH GRINDING
(See ORAL CARE)

THROAT INFECTIONS
(See also COLDS, INFECTION, LUNG INFECTIONS, ORAL CARE)

Cough
Single Oils:
Cypress, *Eucalyptus polybractea, Eucalyptus radiata, Eucalyptus globulus,* lemon, frankincense, ravensara, thyme, oregano, peppermint, myrrh, cedarwood
Cough blend #1:
- 6 drops cypress
- 3 drops *Eucalyptus polybractea*

Blends:
Thieves, Melrose, R.C., Raven, Purification, 3 Wise Men, Exodus II, ImmuPower
EO Applications:
  INHALATION:
    DIRECT, 3-6 times daily
    VAPOR, 2-3 times daily
  INGESTION:
    RICE MILK, 2-4 times daily. It is beneficial to heat the rice milk and sip slowly for more soothing relief.
    SYRUP, 3-5 times daily
  ORAL:
    TONGUE, 2-6 times daily or as often as needed
    GARGLE, 4-8 times daily
  TOPICAL:
    DILUTE 50-50, apply 1-3 drops to throat, chest and back of neck 2-4 times daily
    VITA FLEX, apply 1-3 drops to lung Vita Flex points, 1-3 times daily
    RAINDROP Technique, weekly

Dietary Supplementation:
Super C, Exodus, ImmuGel, Longevity Caps, VitaGreen, ImmuPro, ImmuneTune, Rehemogen

Mountain savory, ravensara, and thyme applied by Raindrop Technique on the spine are beneficial for any and all chest-related infections.

Topical Treatment:
Thieves Antiseptic Spray

Dry Cough
Mix 2 drops lemon and 3 drops Eucalyptus radiata with 1 tsp. agave or maple syrup. Dissolve this mixture into 4 oz. of heated distilled water, and sip slowly. Repeat as often as needed for relief.

Topical Treatment:
Thieves Antiseptic Spray

Laryngitis
Put 1 drop Melrose and 1 drop lemon in 1/2 tsp. agave or maple syrup. Hold in back of mouth for 1-2 minutes, then swallow. Repeat as needed.

Topical Treatment:
Thieves Antiseptic Spray

Sore Throat
Single Oils:
Cypress, *Eucalyptus radiata*, lemon, frankincense, ravensara, thyme, oregano, peppermint, myrrh, sage

Blends:
Thieves, Melrose, Raven

Oral Treatment:
Thieves Antiseptic Spray, Fresh Essence Plus, Thieves Lozenges

Sore throat blend #1:
- 2 drops thyme
- 2 drops cypress
- 1 drop Eucalyptus radiata
- 1 drop peppermint
- 1 drop myrrh

Sore throat blend #2:
- 2 drops Eucalyptus globulus
- 5 drops lemon
- 2 drops wintergreen or birch

EO Applications:

INHALATION:
DIRECT, 3-6 times daily
VAPOR, 2-3 times daily

INGESTION:
RICE MILK, 2-4 times daily. It is beneficial to heat the rice milk and sip slowly for more soothing relief.
SYRUP, 3-5 times daily

ORAL:
TONGUE, 2-6 times daily or as often as needed
GARGLE, 4-8 times daily

TOPICAL:
DILUTE 50-50, apply 1-3 drops to throat, chest and back of neck 2-4 times daily
COMPRESS, warm, on chest area 2-3 times daily
VITA FLEX, apply 1-3 drops to lung Vita Flex points, 1-3 times daily
RAINDROP Technique, weekly

Dietary Supplementation:
Super C, Super C Chewable, Longevity Caps, Thieves lozenges, ImmuPro, Exodus

Strep Throat
Single Oils:
Eucalyptus globulus, oregano, thyme, frankincense, myrrh, and mountain savory, white fir, Douglas fir
Dilute 1:1 with vegetable oil and apply 2-4 drops on tongue.

Blends:
Thieves, Exodus II, ImmuPower, Di-Tone, Melrose, Raven

Oral Treatment:
Thieves Antiseptic Spray, Fresh Essence
Strep throat blend:
- 1 drops cinnamon
- 6 drops lavender
- 2 drops hyssop

EO Applications:
  INHALATION:
    DIRECT, 3-6 times daily
    VAPOR, 2-3 times daily
  INGESTION:
    RICE MILK, 2-4 times daily. It is beneficial to heat the rice milk and sip slowly for more soothing relief.
    SYRUP, 3-5 times daily
  ORAL:
    TONGUE, 2-6 times daily or as often as needed
    GARGLE, 4-8 times daily
  TOPICAL:
    DILUTE 50-50, apply 1-3 drops to throat, chest and back of neck 2-4 times daily
    COMPRESS, warm, on chest area 2-3 times daily
    VITA FLEX, apply 1-3 drops to lung Vita Flex points, 1-3 times daily
    RAINDROP Technique, weekly

Dietary Supplementation:
ImmuPro, ImmuneTune, Super C, Longevity Caps, Super C Chewable, VitaGreen, Royalphilus, Essential Omegas, Rehemogen, Exodus, Cleansing Trio, Thieves Spray, Thieves Lozenges.

Regimen for strep throat:
- ImmuneTune: 2-4 capsules, 3 times daily
- Super C: 2-3 tablets, 3 times daily
- Use Raindrop Technique with ImmuPower and/or Exodus II along sides of spine, weekly
- Gargle every hour with Fresh Essence Plus
- Spray throat with colloidal silver/lemon solution.

Tonsillitis

The tonsils are infection-fighting lymphatic tissues (immune cells) that surround the throat. When these become infected streptococcal bacteria they become inflamed, causing a condition known as tonsillitis.

It became popular in the 1960's and 1970's to have the tonsils removed when they became infected. However, tonsillectomies have become much less frequent as researchers have discovered the important role tonsils play in protecting and fighting infectious diseases and optimizing immune response.

The pharyngeal tonsils located at the back of the throat (known as the adenoids) can also become infected—a condition known as adenitis.

Single Oils:
Clove, tea tree, goldenrod, oregano, mountain savory, ravensara, thyme

Blends:
Exodus II, Thieves, Melrose, Exodus II, ImmuPower

Topical Treatment:
Thieves Antiseptic Spray, Fresh Essence

EO Applications:
  INGESTION:
    RICE MILK, 2-4 times daily. It is beneficial to heat the rice milk and sip slowly for more soothing relief.
    SYRUP, 3-5 times daily
  ORAL:
    TONGUE, 2-6 times daily or as often as needed
    GARGLE, 4-8 times daily
  TOPICAL:
    DILUTE 50-50, apply 1-3 drops to throat, chest and back of neck 2-4 times daily
    COMPRESS, warm, on chest area 2-3 times daily

VITA FLEX, apply 1-3 drops to lung Vita Flex points, 1-3 times daily
RAINDROP Technique, weekly

Dietary Supplementation:
ImmuGel, Super C Chewable, AD&E

THRUSH
(See FUNGAL INFECTIONS)

THYROID PROBLEMS

Located at the base of the neck just below the Adam's apple, the thyroid is the energy gland of the human body. It produces T3 and T4 thyroid hormones that control the body's metabolism. The thyroid also controls other vital functions such as digestion, circulation, immune function, hormone balance, and emotions.

The thyroid gland is actually controlled by the pituitary gland which signals the thyroid when to produce thyroid hormone. The pituitary gland, in turn, is directed by chemical signals sent by the hypothalamus gland which monitors hormone levels in the blood stream.

A lack of thyroid hormone does not necessarily mean that the thyroid is not functioning properly (although in many cases, this may be the case). In some instances, the pituitary may be malfunctioning because of its failure to release sufficient TSH (thyroid stimulating hormone) to spur the thyroid to make thyroid hormone.

Other cases of thyroid hormone deficiency may be due to the hypothalamus failing to release sufficient TRH (thyrotropin releasing hormone).

In cases where thyroid hormone deficiency is caused by a malfunctioning pituitary or hypothalamus, better results may be achieved by using supplements or essential oils that stimulate the pituitary or hypothalamus, such as Ultra Young or Cedarwood.

People with type A blood have more of a tendency to have weak thyroid function.

Hyperthyroid (Graves Disease)

When the thyroid becomes overactive and produces excess thyroid hormone, the following symptoms occur:

Symptoms of hyperthyroidism:
- Anxiety
- Restlessness
- Insomnia
- Premature gray hair
- Diabetes mellitus
- Arthritis
- Vitiligo (loss of skin pigment)

Graves disease, unlike Hashimoto's disease, is an autoimmune disease which results in an excess of thyroid hormone production.

MSM has been studied for its ability to reverse many kinds of autoimmune diseases. MSM is a key component of Sulfurzyme.

Single Oils:
Myrrh, spruce, blue tansy, lemongrass

Blends:
EndoFlex

Dietary Supplementation:
Sulfurzyme, Essential Omegas, Thyromin, VitaGreen, Mineral Essence

Hypothyroid (Hashimoto's Disease)
(see also HYPOGLYCEMIA)

This condition occurs when the thyroid is underactive and produces insufficient thyroid hormone. Approximately 40 percent of the U.S. population suffers from this disorder to some degree, and these people tend to also suffer from hypoglycemia (low blood sugar).

Hashimoto's disease, like Graves disease, is an autoimmune condition. It affects the thyroid, differently, however, limiting its ability to produce thyroid hormone.

The following symptoms occur:
- Fatigue
- Yeast infections (Candida)

- Lack of energy
- Reduced immune function
- Poor resistance to disease
- Recurring infections

Single Oils:
Ledum, lemongrass, myrtle, peppermint, spearmint, myrrh, clove

Blends:
EndoFlex

EO Applications:
  TOPICAL:
    DILUTE 50-50, apply 3-5 drops over the thyroid (lower front of the neck on both sides of the trachea), 1-3 times daily
    VITA FLEX, apply 1-3 drops on the thyroid Vita Flex points of the feet (located on the inside edge of the ball of the foot, just below the base of the big toe.)
  INGESTION:
    CAPSULE, 00 size, 1 capsule twice a day

Dietary Supplementation:
Thyromin, VitaGreen, Sulfurzyme, Essential Omegas

TINNITUS (Ringing in Ears)
(See HEARING IMPAIRMENT)

TOOTHACHE
(See ORAL CARE)

TONSILLITIS
(See COLDS AND THROAT INFECTIONS)

TOXEMIA
(See INFECTION)

When toxins or bacteria begin to accumulate in the bloodstream, a condition called toxemia is created. When toxemia occurs during late pregnancy, it is referred to as "preeclampsia."

Single Oils:
Clove, tangerine, orange, cypress

Blends:
Citrus Fresh, Inner Child, Purification

EO Applications:
  INGESTION:
    CAPSULE, 00 size, 1 capsule 2 times a day

Dietary Supplementation:
ICP, ComforTone, Exodus, Super C, Berry Young Juice, Essential Manna (rich in potassium).
NOTE: Best results are achieved by eliminating all sugar, white flour, breads, pasta, and fried foods.

TRAUMA (EMOTIONAL)
(See SHOCK)

Emotional trauma can be generated from events that involve loss, bereavement, accidents, or misfortunes. Essential oils, through their ability to tap the emotional and memory center of the brain, may facilitate the processing and release of emotional trauma in a way that minimizes psychological turmoil.

Blends:
Trauma Life, Hope, Forgiveness, Release, Envision, Valor

EO Applications:
  TOPICAL:
    DILUTE 50-50, massage 2-4 drops to temples, forehead, crown and shoulders 1-3 times daily
  INHALATION:
    DIRECT, 1-3 times daily as needed

Dietary Supplementation:
Essential Omegas, Super C, Mineral Essence

TUBERCULOSIS
(See also LUNG INFECTION)

Tuberculosis (TB) is a highly contagious lung disease caused by *Mycobacterium tuberculosis*. the germs are spread via coughs, sneezes, and physical contact. The most worrisome aspect of this disease is it latency. Those infected may harbor the germ for years, yet display no outward or visible signs of infection. However, when the immune systems become challenged or downregulated due to stress, candida, diabetes, corticosteroid use, or other factors, the bacteria can become reactivated and develop into full-blown TB.

Prior to the 1940's, tuberculosis was one of the leading causes of the death in the United States. After the introduction of anti-TB drugs following World War II, incidences of the disease dwindled. However, the incidence of TB has recently staged a surprising resurgence, with the number of TB cases increasing dramatically since 1984. In 1993 over 25,000 cases of TB were reported.

Because many essential oils have broad-spectrum antimicrobial properties, they can be diffused to prevent the spread of airborne bacteria like *Mycobacterium tuberculosis*. Essential oils and blends such as Thieves, Purification, Raven, R.C., and Sacred Mountain are extremely effective for killing this type of germs.

Many essential oils have also been shown to be immune-stimulating. Lemon oil has been shown to increase lymphocyte production—a pivotal part of the immune system.

Single Oils:
Ravensara, rosemary, lemon, cinnamon, thyme, sandalwood, *Eucalyptus radiata,* clove, oregano, mountain savory, peppermint, spearmint, myrtle, Idaho balsam fir

Blends:
Raven, R.C., Sacred Mountain, Thieves, ImmuPower, Inspiration

EO Applications:
  INHALATION:
    DIFFUSION, 1 hour, twice a day and at night.
    DIRECT, 3-5 times daily
  TOPICAL:
    DILUTE 50-50, apply 6-10 drops on chest and upper back 1-3 times daily
    COMPRESS, warm, on chest and upper back, twice daily
  INGESTION:
    CAPSULE, 00 size, 1 capsule 3 times daily for 10 days

Dietary Supplementation:
ImmuPro, Super C Chewable, Exodus, Longevity Caps, VitaGreen, ImmuneTune, Cleansing Trio

Tuberculosis-specific regimen:
1. Alternate diffusing Raven and R.C. as often as possible during the day
2. Mix the following in 2 Tbsp. V-6 Oil Complex. Insert into rectum with bulb syringe and retain overnight. Do this nightly for 7 nights; rest for 4 nights; then repeat.
   - 2 drops sage
   - 4 drops myrrh
   - 5 drops clove
   - 6 drops ravensara
   - 15 drops frankincense
3. Put 20 drops Raven in a capsule and swallow 3 times daily for 10 days.
4. Rub 4-6 drops Thieves on the bottom of the feet nightly
5. Rub ImmuPower up the spine daily and apply as a compress on back and chest twice a day. Use Raindrop Technique.
6. Take 3-4 capsules Exodus 3 times daily for 21 days. Discontinue use for 7 days before resuming use.

TUMORS
(See CANCER)

TYPHOID FEVER

Typhoid fever is an infectious disease caused by a bacteria known as *Salmonella typhi*. Usually contracted through infected food or water, typhoid is common in lesser-developed countries.

Some people infected with typhoid fever display no visible symptoms of disease, while others become seriously ill. Both people who recover from typhoid fever and those who remain symptomless are carriers for the disease, and can infect others through the bacteria they shed in their feces.

To avoid contracting typhoid fever—especially when traveling overseas—it is essential to drink purified or distilled water and to thoroughly cook foods. Fresh vegetables can be carriers of the bacteria, especially if they have been irrigated with water that has come into contact with human waste.

Symptoms:
- Sustained, high fever (101° to 104° F).
- Stomach pains
- Headache
- Rash of reddish spots
- Impaired appetite
- Weakness

Single Oils:
Ravensara, cinnamon, cassia, peppermint, black pepper, mountain savory, clove, thyme

EO Applications:
  TOPICAL:
   DILUTE 50-50, massage 4-6 drops on lower abdomen, 2-4 times daily
  INGESTION:
   CAPSULE, 00 size, 1 capsule 2 times daily for 10 days

Dietary Supplementation:
ImmuPro

ULCERS (Stomach)
(See DIGESTIVE PROBLEMS)

URINARY TRACT/BLADDER INFECTION
(See also KIDNEY DISORDERS)

Infections and inflammation of the urinary tract are caused by bacteria that travel up the urethra. This disorder is more common in women than men because of the woman's shorter urethra. If the infection travels up the ureters and reaches the kidneys, kidney infection can result.

Symptoms:
- Frequent urge to urinate with only a small amount of urine coming out
- Strong smelling urine
- Blood in urine
- Burning or stinging during urination

Bladder infection (known as cystitis or interstitial cystitis) is marked by the following symptoms:
- Tenderness or chronic pain in bladder and pelvic area
- Frequent urge to urinate
- Pain intensity fluctuates as bladder fills or empties
- Symptoms worsen during menstruation

Single Oils:
Oregano, mountain savory, tea tree, thyme, cistus, juniper, rosemary, clove

Blends:
Di-Tone, EndoFlex, R.C., Melrose, Purification, Inspiration, Thieves

EO Applications:
  INGESTION:
   CAPSULE, 0 size, 1 capsule 2 times daily
  TOPICAL:
   COMPRESS, warm, over bladder, 1-2 times daily

Dietary Supplementation:
K&B tincture, ImmuPro, AlkaLime
Use K&B tincture (2-3 droppers in distilled water) 3-6 times daily. K & B Tincture helps strengthen and tone weak bladder, kidneys, and urinary tract (see KIDNEY DISORDERS).

Take 1 tsp. of AlkaLime daily, in water only, 1 hour before or after meal.

UTERINE CANCER
(See CANCER)

VAGINAL YEAST INFECTION
(See FUNGAL INFECTIONS or ANTISEPTIC)

Vaginal yeast infections are usually caused from overgrowth of fungi like *Candida albicans*. These naturally-occurring intestinal yeast and fungi are normally kept under control by the immune system, but when excess sucrose is consumed or antibiotics are used, these organisms convert from relatively harmless yeast into an invasive, harmful fungus that secretes toxins as part of its life cycle.

Vaginal yeast infections are just one symptom of systemic fungal infestation. While the yeast infection can be treated locally, the underlying problem of systemic candidiasis may still remain unless specific dietary and health practices are used.

Single Oils:
Myrrh, mountain savory, oregano, tea tree, thyme

Blends:
Melrose, 3 Wise Men, Inspiration

Topical Treatment:
Fresh Essence Plus

EO Applications:
  RETENTION:
    TAMPON, 3 times a week, soaked in Fresh Essence Plus

VARICOSE VEINS (SPIDER VEINS)
(See CIRCULATION DISORDERS)

VASCULAR CLEANSING
(See HEAVY METALS and CIRCULATION DISORDERS)

VITILIGO
(See SKIN DISORDERS)

WARTS (GENITAL)
(See SEXUALLY TRANSMITTED DISEASES)

WEST NILE VIRUS

(See INSECT BITES)

WHOOPING COUGH
(See COLDS, FLU, or INFECTION)

WOUNDS, SCRAPES, OR CUTS
(See SKIN DISORDERS and ANTISEPTIC)

When selecting oils to for surface injuries, treat the whole person, not just the cut. Think through the cause and type of injury and select oils for each aspect of the trauma. For instance, a wound could encompass muscle damage, nerve damage, ligament damage, inflammation, infection, bone injury, fever, and possibly an emotion. Therefore, select an oil or blend that treats each of these.

Melaleuca alternifolia (Tea tree oil)

During World War II, melaleuca was found to have very strong antibacterial properties and worked well in preventing infection in open wounds. Melrose is a blend containing two types of melaleuca oil, making it an exceptional antiseptic and tissue regenerator.

Single Oils:
Lavender, tea tree, rosemary, *Eucalyptus globulus,* cypress, wintergreen/ birch, thyme, oregano, German chamomile, lavandin, mountain savory, peppermint

Blends:
Melrose, Purification, Thieves, 3 Wise Men

Topical Treatment:
Thieves Antiseptic Spray, LavaDerm Spray
  Bruise and scrape blend
  (may be used on infants and children):
  - 3 drop helichrysum
  - 3 drop lavender
  Infected cuts blend:
  - 7 drops geranium
  - 5 drops peppermint
  - 10 drops tea tree
  - 8 drops orange

EO Applications:
  TOPICAL:
  DILUTE 50-50, apply 2-6 drops on location, 1-4 times daily as needed
  NOTE: Peppermint may sting when applied to an open wound. To reduce discomfort, dilute with lavender oil or mix in a sealing ointment before applying. When applied to a wound or cut that has a scab, peppermint will soothe, cool, and reduce inflammation in damaged tissue.

To reduce bleeding
Single Oils:
Geranium, cypress, helichrysum, lemon, rose, rose hip seed

Blends:
Melrose, Thieves
Wound compress blend:
  - 5 drops geranium
  - 5 drops lemon
  - 5 drops German chamomile

First-Aid Spray
- 5 drops lavender
- 3 drops tea tree (Melaleuca alternifolia)
- 2 drops cypress

Mix above oils thoroughly in 1/2 teaspoon of salt. Add this to 8 ounces of distilled water and shake vigorously. Put in a spray bottle. Spray minor cuts and wounds before applying bandage. Repeat 2-3 times daily for 3 days. Complete the healing process by applying a drop or two of tea tree oil to the wound daily for the next few days.

EO Applications:
  TOPICAL:
  COMPRESS, cold, 1-2 times until bleeding stops

To reduce scarring:
Single Oils:
Lavender, frankincense, lemongrass, rose hip seed, geranium, helichrysum, myrrh,

Blends:
Scar Prevention blend #1:
  - 10 drops helichrysum
  - 6 drops lavender
  - 8 drops lemongrass
  - 4 drops patchouly
Scar Prevention blend #2:
  - 3 drops lavender
  - 3 drops lemongrass
  - 3 drops geranium

EO Applications:
  TOPICAL:
  DILUTE 50-50, apply 2-4 drops on wound, 2-5 times daily

To promote healing:
Single Oils:
Lavender, patchouly, tea tree, neroli, myrrh, helichrysum, sandalwood, Idaho tansy
Blends:
Purification, Melrose
EO Applications:
   TOPICAL:
      DILUTE 50-50, apply 2-4 drops on wound 2-5 times daily.
Single Oils:
Thyme, tea tree, mountain savory, oregano
Blends:
Melrose, Purification, Thieves, ImmuPower
EO Applications:
   TOPICAL:
      DILUTE 50-50, apply 2-4 drops on wound 2-5 times daily.
Topical Treatment:
Thieves Antiseptic Spray

WORMS
(See PARASITES)

WRINKLES
(See SKIN DISORDERS)

YEAST INFECTION
(See HORMONES, VAGINAL YEAST INFECTION, or ANTISEPTIC)

Endnotes

1. Taiwan Huang, Fang, Hung, Wu, Tsai "Cyclic monoterpene extract from cardamom oil as a skin permeation enhancer for indomethacin: in vitro and in vivo studies." *Biological and Pharmaceutical Bulletin* 1999 Jun;22(6):642-6.
2. Ogiso, Iwaki, Paku "Effect of various enhancers on transdermal penetration of indomethacin and urea, and relationship between penetration parameters and enhancement factors." *Journal of Pharmaceutical Sciences.* 1995 Apr;84(4):482-8.
3. Galli RL et al., "Fruit polyphenolics and brain aging: nutritional interventions targeting age-related neuronal and behavioral deficits." *Ann N Y Acad Sci.* 2002 Apr; 959: 128-32.
4. Bickford PC et al., "Antioxidant-rich diets improve cerebellar physiology and motor learning in aged rats." *Brain Res.* 2000 Jun 2; 866(1-2): 211-7.
5. Hay, Jamieson, Ormerod "Randomized trial of aromatherapy. Successful treatment for alopecia areata." *Archives of Dermatology.* 1998 Nov;134(11):1349-52.
6. Kalish, Gilhar "Alopecia areata: autoimmunity--the evidence is compelling." *The Journal of Investigative Dermatology Symposium Proceedings* 2003 Oct;8(2):164-7.
7. Jean Valnet, MD, "The Practice of Aromatherapy: A Classic Compendium of Plant Medicines & Their Healing Properties," *Healing Arts Press*, 1990, p. 197.
8. Gobel et al., "Effect of peppermint and eucalyptus oil preparations on neurophysiological and experimental algesimetric headache parameters." *Cephalalgia.* 1994 Jun;14(3):228-34; discussion 182.
9. Haze S, Sakai K, Gozu Y, "Effects of fragrance on sympathetic activity in normal adults," *Jpn J Pharmacol* 2002 Nov;903):247-53.
10. Koo HN et al., "Inhibition of heat shock-induced apoptosis by peppermint oil in astrocytes," *J Mol Neurosci* 2001 Dec;17(3):391-6.
11. Dember, Warm, 1994. USA. Parasuraman, Compendium of Olfactory Research
12. Crowell P. Prevention and therapy of cancer by dietary monoterpenes. J Nutr. 1999 Mar;129(3):775S-778S.
13. Uemura N, Okamoto S, Yamamoto S, "H. pylori infection and development of gastric cancer," *Keio J Med* 2002 Dec;51 Suppl 2:63-8.
14. de Castillo et al., "Bactericidal activity of lemon juice and lemon derivatives against Vibrio cholerae," *Biol Pharm Bull* 2000 Oct;23(10):1235-8.
15. Dimitrova et al., "effect of Melissa officinalis L. extracts," *Acta Microbiol Bulg* 1993;29-:65-72.
16. Koytchev R, et al., "Balm mint extract (Lo-701) for topical treatment of recurring herpes labialis," *Phytomedicine* 1999 Oct;6(4):225-30.
17. Davies SJ, Harding LM, Baranowski AP, "A novel treatment of postherpetic neuralgia using peppermint oil," *Clin J Pain* 2002 May-Jun;18(3):200-2
18. Carson CF et al., "Melaleuca alternifolia (tea tree) oil gel (6%) for the treatment of recurrent herpes labialis," *J Antimicrob Chemother* 2001 Sep;48(3):450-1.
19. Nasel et al., Functional imaging of effects of fragrances on the human brain after prolonged inhalation, *Chem Senses,* 1995 Jun;20(3):349-50.
20. Komori, Fujiward, Tanida, Nomura, Yokoyama "Effects of citrus fragrance on immune function and depressive states". *Neuroimmunomodulation.* 1995 May-Jun;2(3):174-80.
21. Weiss HJ, et al., "The effect of salicylates on the hemostatic properties of platelets in man," *J Clin Invest* 1968 Sep;47(9):2169-80.
22. Fawell WN, Thompson G, "Nutmeg for diarrhea of medullarly carcinoma of thyroid," *N Eng J Med* 1973 Jul 12;289(2):108-9.

23. "Antifungal activity of the essential oil of *Melaleuca alternifolia* (tea ree oil) against pathogenic fungi in vitro." *Skin Pharmacol.* 1996;9(6):388-94.

24. Veal L, "The potential effectiveness of essential oils as a treatment for headlice, Pediculus humanus capitis," *Complement Ther Nurs Midwifery* 1996 Aug;2(4):97-101.

25. Gobel H, et al., *Effectiveness of Oleum menthae piperitae and paracetamol in therapy of headache of the tension type.* Nervenarzt. 1996 Aug; 67(8): 672-81.

26. Gobel H, Schmidt G, Soyka D. *Effect of peppermint and eucalyptus oil preparations on neurophysiological and experimental algesimetric headache parameters.* Cephalalgia. 1994 Jun; 14(3): 228-34; discussion 182.

27. Weydert JA, et al., "Systematic review of treatments for recurrent abdominal pain," *Pediatrics* 2003 Jan;111(1):e1-11.

28. Logan AC, Beaulne TM, "The treatment of small intestinal bacterial overgrowth with enteric-caoated peppermint oil: a case report," *Altern Med Rev,* 2002 Oct;7(5):410-7.

29. Sagduyu K, "Peppermint oil for irritable bowel syndrome," *Psychosomatics* 2002 Nov-Dec;43(6):508-9.

30. Yang, Kinoshita, Koyama, Takahashi, Tai, Nunoura, "Anti-emetic principles of Pogostemon cablin" (Blanco) 1999 *Watanabe Phytomedicine* Vol. 6(2), pp 89-93.

31. Baulieu E, Schumacher M, Progesterone as a neuroactive neurosteriod, with special reference to the effect of progesterone on myelination, *Steroids* 2000 Oct-Nov;65(10-11):605-12.

32. Gupta M, Mazumder UK, Bhawal SR, "CNS activity of Vitex negundo Linn. in mice," *Indian J Exp Biol* 1999 Feb;37(2):143-6.

33. Nasel, C. et al. "Functional imaging of effects of fragrances on the human brain after prolonged inhalation." Chemical Senses. 1994;19(4):359-64

34. Hirsch AR. Inhalation of Odorants for Weight Reduction, *Int J Obes,* 1994, page 306

35. "Effect of Peppermint and Eucalyptus Oil Preparations on Neurophysiological and experimental algesimetric headache parameters" 1994 Germany Gobel, Schmidt, Soyka Cephalalgia Jun;14(3):228-34; discussion 182.

36. Skakkebaek NE, "Endocrine disrupters and testicular dysgenesis syndrome," *Horm Res* 2002;57 Suppl 2:43.

37. Zhang X, et al., "Effect of the extracts of pumpkin seeds on the urodynamics of rabbits: an experimental study," *J Tongji Med Univ* 1994:14(4):235-8.

38. Benencia F, et al. "Antiviral activity of sandalwood oil against herpes simplex viruses-1 and -2." *Phytomedicine.* 1999;6(2):119-23

39. Pénoël, Daniel, MD. and Rose Marie, *Natural Home Health Care Using Essential Oils, Essential Science Publishing,* 1998. pp. 166-167

40. Bassett IB, et al. "A comparative study of tea-tree oil versus benzoyl peroxide in the treatment of acne." *Med J Aust.* 1990;153(8):455-8.

41. Toyoda M, Morohashi M, "Pathenogenesis of acne," *Med Electron Microsc* 2001 Mar;34(1):29-40.

Appendix A

Application Codes

NEAT = straight, undiluted
Dilution usually NOT required; suitable for all but the most sensitive skin. Safe for children over 2 years old.

50-50 = Dilute 50-50
Dilution recommended at 50-50 (1 part essential oils to 1 part vegetable or massage oil) for topical and internal use, especially when used on sensitive areas — face, neck, genital area, underarms, etc. Keep out of reach of children.

PH = Photosensitizing
Avoid using on skin exposed to direct sunlight or UV rays (i.e. sunlamps, tanning beds, etc.)

20-80 = Dilute 20-80
Always dilute 20-80 (1 part essential oils to 4 parts vegetable or massage oil) before applying to the skin or taking internally. Keep out of reach of children.

Singles

Angelica	**PH**	**50-50**
Anise		**50-50**
Basil		**50-50**
Bergamot	**PH**	**50-50**
Benzoin		**50-50**
Cajeput		**50-50**
Cedar, Western Red		**50-50**
Cardemom		**50-50**
Carrot Seed		**NEAT**
Cassia		**20-80**
Celery Seed		**NEAT**
Cedarwood		**NEAT**
Chamomile, German		**NEAT**
Chamomile, Roman		**NEAT**
Cinnamon Bark		**20-80**
Cistus		**NEAT**
Citronella		**50-50**
Citrus Hystrix	**PH**	**50-50**
Clary Sage		**50-50**
Clove		**20-80**
Coriander		**50-50**
Cumin		**50-50**
Cypress		**50-50**
Davana		**NEAT**
Dill		**50-50**
Elemi		**NEAT**
Eucalyptus dives		**50-50**
Eucalyptus globulus		**50-50**
Eucalyptus polybractea		**50-50**
Eucalyptus radiata		**50-50**
Fennel		**NEAT**
Fir, Douglas		**50-50**
Fir, Idaho Balsam		**50-50**
Fir, White		**50-50**
Fleabane		**50-50**
Frankincense		**50-50**
Galbanum		**NEAT**
Geranium		**50-50**

Oil	Dilution
Ginger	50-50
Goldenrod	50-50
Grapefruit **PH**	50-50
Helichrysum	50-50
Hyssop	20-80
Jasmine	NEAT
Juniper	50-50
Laurus nobilis	50-50
Lavandin	50-50
Lavender	NEAT
Ledum	NEAT
Lemon **PH**	50-50
Lemongrass	20-80
Lime **PH**	50-50
Mandarin	50-50
Manuka	NEAT
Marjoram	50-50
Melaleuca ericifolia	50-50
Melissa	NEAT
Mountain Savory	50-50
Myrrh	NEAT
Myrtle	50-50
Neroli	NEAT
Niaouli	50-50
Nutmeg	50-50
Orange **PH**	50-50
Oregano	20-80
Palmarosa	50-50
Patchouli	NEAT
Pepper, Black	50-50
Peppermint	50-50
Petitgrain	NEAT
Pine	50-50
Ravensara	50-50
Rose	NEAT
Rosemary CT cineol	50-50
Rosemary CT verbenon	50-50
Rosewood	NEAT
Sage	50-50
Sandalwood	NEAT
Spearmint	50-50
Spikenard	NEAT
Spruce	50-50
Tangerine **PH**	50-50
Tansy	50-50
Tansy, Blue	NEAT
Tarragon	50-50
Tea Tree	50-50
Thyme	20-80
Tsuga	50-50
Valerian Root	NEAT
Vetiver	NEAT
Wintergreen	50-50
Yarrow	NEAT
Ylang Ylang	NEAT

Blends

Blend	Dilution
Abundance	50-50
Acceptance	NEAT
Aroma Life	NEAT
Aroma Siez	50-50
Australian Blue	NEAT
Awaken	NEAT
Believe	50-50
Brain Power	NEAT
Chivalry	50-50
Christmas Spirit	50-50
Citrus Fresh	50-50
Clarity	NEAT
Di-Tone	NEAT
Dragon Time	NEAT
Dream Catcher	NEAT
EndoFlex	NEAT
En-R-Gee	50-50
Envision	NEAT
Evergreen Essence	50-50
Exodus II	50-50
Forgiveness	NEAT
Gathering	NEAT
Gentle Baby	NEAT
Gratitude	50-50
Grounding	NEAT

Harmony	**NEAT**	M-Grain	**50-50**
Highest Potential	**50-50**	PanAway	**50-50**
Hope . . . . **NEAT**		Peace & Calming	**NEAT**
Humility	**NEAT**	Present Time	**NEAT**
ImmuPower	**50-50**	Purification	**NEAT**
Inner Child	**NEAT**	R.C.	**NEAT**
Inspiration	**NEAT**	R.C.	**50-50**
Into The Future	**NEAT**	Release	**50-50**
Joy . . . . **PH** . . . . **NEAT**		Relieve It	**50-50**
Juva Cleanse	**NEAT**	Sacred Mountain	**NEAT**
JuvaFlex	**50-50**	SARA	**NEAT**
Legacy	**20-80**	Sensation	**NEAT**
Live With Passion	**NEAT**	Surrender	**NEAT**
Longevity	**20-80**	Thieves	**20-80**
Magnify Your Purpose	**NEAT**	3 Wise Men	**NEAT**
Melrose	**50-50**	Trauma Life	**NEAT**
Mister	**NEAT**	Valor	**NEAT**
Motivation	**NEAT**	White Angelica . . . . **PH** . . . . **NEAT**	

Appendix B

Body Systems Chart

Product Type Key

- **S** Essential Oil Single
- **B** Essential Oil Blend
- **D** Dietary Supplement
- **P** Personal Care/Hair and Skin
- **L** Lotions/Creams/Massage Oils
- **G** Bath and Shower Gels/Soaps
- **E** Essential Waters
- **F** Powergize Fitness
- **O** Oral Care

	Product Type	Nervous System	Cardiovascular System	Respiratory System	Digestive/Elimination	Immune/Anti-infectious	Glandular/Hormonal	Emotional Balance	Muscle & Bone	Anti Aging	Oral Hygiene	Skin and Hair
Abundance	B			■		■		■				
Acceptance	B	■						■				
A D & E	D	■				■						■
Agave Syrup	F						■		■			
AlkaLime	D		■		■				■			
Allerzyme Capsules	D			■	■							
Amino Tech	F								■			
Angelica	S	■						■				
Animal Scents Pet Shampoo	G											■
Animal Scents Pet Ointment	L											■
Anise	S				■					■		
Aroma Life	B		■									
Aroma Siez	B			■					■			
AromaSilk Lavender Volume Wash	P											■
AromaSilk Lavender Volume Rinse	P											■
AromaSilk Lemon-Sage Clarifying Wash	P											■
AromaSilk Lemon-Sage Clarifying Rinse	P											■
AromaSilk Rosewood Moisturizing Wash	P											■
AromaSilk Rosewood Moisturizing Rinse	P											■
ArthroTune	D								■			
AuraLight	D	■					■	■				
Australian Blue	B							■				
Awaken	B							■				
Basil	S		■						■			

Product Type Key

- **S** Essential Oil Single
- **B** Essential Oil Blend
- **D** Dietary Supplement
- **P** Personal Care/Hair and Skin
- **L** Lotions/Creams/Massage Oils
- **G** Bath and Shower Gels/Soaps
- **E** Essential Waters
- **F** Powergize Fitness
- **O** Oral Care

Product	Product Type	Nervous System	Cardiovascular System	Respiratory System	Digestive/Elimination	Immune/Anti-infectious	Glandular/Hormonal	Emotional Balance	Muscle & Bone	Anti Aging	Oral Hygiene	Skin and Hair
Basil Essential Water	E								■			
Bath Gel Base	G											■
Be-Fit	F								■			
Bergamot	S				■			■				■
Berry Young Juice	F					■				■		
BerryGize Bars	F					■				■		
Birch	S								■			
Body Gize	D				■	■			■			
Boswellia Wrinkle Crème	P									■		■
Brain Power	B	■						■				
Cajeput	S		■	■								
CarboZyme	D				■							
Cardamom	S				■							
CardiaCare	D		■									
Carrot Seed Oil	S	■	■									■
Cassia	S		■		■					■	■	
Cedar Essential Water	E							■				■
Cedar, Canadian Red	S			■				■				■
Cedar, Western Red	S											■
Cedarwood	S	■		■								
Cel-Lite Magic	L											■
Celery Seed	S				■							
Chamomile Moisturizing Bar Soap	G											■
Chamomile, German	S	■						■				■
Chamomile, German Essential Water	E	■										■
Chamomile, Roman	S	■						■				■
Chelex	D				■							
Chivalry	B							■				
Christmas Spirit	B	■	■					■				
Cinnamint Lip Balm	P											■

Product Type Key

- **S** Essential Oil Single
- **B** Essential Oil Blend
- **D** Dietary Supplement
- **P** Personal Care/Hair and Skin
- **L** Lotions/Creams/Massage Oils
- **G** Bath and Shower Gels/Soaps
- **E** Essential Waters
- **F** Powergize Fitness
- **O** Oral Care

Product	Product Type	Nervous System	Cardiovascular System	Respiratory System	Digestive/Elimination	Immune/Anti-infectious	Glandular/Hormonal	Emotional Balance	Muscle & Bone	Anti Aging	Oral Hygiene	Skin and Hair
Cinnamon Bark	S					■						
Cistus	S					■					■	
Citronella	S								■			■
Citrus Fresh	B				■			■				
Citrus Hystrix	S						■	■				
Clarity	B	■						■				
Clary Sage	S						■					
Clary Sage Essential Water	E						■					■
Clove	S		■	■	■	■					■	■
CMG	D								■			
ComforTone	D				■	■						
Coral Sea Powder	D								■	■		
Coriander	S				■		■					
Cortistop, Women's	D						■					
Cumin	S				■	■						
Cypress	S		■						■			
Cypress, Blue	S					■						
Dentarome	O										■	
Dentarome Plus	O										■	
Dentarome Ultra	O		■								■	
Detoxzyme Capsules	D				■	■						
Di-Tone	B				■							
Dill	S				■							
Dragon Time	B						■	■				
Dragon Time Bath Gel	G						■	■				
Dream Catcher	B							■				
Elemi	S											■
En-R-Gee	D	■						■				
Endo Balance	D						■	■			■	
Endo Balance Moisturizing Crème	L						■					■

Product Type Key

- **S** Essential Oil Single
- **B** Essential Oil Blend
- **D** Dietary Supplement
- **P** Personal Care/Hair and Skin
- **L** Lotions/Creams/Massage Oils
- **G** Bath and Shower Gels/Soaps
- **E** Essential Waters
- **F** Powergize Fitness
- **O** Oral Care

	Product Type	Nervous System	Cardiovascular System	Respiratory System	Digestive/Elimination	Immune/Anti-infectious	Glandular/Hormonal	Emotional Balance	Muscle & Bone	Anti Aging	Oral Hygiene	Skin and Hair
EndoFlex	B						■					
EndoPro Essential Oil Caps	D						■					
Envision	B							■				
Essentialzyme	D				■				■			
Essential Manna	D				■	■			■			
Essential Omegas	D	■	■									■
Estro	D						■					
Eucalyptus citriodora	S			■								
Eucalyptus Essential Water	E			■					■	■		
Eucalyptus globulus	S			■					■		■	
Eucalyptus polybrachta	S			■								
Eucalyptus radiata	S			■								■
Evening Peace Bath Gel	G											■
Evergreen Essence	B							■				
Exodus	D					■						
Exodus II	B					■						
Femagen	G						■					
Fennel	S				■		■					
FiberZyme	D				■							
Fir, Douglas	S			■					■			
Fir, White	S			■					■	■	■	
Fir, White Essential Water	E											■
Fleabane, Canadian (Conyza)	S		■				■					
Forgiveness	B							■				
Frankincense	S	■				■		■		■		■
Fresh Essence	O				■						■	
Fresh Essence Plus	O				■						■	
Galbanum	S					■						
Gathering	B							■				
Genesis Lotion	L											■

Product Type Key

- **S** Essential Oil Single
- **B** Essential Oil Blend
- **D** Dietary Supplement
- **P** Personal Care/Hair and Skin
- **L** Lotions/Creams/Massage Oils
- **G** Bath and Shower Gels/Soaps
- **E** Essential Waters
- **F** Powergize Fitness
- **O** Oral Care

Product	Product Type	Nervous System	Cardiovascular System	Respiratory System	Digestive/Elimination	Immune/Anti-infectious	Glandular/Hormonal	Emotional Balance	Muscle & Bone	Anti Aging	Oral Hygiene	Skin and Hair
Gentle Baby	B							■				■
Geranium	S							■				■
Ginger	S	■			■							
Goldenrod	S		■				■					
Grapefruit	S		■							■		
Grounding	B							■				
Harmony	B							■				
Helichrysum	S		■						■			
Highest Potential	B							■				
Hope	B							■				
H2Oils, Lemon	D			■				■				
H2Oils, Lemon/Grapefruit	D			■				■				
H2Oils, Lemon/Orange	D			■				■				
H2Oils, Peppermint	D			■				■				
HRT	D		■									
Humility	B							■				
Hyssop	S	■	■	■								
ICP	D		■		■							
Idaho Balsam Fir	S	■			■		■					
ImmuGel	D					■						
ImmuneTune	D					■					■	
ImmuPower	B					■						
ImmuPro	D					■						
Inner Child	B							■				
Inspiration	B							■				
Into the Future	B							■				
Jasmine Absolute	S						■	■				
Joy	B							■				
Juniper	S				■			■				
Juniper Essential Water	E							■	■			■

Product Type Key

- **S** Essential Oil Single
- **B** Essential Oil Blend
- **D** Dietary Supplement
- **P** Personal Care/Hair and Skin
- **L** Lotions/Creams/Massage Oils
- **G** Bath and Shower Gels/Soaps
- **E** Essential Waters
- **F** Powergize Fitness
- **O** Oral Care

Product	Product Type	Nervous System	Cardiovascular System	Respiratory System	Digestive/Elimination	Immune/Anti-infectious	Glandular/Hormonal	Emotional Balance	Muscle & Bone	Anti Aging	Oral Hygiene	Skin and Hair
JuvaFlex	B				■			■				
JuvaTone	D				■	■						
Juva Cleanse	B				■					■		
Juva Power	D				■					■		
Juva Spice	D				■					■		
K & B	D				■							
KidScents Bath Gel	G											■
KidScents Lotion	L											■
KidScents Shampoo	P											■
KidScents Toothpaste	O										■	
Laurel nobilus	S			■	■	■						
LavaDerm Cooling Mist	P							■				■
Lavandin	S		■	■					■			
Lavender	S	■	■					■				■
Lavender Essential Water	E	■										■
Lavender-Rosewood Moisturizing Bar Soap	G											■
Lavender Volume Hair & Scalp Wash	P											■
Lavender Volume Nourishing Rinse	P											■
Ledum	S				■	■				■		■
Legacy	B							■				
Lemon	S			■	■	■				■		
Lemon-Sage Clarifying Hair & Scalp Wash	P											■
Lemon-Sage Clarifying Nourishing Rinse	P											■
Lemon-Sandalwood Cleansing Bar Soap	G											■
Lemongrass	S				■				■			
Lime	S			■	■	■				■		
Live with Passion	B	■						■				
Longevity	B									■		
Longevity Essential Oil Caps	D		■							■		
LypoZyme	D				■							

232

Product Type Key

- **S** Essential Oil Single
- **B** Essential Oil Blend
- **D** Dietary Supplement
- **P** Personal Care/Hair and Skin
- **L** Lotions/Creams/Massage Oils
- **G** Bath and Shower Gels/Soaps
- **E** Essential Waters
- **F** Powergize Fitness
- **O** Oral Care

	Product Type	Nervous System	Cardiovascular System	Respiratory System	Digestive/Elimination	Immune/Anti-infectious	Glandular/Hormonal	Emotional Balance	Muscle & Bone	Anti Aging	Oral Hygiene	Skin and Hair
M-Grain	B	■										
Magnify Your Purpose	B	■						■				
Mandarin	S				■						■	■
Marjoram	S		■						■			
Massage Oil Base	L								■			■
Master Formula vitamins	D	■	■			■		■				
Mega Cal	D		■						■			
Melaleuca alternifolia	S			■		■			■			■
Melaleuca ericifolia	S			■								■
Melaleuca-Geranium Moisturizing Bar Soap	G											■
Melaleuca quinquenervia	S			■					■			
Melissa	S								■	■		■
Melissa Essential Water	E	■										■
Melrose	B			■								■
Mineral Essence	D	■	■			■	■	■	■			
Mighty Mist	D									■		
Mighty Vites	D									■		
Mint Condition	D				■							
Mister	B						■					
Morning Start Shower Gel	G											■
Morning Start Moisturizing Bar Soap	G							■				■
Motivaton	B	■						■				
Mountain Essence Essential Water	E			■								■
Mountain Savory	S					■						
Mugwort	S				■							
Myrrh	S	■				■	■					■
Myrtle	S			■	■		■		■			
Neroli	S				■							■
NeuroGen	D	■					■		■			
Niaouli	S			■								

Product Type Key

- **S** Essential Oil Single
- **B** Essential Oil Blend
- **D** Dietary Supplement
- **P** Personal Care/Hair and Skin
- **L** Lotions/Creams/Massage Oils
- **G** Bath and Shower Gels/Soaps
- **E** Essential Waters
- **F** Powergize Fitness
- **O** Oral Care

	Product Type	Nervous System	Cardiovascular System	Respiratory System	Digestive/Elimination	Immune/Anti-infectious	Glandular/Hormonal	Emotional Balance	Muscle & Bone	Anti Aging	Oral Hygiene	Skin and Hair
Nutmeg	S	■				■	■					
Onycha	S		■					■				
Orange	S				■	■				■		■
Orange Blossom Facial Wash	P											■
Oregano	S		■			■			■	■		
Ortho Sport	L								■			
Ortho Ease	L								■			■
Palmarosa	S		■					■				■
PanAway	B	■							■			
ParaFree Liquid and Softgel	D				■	■						
Patchouly	S											■
PD 80/20	D					■	■	■				
Peace & Calming	B	■						■				
Pepper, Black	S	■			■							
Peppermint	S	■		■	■				■		■	
Peppermint-Cedarwood Moisturizing Bar Soap	G								■			■
Peppermint Essential Water	E				■				■		■	
Petitgrain	S							■				
Pine	S			■				■				
PolyZyme	D				■				■	■		
Power Meal	F		■		■	■			■			
Prenolone	D	■					■	■	■	■		
Prenolone +	D	■					■	■	■	■		
Present Time	B							■				
ProGen	D						■					
Progressence												
Protec	D						■			■		
Purification	B				■			■				■
R.C.	B			■								■
Ravensara	S			■		■						

Product Type Key

- **S** Essential Oil Single
- **B** Essential Oil Blend
- **D** Dietary Supplement
- **P** Personal Care/Hair and Skin
- **L** Lotions/Creams/Massage Oils
- **G** Bath and Shower Gels/Soaps
- **E** Essential Waters
- **F** Powergize Fitness
- **O** Oral Care

Product	Product Type	Nervous System	Cardiovascular System	Respiratory System	Digestive/Elimination	Immune/Anti-infectious	Glandular/Hormonal	Emotional Balance	Muscle & Bone	Anti Aging	Oral Hygiene	Skin and Hair
RC	B			■								
Regenolone	D	■					■		■			■
Rehemogen	D		■		■							
Relaxation	B							■				■
Release	B							■				
Relieve It	B								■			
Rose	S							■				■
Rose Ointment	P											■
Rosemary CT cineol	S		■		■				■			
Rosewood	S											■
Rosewood Moisturizing Hair & Scalp Wash	P											■
Rosewood Moisturizing Nourishing Rinse	P											■
Royaldophilus	D				■	■						
Sacred Mountain	B							■				
Sacred Mountain Bar Soap for Oily Skin	G							■				■
Sage	S				■	■						
Sage Lavender	S				■	■						
Sandalwood	S	■							■	■		■
Sandalwood Moisture Crème	P											■
Sandalwood Toner	P											■
SARA	B							■				
Satin Body Lotion	L											■
Satin Facial Scrub-Juniper	P											■
Satin Facial Scrub-Mint	P											■
Sensation	B						■	■				
Sensation Bath and Shower Gel	G											■
Sensation Hand and Body Lotion	L											■
Sensation Massage Oil	L											■
Spearmint	S				■				■			
Spearmint Essential Water	E										■	■

Product Type Key

- **S** Essential Oil Single
- **B** Essential Oil Blend
- **D** Dietary Supplement
- **P** Personal Care/Hair and Skin
- **L** Lotions/Creams/Massage Oils
- **G** Bath and Shower Gels/Soaps
- **E** Essential Waters
- **F** Powergize Fitness
- **O** Oral Care

Product	Product Type	Nervous System	Cardiovascular System	Respiratory System	Digestive/Elimination	Immune/Anti-infectious	Glandular/Hormonal	Emotional Balance	Muscle & Bone	Anti Aging	Oral Hygiene	Skin and Hair
Spikenard	S							■				■
Spruce	S	■		■				■				
Stevia Extract	D		■		■	■						
Stevia Select Powder	D		■		■	■						
Sulfurzyme Capsules or Powder	D	■				■			■	■		■
Sunsation Suntan Oil	L											■
Super B	D	■	■						■			
Super C	D			■		■				■		
Super C Chewable	D					■				■		
Super Cal	D	■	■						■	■		
Surrender	B	■						■				
Tangerine	S				■			■		■		■
Tansy, Blue	S	■										
Tansy, Idaho	S					■						
Tansy, Idaho Essential Water	P											■
Tarragon	S	■			■							
Tender Tush Ointment	P											■
Tea Tree	S			■							■	
ThermaBurn	D								■			
ThermaMist	D				■				■			
Thieves	B					■				■	■	
Thieves Cleaner	P					■						
Thieves Cleansing Bar Soap	P											■
Thieves Cleansing Spray	P					■						
Thieves Lozenges	O			■							■	
Thieves Wipes	P					■						
3 Wise Men	B							■				
Thyme	S					■				■	■	
Thyme Essential Water	E				■						■	■
Thyromin	D						■					

Product Type Key

- **S** Essential Oil Single
- **B** Essential Oil Blend
- **D** Dietary Supplement
- **P** Personal Care/Hair and Skin
- **L** Lotions/Creams/Massage Oils
- **G** Bath and Shower Gels/Soaps
- **E** Essential Waters
- **F** Powergize Fitness
- **O** Oral Care

Product	Product Type	Nervous System	Cardiovascular System	Respiratory System	Digestive/Elimination	Immune/Anti-infectious	Glandular/Hormonal	Emotional Balance	Muscle & Bone	Anti Aging	Oral Hygiene	Skin and Hair
Trauma Life	B							■				
Tsuga	S		■	■								
UltraSeptic Spray	P										■	■
Ultra Young	D					■	■			■		
Ultra Young +	D					■	■			■		
V-6 Mixing Oil	L								■			■
Valerian	S	■										
Valor	B	■						■	■			■
Valor Moisturizing Bar Soap	P	■										■
Vetiver	S	■					■	■				■
VitaGreen	D	■	■		■	■			■			
WheyFit	F								■	■		
White Angelica	B							■				
Wintergreen	S								■			
Wolfberry Crisp Bars	F				■	■			■	■		
Wolfberry Eye Crème	P									■		■
Yarrow	S					■	■					■
Yarrow, Blue	S						■	■				
Ylang Ylang	S		■				■	■				

237

Safety Data Legend:

A	Anti-coagulant – May enhance the effects of blood thinners; avoid using with Aspirin, heparin, Warfarin, etc)	HBP+	**Avoid** if dealing with **high blood pressure**
CH	Do not use on children younger than 18 months of age	P	Use with **caution** during pregnancy
		P+	**Avoid** during pregnancy
CH+	Do not use on children younger than 5 years of age	PH	**Photosensitivity** – direct exposure to sunlight within 24 hours after use could cause dermatitis (test first)
DS	Dietary supplement		
E	Use with **caution** if susceptible to **epilepsy** (small amounts or in dilution)	PH+	**Extreme Photosensitivity** – direct exposure to sunlight after use within 72 hours can cause severe dermatitis (avoid exposing affected area of skin to direct sunlight for 48-72 hours)
E+	**Avoid** if susceptible to **epilepsy** (can trigger a seizure)		
FA	Food additive	SI	Could possibly result in **skin irritation** (dilution may be necessary)
FL	Flavoring agent		
GRAS	Generally regarded as safe	SI+	Can cause **extreme skin irritation** (dilution highly recommended)
HBP	Use with **caution** if dealing with **high blood pressure** (small amounts)		

Appendix C

Single Oil Data

Single Oil Name	Botanical Name	Safety Data	Products containing single oil
Angelica	*Angelica archangelica* (Umbelliferae)	GRAS, FA, P, PH, DS	Awaken, Forgiveness, Grounding, Harmony, Live with Passion, Surrender
Anise	*Pimpinella anisum* (Umbelliferae)	GRAS, FA, DS	Awaken, Di-Tone, Dream Catcher, ICP, Essentialzyme, ParaFree, Power Meal, Polyzyme, Detoxzyme, Allerzyme, Lipozyme, Fiberzyme, ComforTone
Basil	*Ocimum basilicum* (Labiatae)	GRAS, FA, E+, CH, P+, SI, DS	Aroma Siez, Clarity, M-Grain ArthroTune, Super Cal
Bergamot	*Citrus bergamia* (Rutaceae)	GRAS, FA, SI, DS, CH+	Awaken, Chivalry, Clarity, Forgiveness, Gentle Baby, Harmony, Joy, White Angelica, Progessence, Genesis Lotion, Prenolone, Prenolone+, Regenolone, NeuroGen, Rosewood Shampoo/ Conditioner, Dream Catcher, Dragon Time Bath Gel, Evening Peace Bath Gel
Blue Cypress	*Callitris intratropica*		Brain Power, Highest Potential
Cajeput	*Melaleuca leucadendra* (Myrtaceae)	SI	
Calamus	*Acorus calamus* (Araceae)	SI, P+, CH+	Exodus II
Cardamom	*Elettaria cardamomum* (Zingiberaceae)	GRAS, FA, DS SI	Clarity
Carrot Seed Oil	*Daucus carota* (Umbelliferae)	GRAS, FA, DS	Rose Ointment
Cassia	*Cinnamomum cassia* (Lauraceae)	GRAS, FA, DS, P, CH, SI+	Exodus II, Oils of Ancient Scripture
Cedar, Canadian Red	*Thuja plicata* (Cupressaceae)		KidScents Lotion
Cedar, Western Red	*Thuja plicata* (Cupressaceae)	SI	Evergreen Essence

Single Oil Name	Botanical Name	Safety Data	Products containing single oil
Cedarwood	*Cedrus atlantica* (Pinaceae)		Australian Blue, Brain Power, SARA, Grounding, Highest Potential, Inspiration, Into the Future, Oils of Ancient Scripture, KidScents Lotion, Live with Passion, Sacred Mountain, Sacred Mountain Bar Soap, Peppermint-Cedarwood Bar Soap, Cel-Lite Magic
Celery Seed		P, SI, DS	JuvaCleanse
Chamomile (German/Blue)	*Matricaria chamomilla/recutita* (Compositae)	GRAS, FA, DS	EndoFlex, Surrender, K&B Tincture, JuvaTone, ComforTone
Chamomile (Roman)	*Chamaemelum nobile* (Compositae)	GRAS, FA, DS	Awaken, Chivalry, Clarity, Forgiveness, Gentle Baby, Harmony, Joy, JuvaFlex, Surrender, M-Grain, Motivation, Genesis Lotion, Lemon Sage Shampoo/Conditioner, Sandalwood Toner, Satin Body Lotion, Wolfberry Eye Creme, Dragon Time Bath Gel, Evening Peace Bath Gel, Chelex Tincture, K&B Tincture, Tender Tush Ointment, Rehemogen Tincture
Cinnamon Bark	*Cinnamomum verum* (Lauraceae)	GRAS, FA, DS, P, SI+, CH	Abundance, Christmas Spirit, Exodus II, Gathering, Highest Potential, Magnify Your Purpose, Oils of Ancient Scripture, Thieves, Cinnamint Lip Balm, Thieves Bar Soap, ImmuGel, Mineral Essence, Carbozyme, Fresh Essence Plus, Dentarome Plus/Ultra Toothpaste, Thieves Antiseptic Spray, Thieves Wipes, Thieves Household Cleaner
Cistus	*Cistus ladanifer* (Cistaceae)	FA	ImmuPower, ImmuneTune, KidScents Lotion
Citronella	*Cymbopogon nardus* (Gramineae)	GRAS, FA, DS, P, SI	Purification, Sunsation Suntan Oil
Citrus Hystrix		DS, SI, PH, CH	Trauma Life

Single Oil Name	Botanical Name	Safety Data	Products containing single oil
Clary Sage	*Salvia sclarea* (Labiatae)	GRAS, FA, P, DS	Into the Future, Live with Passion, Progessence, Lavender Shampoo/Conditioner, Prenolone, Prenolone+, Rosewood Shampoo/Conditioner, Dragon Time EO/Bath Gel/Massage Oil, EveningPeace Bath Gel, Estro Tincture, Cel-Lite Magic, Cortistop WOMEN
Clove	*Syzygium aromaticum* (Myrtaceae)	GRAS, FA, DS, A, SI+	Abundance, BLM, BLM Powder, K&B Tincture, Carbozyme, En-R-Gee, ImmuPower, Longevity, Longevity Caps, Melrose, PanAway, Thieves, Dentarome Plus/Ultra Toothpaste, Fresh Essence Plus, Kidscent Toothpaste, Thieves Bar Soap, Essential Omegas, ImmuGel, ParaFree, Essentialzyme, Thieves Wipes, Thieves Household Cleaner, Thieves Antiseptic Spray, AromaGuard Stick Deodorant
Coriander	*Coriandrum sativum L.* (Umbelliferae)	GRAS, FA, DS	
Cumin	*Cuminus cyminum* (Umbelliferae)	GRAS, FA, DS, SI	ImmuPower, Protec, ParaFree, Detoxzyme
Cypress	*Cupressus sempervirens* (Cupressaceae)		Aroma Life, Aroma Siez, RC, H-R-T Tincture, Cel-Lite Magic, ArthroTune, BodyGize, Power Meal, Super Cal
Davana	*Artemisia pallens* (Compositae)		Trauma Life
Dill	*Anethum graveolens* (Umbelliferae)	GRAS, FA, DS, E	
Elemi	*Canarium luzonicum* (Burseraceae)		Ortho Sport
Eucalyptus citriodora	*Eucalyptus citriodora* (Myrtaceae)		RC
Eucalyptus dives	*Eucalyptus dives* (Myrtaceae)	SI, P	
Eucalyptus globulus	*Eucalyptus globulus* (Myrtaceae)	FA, FL, DS	RC, Fresh Fresh Essence Plus Mouthwash, Dentarome Plus/Ultra Toothpaste, Chelex Tincture, Ortho Sport
Eucalyptus polybractea	*Eucalyptus polybractea* (Myrtaceae)		

Single Oil Name	Botanical Name	Safety Data	Products containing single oil
Eucalyptus radiata	*Eucalyptus radiata* (Myrtaceae)		RC, Thieves, AromaGuard Stick Deodorant, Thieves Bar Soap, Carbozyme, Thieves Antiseptic Spray, Dentarome Plus/Ultra Toothpaste, Fresh Essence Plus Mouthwash, Thieves Wipes, Thieves Household Cleaner
Fennel	*Foeniculum vulgare* (Umbelliferae)	GRAS, FA, DS, E, P	Allerzyme, Di-Tone, JuvaFlex, Mister, Progessence, Detoxzyme, Lipozyme,
			Fiberzyme, Prenolone, Prenolone+, Dragon Time EO/Bath Gel/Massage Oil,
			Estro Tincture, K&B Tincture, ICP, Essentialzyme, ParaFree, Power Meal, ProGen, Cortistop WOMEN
Fir, Douglas	*Pseudotsuga menziesii* (Pinaceae)	SI	Regenolone
Fir, Idaho Balsam	*Abies grandis* (Pinaceae)	FA, FL, SI, DS	Gratitude, BLM, BLM Powder, Sacred Mountain, Believe, En-R-Gee, Sacred Mountain Bar Soap
Fir, White	*Abies grandis* (Pinaceae)	SI	Arthrotune, ImmuneTune, AromaGuard Stick Deodorant, Evergreen Essence, Grounding, Australian Blue, Into the Future
Fleabane	*Conyza canadensis* (Compositae)		Progessence, ProMist, ThermaBurn, Ultra Young, Ultra Young Plus, Cortistop MEN, Cortistop WOMEN
Frankincense	*Boswellia carteri* (Burseraceae)	FA, FL, DS	Abundance, Acceptance, Awaken, Believe, Brain Power, Chivalry, Exodus II, Forgiveness, Gathering, Harmony, Humility, ImmuPower, Gratitude, Inspiration, Into the Future, Longevity, Oils of Ancient Scripture, 3 Wise Men, Trauma Life, Valor, Valor Bar Soap, Boswellia Wrinkle Creme, Protec, Wolfberry Eye Creme, Exodus, ThermaBurn, Cortistop MEN, Cortistop WOMEN, Tender Tush Ointment
Galbanum	*Ferula gummosa* (Umbelliferae)	FA, FL, DS	Chivalry, Exodus II, Gathering, Gratitude Highest Potential, Oils of Ancient Scripture

Single Oil Name	Botanical Name	Safety Data	Products containing single oil
Geranium	*Pelargonium graveolens* (Geraniaceae)	GRAS, FA, DS, FL	Acceptance, Chivalry, Clarity, EndoFlex, Envision, Forgiveness, Gathering, Highest Potential, Gentle Baby, Harmony, Humility, Joy, JuvaFlex, Release, SARA, Trauma Life, White Angelica, AromaGuard Stick Deodorant, Boswellia, Wrinkle Creme, Progessence, Genesis Lotion, Lemon-Sage Shampoo/Conditioner, Prenolone, Prenolone+, Rosewood Shampoo/Conditioner, KidScents Lotion, Satin Body Lotion, Wolfberry Eye Creme, Dragon Time Bath Gel, Evening Peace Bath Gel, Melaleuca-Geranium Bar Soap, K&B Tincture, JuvaTone, KidScents Liquid Soap
Ginger	*Zingiber officinale* (Zingiberaceae)	GRAS, FA, DS, A, PH	Abundance, Allerzyme, Di-Tone, Live with Passion, ComforTone, ICP, Mint Condition, Magnify Your Purpose, Lipozyme, Fiberzyme
Goldenrod	*Solidago canadensis* (Asteraceae)	DS	
Grapefruit	*Citrus x paradisi* (Rutaceae)	GRAS, FA, DS	Citrus Fresh, Cel-Lite Magic Bodygize, Power Meal, ProMist, Super C, ThermaMist
Helichrysum	*Helichrysum italicum* (Compositae)	GRAS, FA, DS	Aroma Life, Brain Power, Forgiveness, Awaken, JuvaFlex, JuvaCleanse, Live with Passion, M-Grain, PanAway, Trauma Life, Chelex Tincture, ArthroTune, CardiaCare
Hyssop	*Hyssopus officinalis* (Labiatae)	GRAS, FA, DS, E+, HBP+, P+	Chivalry, Exodus II, Harmony, ImmuPower, Relieve It, White Angelica, Exodus, Oils of Ancient Scripture
Jasmine Absolute	*Jasminum officinale* (Oleaceae)		Awaken, Chivalry, Clarity, Dragon Time, Forgiveness, Gentle Baby, Harmony, Highest Potential, Inner Child, Joy, Into the Future, Live with Passion, Lavender Shampoo/Conditioner, Genesis Lotion, Satin Body Lotion, Dragon Time Bath Gel/Massage, Evening Peace Bath Gel, Sensation EO/Lotion/Bath Gel/Message Oil

Single Oil Name	Botanical Name	Safety Data	Products containing single oil
Juniper	*Juniperus osteosperma* and/or *J. scopulorum* (Cupressaceae)	GRAS, FA, DS SI	Awaken, Di-Tone, Dream Catcher, En-R-Gee, Grounding, Hope, Into the Future, 3 Wise Men, NeuroGen, Cel-Lite Magic, Ortho Ease, Morning Start Bath Gel, Morning Start Bar Soap, K&BTincture, Lipozyme, Fiberzyme, Allerzyme, Arthro Tune
Laurel	*Laurus nobilis* (Lauraceae)	GRAS, FA, DS, SI	Exodus, ParaFree
Lavandin	*Lavandula x hybrida* (Labiatae)	GRAS, FA, DS,	Purification, Release
Lavender	*Lavandula angustifolia* CT linalol (Labiatae)	GRAS, FA, DS	Aroma Siez, Awaken, Brain Power, RC, Chivalry, Envision, Forgiveness, Gentle Baby, Harmony, Gathering, Highest Potential, M-Grain, Mister, Motivation, SARA, Surrender, Trauma Life, ProGen, LavaDerm Cooling Mist, AromaGuard Stick Deodorant, Lavender Shampoo/ Conditioner, Tender Tush Ointment, Orange Blossom Facial Wash, Sunsation Suntan Oil, Sandalwood Moisture Creme, Wolfberry Eye Creme, Juniper Satin Scrub, Lavender Rosewood Bar Soap, Dragon Time EO/Bath Gel/Massage Oil Estro Tincture, Relaxation Massage Oil
Ledum	*Ledum groenlandicum* (Ericaceae)	DS	JuvaCleanse
Lemon	*Citrus limon* (Rutaceae)	GRAS, FA, DS, PH, SI	
Lemon	*Citrus limon* (Rutaceae)	GRAS, FA, DS, PH, SI	Chivalry, Citrus Fresh, Clarity, Thieves, Forgiveness, Gentle Baby, Harmony, Joy, RC, Surrender, Genesis Lotion, Lavender Shampoo/Conditioner, Lemon-Sage Shampoo/ Conditioner, KidScents Shampoo, Orange Blossom Facial Wash, Dragon Time Bath Gel, Evening Peace Bath Gel, AromaGuard Stick Deodorant, Thieves Bar Soap, Lemon-Sandalwood Bar Soap, H-R-T Tincture, AlkaLime, AminoTech, Bodygize, CardiaCare, Carbozyme, ImmuGel, ImmuneTune, JuvaTone, MegaCal, Mineral Essence, Power Meal, Super C, Super C Chewable, WheyFit, VitaGreen, KidScents Detangler, Dentarome Plus/Ultra Toothpaste, Fresh Essence Plus Mouthwash, Thieves Antiseptic Spray, Thieves Wipes, Thieves Household Cleaner

Single Oil Name	Botanical Name	Safety Data	Products containing single oil
Lemongrass	*Cymbopogon flexuosus* (Gramineae)	GRAS, FA, DS, CH, SI+	ICP, Di-Tone, En-R-Gee, Inner Child, Purification, NeuroGen, Sunsation Suntan Oil, Morning Start Bath Gel, Morning Start Bar Soap, Ortho Ease, Ortho Sport, Bodygize, Allerzyme, Be-Fit, Lipozyme, Fiberzyme, VitaGreen
Lime	*Citrus aurantifolia* (Rutaceae)	GRAS, FA, DS, PH+	Lemon-Sage Shampoo/Conditioner AlkaLime, Super C, AminoTech, Master Formula Children's
Mandarin	*Citrus reticulata* (Rutaceae)	GRAS, FA, DS, PH	Awaken, Citrus Fresh, Joy, Dragon Time Bath Gel, Master Formula Children's, Super C, Bodygize
Marjoram	*Origanum majorana* (Labiatae)	GRAS, FA, DS, P	Aroma Life, Aroma Siez, Dragon Time, M-Grain, RC, Dragon Time Bath Gel, Ortho Ease, Ortho Sport ArthroTune, CardiaCare, Super Cal
Melaleuca ericifolia (formerly Rosalina)	*Melaleuca ericifolia* (Myrtaceae)		Melaleuca-Geranium Bar Soap
Melissa	*Melissa officinalis* (Labiatae)	GRAS, FA, DS	Brain Power, Forgiveness, Hope, Humility, Live with Passion, White Angelica, VitaGreen
Mountain Savory	*Satureja montana* (Labiatae)	GRAS, FA, DS, CH, SI+	ImmuPower, Surrender
Mugwort		GRAS, FA, DS P, CH	Comfortone
Myrrh	*Commiphora myrrha* (Burseraceae)	FA, FL, DS	Abundance, Chivalry, Exodus II, Protec, Gratitude, Hope, Humility, Oils of Ancient Scripture, 3 Wise Men, White Angelica, Boswellia Wrinkle Creme, Rose Ointment, Sandalwood Moisture Creme, Sandalwood Toner, Thyromin
Myrtle	*Myrtus communis* (Myrtaceae)	FA, FL, DS	EndoFlex, Inspiration, Mister, Purification, RC, JuvaTone, ProGen, ThermaBurn, Thyromin
Neroli	*Citrus aurantium bigaradia* (Rutaceae)	GRAS, FA, DS	Acceptance, Awaken, Humility, Inner Child, Live with Passion, Present Time
Niaouli	*Melaleuca quinquenervia* (Myrtaceae)		Melrose, AromaGuard Stick Deodorant

Single Oil Name	Botanical Name	Safety Data	Products containing single oil
Nutmeg	*Myristica fragrans* (Myristicaceae)	GRAS, FA, DS, SI, E, P, CH+	EndoFlex, En-R-Gee, Magnify Your Purpose, Royal Essence Tincture, Be-Fit, ParaFree, Power Meal, ThermaBurn
Onycha	*Styrax benzoin* (Styracaceae)		Oils of Ancient Scripture
Orange	*Citrus aurantium* (Rutaceae)	GRAS, FA, DS, PH	Abundance, Christmas Spirit, Chivalry, Citrus Fresh, Envision, Harmony, Inner Child, Peace & Calming, SARA, Bodygize, Essential Omegas, ImmuneTune, ImmuPro, Mighty Vites, Longevity, Longevity Caps, Power Meal, Super C, Wolfberry Bar
Oregano	*Origanum compactum* (Labiatae)	GRAS, FA, DS, SI+	ImmuPower, Regenolone, Ortho Sport Massage Oil, ImmuGel
Palmarosa	*Cymbopogon martinii* (Gramineae)	GRAS, FA, DS	Awaken, Chivalry, Clarity, Forgiveness, Gentle Baby, Harmony, Joy, Genesis Lotion, Rose Ointment, Dragon Time Bath Gel, Evening Peace Bath Gel
Patchouly	*Pogostemon cublin* (Labiatae)	FA, FL, DS	Abundance, Allerzyme, Di-Tone, Live with Passion, Magnify Your Purpose, Peace & Calming, Orange Blossom Facial Wash, Lipozyme, Fiberzyme, Rose Ointment
Pepper (black)	*Piper nigrum* (Piperaceae)	GRAS, FA, DS, SI	Dream Catcher, En-R-Gee, Relieve It, Cel-Lite Magic, ArthroTune
Peppermint	*Mentha piperita* (Labiatae)	GRAS, FA, DS, SI+, HB, P, CH+	Allerzyme, Aroma Siez, Clarity, Di Tone, M-Grain, Mister, PanAway, Raven, RC, Relieve It, AromaGuard Stick Deodorant, Cinnamint Lip Balm, Mint Condition Dentarome Plus/Ultra Toothpaste, Detoxzyme, Fresh Essence Plus Mouthwash, Lipozyme, Fiberzyme, Peppermint Satin Scrub MINT, NeuroGen, Regenolone, Satin Body Lotion, Morning Start Bath Gel, Peppermint-Cedarwood Bar Soap, Morning Start Bar Soap, Ortho Ease, Ortho Sport, Relaxation Massage Oil, Polyzyme, BLM Powder, Cortistop MEN, Cortistop WOMEN, ComforTone, Thyromin, Satin Scrub, Essential Manna (Carob Mint), Essentialzyme, Mineral Essence, Pro-Gen, ProMist, ThermaMist

Single Oil Name	Botanical Name	Safety Data	Products containing single oil
Petitgrain	*Citrus aurantium* (Rutaceae)	GRAS, FA, DS	
Pine	*Pinus sylvestris* (Pinaceae)	FA, FL, SI, DS	Evergreen Essence, Grounding, RC, Lemon-Sage Shampoo/Conditioner, ImmuneTune
Pine, Ponderosa	*Pinus ponderosa* (Pinaceae)	SI	Evergreen Essence
Ravensara	*Ravensara aromatica* (Lauraceae)		ImmuPower, Respiratory S, ImmuneTune
Rose	*Rosa damascena* (Rosaceae)	GRAS, FA, DS	Awaken, Chivalry, Envision, Forgiveness, Gathering, Gentle Baby, Harmony, Joy, Humility, Highest Potential, SARA, Trauma Life, White Angelica, Rose Ointment
Rosemary	*Rosmarinus officinalis* CT cineol (Labiatae)	GRAS, FA, DS, E+, HBP, P+ CH+	Clarity, En-R-Gee, JuvaFlex, Melrose, Purification, Thieves, Morning Start Bath Gel, VitaGreen, AromaGuard Stick Deodorant, Thieves Bar Soap, Morning Start Bar Soap, Chelex Tincture, Rehemogen Tincture, Sandalwood Moisture Creme, Be-Fit, Carbozyme, ComforTone, Polyzyme, ICP, ImmuGel, JuvaTone, Orange Blossom Facial Wash, Fresh Essence Plus Mouthwash, Dentarome Plus/Ultra Toothpaste, Thieves Antiseptic Spray, Thieves Wipes, Thieves Household Cleaner
Rosewood	*Aniba rosaeodora* (Lauraceae)		Acceptance, Awaken, Believe, Chivalry, Clarity, Forgiveness, Gentle Baby, Joy, Gratitude, Harmony, Humility, Valor, Inspiration, Magnify Your Purpose, White Angelica, Genesis Lotion, Rose Ointment, AromaGuard Stick Deodorant, Rosewood Shampoo/Conditioner, KidScents Lotion, Sandalwood Moisture Creme, Sandalwood Toner, Satin Body Lotion, Wolfberry Eye Creme, Dragon Time Bath Gel, Evening Peace Bath Gel, Sensation EO/Lotion/Bath Gel/Massage Oil, Lavender Rosewood Bar Soap, Valor Bar Soap, H-R-T Tincture, Relaxation Massage Oil, Tender Tush Ointment

Single Oil Name	Botanical Name	Safety Data	Products containing single oil
Sage	*Salvia officinalis* (Labiatae)	GRAS, FA, DS, E+, P+, CH+	Chivalry, EndoFlex, Envision, Magnify Your Purpose, Mister, Protec, Lemon Sage Shampoo/Conditioner, Dragon Time Massage Oil/Bath Gel, K&B Tincture, Progen
Sage Lavender	*Salvia lavandulifolia*		Awaken, Chivalry, Harmony
Sandalwood	*Santalum album* (Santalaceae)	FA, FL, DS	Acceptance, Awaken, Brain Power, Chivalry, Dream Catcher, Forgiveness, Gathering, Harmony, Highest Potential, Inner Child, Inspiration, Live with Passion, Magnify Your Purpose, Oils of Ancient Scripture, Release, 3 Wise Men, Trauma Life, White Angelica, Boswellia Wrinkle Creme, Rosewood Shampoo/ Conditioner, Sandalwood Moisture Creme, Sandalwood Toner, Satin Body Lotion, Evening Peace Bath Gel, Lemon-Sandalwood Bar Soap, Ultra Young, Ultra Young Plus, Tender Tush Ointment
Spearmint	*Mentha spicata* (Labiatae)	GRAS, FA, DS SI, CH+	Citrus Fresh, EndoFlex, Cinnamint Lip Balm, Fresh Essence Plus Mouthwash, Relaxation Massage Oil, Mint Condition, ProMist, ThermaBurn, ThermaMist, Thyromin
Spikenard	*Nardostachys jatamansi* (Valerianaceae)		Exodus II, Humility, Exodus, Oils of Ancient Scripture
Spruce	*Picea mariana* (Pinaceae)	FA, FL, DS SI	Abundance, Christmas Spirit, Chivalry, Envision, Gathering, Grounding, Harmony, Hope, Highest Potential, Inner Child, Inspiration, Motivation, Present Time, RC, Relieve It, Sacred Mountain, Surrender, 3 Wise Men, Trauma Life, Valor, White Angelica, Sacred Mountain Bar Soap, Valor Bar Soap, ArthroTune
Tangerine	*Citrus nobilis* (Rutaceae)	GRAS, FA, DS SI, PH	Awaken, Citrus Fresh, Dream Catcher, Inner Child, Peace & Calming, Bodygize, Relaxation Massage Oil, ComforTone, KidScents Detangler, KidScents Shampoo
Tansy, Blue	*Tanacetum annum* (Compositae)		Acceptance, Australian Blue, Awaken, Dream Catcher, Highest Potential, JuvaFlex, Peace & Calming, Release, SARA, Valor, Dragon Time Bath Gel, Evening Peace Bath Gel, Valor Bar Soap, JuvaTone, Tender Tush Ointment

Single Oil Name	Botanical Name	Safety Data	Products containing single oil
Tansy, Idaho	*Tanacetum vulgare* (Compositae)	E+, P+. CH+	Awaken, ImmuPower, Into the Future, ParaFree, KidScents Shampoo
Tarragon	*Artemisia dracunculus* (Compositae)	GRAS, FA, DS, E+, P+, CH+	Allerzyme, Di-Tone, ComforTone, ICP, Essentialzyme, Lipozyme, Fiberzyme, KidScents Detangler
Tea Tree	*Melaleuca alternifolia* (Myrtaceae)		Melrose, Purification, AromaGuard Stick Deodorant, Rose Ointment, Sunsation Suntan Oil, Melaleuca-Geranium Bar Soap, Rehemogen Tincture, ParaFree
Thyme, Red	*Thymus vulgaris* (Labiatae)	GRAS, FA, DS, HBP, M, CH	Longevity, Longevity Caps, Kidscent Toothpaste, ImmuGel, ParaFree, Rehemogen, Ortho Ease
Tsuga	*Tsuga canadensis* (Pinaceae)	SI+	
Valerian	*Valeriana officinalis* (Valerianaceae)	FA, FL, DS	Trauma Life
Vetiver	*Vetiveria zizanoides* (Gramineae)	FA, FL, DS	Fresh Essence Plus Mouthwash, Melaleuca-Geranium Bar Soap, Ortho Ease, Ortho Sport, ParaFree
Wintergreen/ Birch	*Gaultheria procumbens* (Ericaceae) *Betula alleghaniensis*	E+, P+, CH+ A	PanAway, Dentarome Plus/Ultra Toothpaste Regenolone, Be-Fit, Super Cal, ArthoTune, Rosewood Shampoo/Conditioner, BLM, BLM Powder, Ortho Ease, Ortho Sport
Yarrow	*Achillea millefolium* (Compositae)		Dragon Time, Mister, Dragon Time Massage Oil, Prenolone/Prenolone+, ProGen
Ylang Ylang	*Cananga odorata* (Annonaceae)	GRAS, FA, DS,	Aroma Life, Awaken, Chivalry, Clarity, Dream Catcher, Forgiveness, Gathering, Gentle Baby, Gratitude, Grounding, Harmony, Humility, Australian Blue, Highest Potential, Inner Child, Joy, Motivation, Peace & Calming, Present Time, Release, Sacred Mountain, SARA, White Angelica, Boswellia Wrinkle Creme, Progessence, Genesis Lotion, Lemon Sage Shampoo/Conditioner, Prenolone/ Prenolone+, Satin Body Lotion, CardiaCare, Sensation EO/Lotion/Bath Gel/Massage Oil, Dragon Time Bath Gel/Massage Oil, Evening Peace Bath Gel, Sacred Mountain Bar Soap, H-R-T Tincture, Relaxation Massage Oil

Safety Data Legend:

A	Anti-coagulant – May enhance the effects of blood thinners; avoid using with Aspirin, heparin, Warfarin, etc)	HBP+	**Avoid** if dealing with **high blood pressure**
CH	Do not use on children younger than 18 months of age	P	Use with **caution** during pregnancy
		P+	**Avoid** during pregnancy
CH+	Do not use on children younger than 5 years of age	PH	**Photosensitivity** – direct exposure to sunlight within 24 hours after use could cause dermatitis (test first)
DS	Dietary supplement		
E	Use with **caution** if susceptible to **epilepsy** (small amounts or in dilution)	PH+	**Extreme Photosensitivity** – direct exposure to sunlight after use within 72 hours can cause severe dermatitis (avoid exposing affected area of skin to direct sunlight for 48-72 hours)
E+	**Avoid** if susceptible to **epilepsy** (can trigger a seizure)		
FA	Food additive		
FL	Flavoring agent	SI	Could possibly result in **skin irritation** (dilution may be necessary)
GRAS	Generally regarded as safe		
HBP	Use with **caution** if dealing with **high blood pressure** (small amounts)	SI+	Can cause **extreme skin irritation** (dilution highly recommended)

Appendix D

Oil Blends Data

Blend Name	Single Oil Contents	Safety Data	Uses/Application Areas
Abundance	Myrrh, Cinnamon Bark, Patchouly, Orange, Clove, Ginger, Spruce, Frankincense	SI, CH	Diffuse; wrists, ears, neck, face; wallet/purse; painting; direct inhalation
Acceptance	Geranium, Blue Tansy, Frankincense, Sandalwood, Neroli, Rosewood (Carrier: Almond Oil)		Diffuse; liver, heart, chest, face, ears, neck, thymus, wrists; sacral chakra; direct inhalation
Aroma Life	Cypress, Marjoram, Helichrysum, Ylang Ylang (Carrier: Sesame Seed Oil)		Heart; Vita Flex heart points, under left ring finger, under left ring toe, above left elbow, neck; spine; direct inhalation
Aroma Siez	Basil, Marjoram, Lavender, Peppermint, Cypress	SI, CH	Muscles; neck; heart; Vita Flex points; full body massage; bath; direct inhalation
Australian Blue	Blue Cypress, Ylang Ylang Cedarwood, Blue Tansy, White Fir		Diffuse; chest, heart, forehead, neck, temples, wrists; direct inhalation
Awaken	Lemon, Mandarin, Bergamot, Ylang Ylang, Rose, Rosewood, Geranium, Palmarosa, Roman Chamomile, Jasmine, Hyssop, Frankincense, Sandalwood, Helichrysum, Juniper, Blue Tansy, Tangerine, Black Pepper, Anise, Neroli, Spruce, Lavender, Orange, Angelica, Sage Lavender (Carrier: Almond Oil)	PH	Diffuse; chest, heart, forehead, neck, temples, wrists; full body massage; bath
Believe	Idaho Balsam Fir, Rosewood, Frankincense		Diffuse; heart, forehead, neck, temples, wrists; bath; direct inhalation
Brain Power	Cedarwood, Sandalwood, Frankincense, Melissa, Australian Blue Cypress, Lavender, Helichrysum		Diffuse; neck, throat, nose; inside of cheeks, wrists; direct inhalation

251

Blend Name	Single Oil Contents	Safety Data	Uses/Application Areas
Chivalry	Spruce, Rosewood, Blue Tansy, Frankincense, Mandarin, Bergamot, Lemon, Ylang Ylang, Rose, Palmarosa, Roman Chamomile, Jasmine, Hyssop, Lavender, Orange, Sandalwood, Angelica, Sage Lavender, Idaho Balsam Fir, Myrrh, Galbanum	SI	Diffuse; crown; neck, wrists; direct inhalation
Christmas Spirit	Orange, Cinnamon Bark, Spruce	SI, CH	Diffuse; crown; neck, wrists; heart, temple; bath; direct inhalation
Citrus Fresh	Orange, Tangerine, Mandarin, Grapefruit, Lemon, Spearmint	SI, PH DS	Diffuse; ears, heart, wrists; neck, wrists; full body massage; bath; purify drinking water
Clarity	Basil, Cardamom, Rosemary cineol, Peppermint, Rosewood, Geranium, Lemon, Palmarosa, Ylang Ylang, Bergamot, Roman Chamomile, Jasmine	SI, P, PH+, CH, DS	Diffuse; forehead, neck, temples, wrists, neck; bath direct inhalation
Di-Tone	Tarragon, Ginger, Peppermint, Juniper, Anise, Fennel, Lemongrass, Patchouly	SI, P, E, CH+, DS	Vita Flex points, compress ankles; stomach; abdomen, bottom of throat; direct inhalation
Dragon Time	Clary Sage, Fennel, Lavender, Jasmine, Yarrow, Marjoram	P	Vita Flex points; diffuse; abdomen, lower back, location direct inhalation
Dream Catcher	Sandalwood, Bergamot, Ylang Ylang, Juniper, Blue Tansy, Tangerine, Black Pepper, Anise	PH	Diffuse; forehead, eye brows, temples, ears, throat chakra; neck, wrists; bath; direct inhalation
EndoFlex	Spearmint, Sage, Geranium, Myrtle, Nutmeg, German Chamomile (Carrier: Sesame Seed Oil)	SI, E, CH	Thyroid, kidneys, liver, pancreas, glands; Vita Flex points; direct inhalation
En-R-Gee	Rosemary cineol, Juniper, Nutmeg, Idaho Balsam Fir, Black Pepper, Lemongrass, Clove	SI, E	Diffuse; wrists, ears, neck, temples, feet; full body massage; direct inhalation
Envision	Spruce, Sage, Rose, Geranium, Orange, Lavender	HBP, E, P	Vita Flex points; diffuse; wrists, temples; bath; massage direct inhalation
Evergreen Essence	Colorado Blue Spruce, Ponderosa Pine, Pine, Red Fir Cedar, White Fir, Black Pine Piñon Pine, Lodge Pole Pine	SI	Diffuse; forehead, heart, temples, neck, thymus, direct inhalation

Blend Name	Single Oil Contents	Safety Data	Uses/Application Areas
Exodus II	Cinnamon Bark, Cassia, Calamus, Myrrh, Hyssop, Frankincense, Spikenard, Galbanum (Carrier: Olive Oil)	SI+, P+, CH+	Diffuse; Direct Inhale; Chest, ears, wrist, spine, (Raindrop style); VitaFlex direct inhalation
Forgiveness	Frankincense, Sandalwood, Lavender, Melissa, Angelica, Helichrysum, Rose, Rosewood, Geranium, Lemon, Palmarosa, Ylang Ylang, Bergamot, Roman Chamomile, Jasmine (Carrier: Sesame Seed Oil)		Diffuse; navel, heart, ears, wrists; direct inhalation
Gathering	Galbanum, Frankincense, Sandalwood, Lavender, Cinnamon Bark, Rose, Spruce, Geranium, Ylang Ylang		Diffuse; forehead, heart, temples, neck, thymus, face, chest; direct inhalation
Gentle Baby	Geranium, Rosewood, Palmarosa, Lavender, Roman Chamomile, Ylang Ylang, Rose, Lemon, Bergamot, Jasmine		Diffuse; ankles, lower back, abdomen, feet, face, neck; massage; bath; direct inhalation
Gratitude	Idaho Balsam Fir, Frankincense, Rosewood, Myrrh, Galbanum Ylang Ylang		Diffuse; ears; chest, heart, temples, neck, feet, wrists direct inhalation
Grounding	Juniper, Angelica, Ylang Ylang, Cedarwood, Pine, Spruce, White Fir	SI	Diffuse; brain stem, back of neck, sternum, temples; direct inhalation
Harmony	Hyssop, Spruce, Lavender, Frankincense, Geranium, Ylang Ylang, Orange, Sandalwood, Angelica, Sage Lavender, Rose, Rosewood, Lemon, Palmarosa, Bergamot, Roman Chamomile, Jasmine	P, E+, HBP, PH	Diffuse; Vita Flex points; ears, feet, heart; energy meridians, crown; direct inhalation
Highest Potential	Galbanum, Frankincense, Sandalwood, Lavender, Cinnamon Bark, Rose, Spruce, Geranium, Ylang Ylang, Blue Cypress, Cedarwood, Blue Tansy, White Fir, Jasmine		Diffuse; ears; chest, heart, temples, wrists, neck, feet; direct inhalation
Hope	Melissa, Myrrh, Juniper, Spruce (Carrier: Almond Oil)		Diffuse; ears; chest, heart, temples, solar plexus, neck, feet, wrists; direct inhalation
Humility	Geranium, Ylang Ylang, Frankincense, Spikenard, Myrrh, Rose, Rosewood, Melissa, Neroli (Carrier: Sesame Seed Oil)		Diffuse; heart, neck, temples; direct inhalation

Blend Name	Single Oil Contents	Safety Data	Uses/Application Areas
ImmuPower	Cistus, Frankincense, Hyssop, Ravensara, Mountain Savory, Oregano, Clove, Cumin, Idaho Tansy	SI, P, E, CH	Diffuse; throat, chest, spine, feet; thymus; neck, under arms direct inhalation
Inner Child	Orange, Tangerine, Jasmine, Ylang Ylang, Spruce, Sandalwood, Lemongrass, Neroli	PH, SI	Diffuse; navel, chest, temples nose; direct inhalation
Inspiration	Cedarwood, Spruce, Rosewood, Sandalwood, Frankincense, Myrtle, Mugwort		Diffuse; temples, crown, shoulders, back of neck direct inhalation
Into the Future	Frankincense, Jasmine, Clary Sage, Juniper, Idaho Tansy, White Fir, Orange, Cedarwood, Ylang Ylang, White Lotus (Carrier: Almond Oil)		Diffuse; bath; heart, wrists neck; compress; full body massage; direct inhalation
Joy	Lemon, Mandarin, Bergamot, Ylang Ylang, Rose, Rosewood, Geranium, Palmarosa, Roman Chamomile, Jasmine	PH, CH	Diffuse; heart, ears, neck, thymus, temples, forehead, wrists; bath; compress; massage; direct inhalation
Juva Cleanse	Helichrysum, Celery Seed, Ledum	CH+	Take 1 capsule size 0 1-2 times daily
JuvaFlex	Fennel, Geranium, Rosemary cineol, Roman Chamomile, Blue Tansy, Helichrysum (Carrier: Sesame Seed Oil)	SI	Vita Flex points; feet, spine, liver; full body massage direct inhalation
Legacy	(See LEGACY in Blend section of the *Essential Oils Desk Reference* for complete list of 91 single oils)	SI, CH	Diffuse; forehead, wrists, sternum, feet; neck; direct inhalation
Live with Passion	Melissa, Helichrysum, Clary Sage, Cedarwood, Angelica, Ginger, Neroli, Sandalwood, Patchouly, Jasmine		Diffuse; Wrists, temples, chest, forehead; neck, bath; direct inhalation
Longevity	Clove, Orange, Thyme, Frankincense	DS, CH+	Take 1 capsule size 00 1-2 x daily
M-Grain	Basil, Marjoram, Lavender, Peppermint, Roman Chamomile, Helichrysum	SI, CH	Diffuse; forehead, crown shoulders, neck, temples; Vita Flex points; massage direct inhalation
Magnify Your Purpose	Sandalwood, Nutmeg, Patchouly, Rosewood, Cinnamon Bark, Ginger, Sage	E, P, SI, CH	Vita Flex points; feet, wrists, temples; diffuse; bath; massage direct inhalation

Blend Name	Single Oil Contents	Safety Data	Uses/Application Areas
Melrose	Melaleuca (Alternifolia & Quinquenervia), Rosemary cineol, Clove	SI	Topically on location diffuse; forehead, liver; direct inhalation
Mister	Sage, Fennel, Lavender, Myrtle, Yarrow, Peppermint (Carrier: Sesame Seed Oil)	P+, E, CH	Vita Flex points; ankles, lower pelvis, prostate (dilute); compress; direct inhalation
Motivation	Roman Chamomile, Ylang Ylang, Spruce, Lavender		Diffuse; chest, neck; solar plexus, sternum, feet, navel, ears; wrists, palms; direct inhalation
PanAway	Wintergreen, Helichrysum, Clove, Peppermint	SI, CH	Apply on location of pain; Vitaflex feet; direct inhalation
Peace & Calming	Tangerine, Orange, Ylang Ylang, Patchouly, Blue Tansy	PH	Diffuse; navel, nose, neck, feet; bath; wrists; direct inhalation
Present Time	Neroli, Spruce, Ylang Ylang (Carrier: Almond Oil)		Thymus; neck, forehead direct inhalation
Purification	Citronella, Lemongrass, Rosemary cineol, Melaleuca, Lavandin, Myrtle	SI	Diffuse; Vita Flex points; ears, feet, temples; on location of injury; direct inhalation
Raven	Ravensara, Eucalyptus radiata, Peppermint, Wintergreen, Lemon	SI, CH	Diffuse; compress; Vita Flex points; lungs, throat; pillow; suppository; direct inhalation
R.C.	Eucalyptus (E. globulus, E. radiata, E. australiana, E. citriodora), Myrtle, Marjoram, Pine, Cypress, Lavender, Spruce, Peppermint	CH	Compress; diffuse; chest, back, feet; sinuses, nasal passages; ears, neck, throat; massage; direct inhalation
Release	Ylang Ylang, Lavandin, Geranium, Sandalwood, Blue Tansy (Carrier: Olive Oil)		Compress on liver; ears, feet, Vita Flex points; wrists
Relieve It	Spruce, Black Pepper, Hyssop, Peppermint	SI, P, E, HBP, CH	Apply on location of pain; direct inhalation; Raindrop Technique
Sacred Mountain	Spruce, Ylang Ylang, Cedarwood Idaho Balsam Fir	SI	Diffuse; solar plexus, brain stem, crown, neck ears, thymus, wrists; direct inhalation
SARA	Blue Tansy, Rose, Lavender, Geranium, Orange, Cedarwood, Ylang Ylang, White Lotus (Carrier: Almond Oil)		En-R-Gee centers; Vita Flex points; temples, nose; places of abuse; direct inhalation

Blend Name	Single Oil Contents	Safety Data	Uses/Application Areas
Sensation	Rosewood, Ylang Ylang, Jasmine		Diffuse; apply on location; massage; bath; direct inhalation
Surrender	Lavender, Roman Chamomile, German Chamomile, Angelica, Mountain Savory, Lemon, Spruce	SI, DS	Forehead, rim of ears, nape of neck, chest, solar plexus; bath direct inhalation
Thieves	Clove, Lemon, Cinnamon Bark, Eucalyptus radiata, Rosemary cineol	SI+, P, CH	Diffuse; feet, throat, stomach, intestines; thymus, under arms; direct inhalation
3 Wise Men	Sandalwood, Juniper, Frankincense, Spruce, Myrrh (Carrier: Almond Oil)		Diffuse; crown of head; neck, forehead, solar plexus, thymus direct inhalation
Trauma Life	Citrus Hystrix, Davana, Geranium, Spruce, Helichrysum, Rose, Sandalwood, Frankincense, Lavender, Valerian		Diffuse; spine; feet, chest, ears, neck, forehead direct inhalation
Valor	Spruce, Rosewood, Blue Tansy, Frankincense (Carrier: Almond Oil)		Feet; diffuse; heart, wrists, solar plexus, neck to thymus, spine; direct inhalation
White Angelica	Geranium, Spruce, Myrrh, Ylang Ylang, Hyssop, Bergamot, Melissa, Sandalwood, Rose, Rosewood (Carrier: Almond Oil)	PH	Diffuse; shoulders, crown, chest, ears, neck, forehead, wrists; bath; direct inhalation; compress

Index

Index
Abscesses/Boils:: 200
Absentmindedness: 69
Abuse: 60, 69
Acidosis: 70
Acne: 200
Acupressure: 22
Acupuncture: 22
Addictions: 70
Addison's Disease: 71
Adrenal Gland Imbalance: 71
Adulterated Oils: 13
AFNOR: 11
Agent Orange Exposure: 73
Age-Related Macular
   Degeneration (AMD): 72
Agitation: 60, 73
Aids: 73
Alcoholism: 74
Alkalosis: 74
Allergies: 16, 75
Alopecia Areata (Hair Loss): 75
ALS (Lou Gehrig's Disease): 176
Alzheimer's Disease: 87
Analgesic: 76
Anemia: 85
Aneurysm: 76
Anger: 60
Angina: 142
Anorexia: 77
Anthrax: 77
Antibiotic Reactions: 78
Antiseptic: 78
Anxiety: 60
Apathy: 60
Apnea: 78
Appetite, Loss Of: 79
Application Codes: 223
Argumentative: 60
Arteriosclerosis: 79
Arthritis: 79

Asthma: 81
Athlete's Foot: 131
Attention Deficit Disorder: 81
Auricular Technique: 55
Autism: 82
Backache: 208
Baldness: 83
Bath: 23
Bath Salt: 67
Bed Wetting: 83
Bee Stings: 150
Bell's Palsy: 173
Benign Prostate Hyperplasia
   (BPH): 190
Bible: 6
Black Widow Spider Bite: 150
Bleeding Gums: 182
Blisters: 83
Bloating: 84
Blocked Tear Ducts: 125
Blood Circulation (Poor): 85
Blood Clots: 84
Blood Detoxification: 85
Blood Disorders: 84
Blood Platelets (Low): 85
Blood Pressure, High: 102
Blood Pressure, Low: 102
Blurred Vision: 125
Body Massage: 67
Body Systems: 227
Boils: 83
Bone (Bruised, Broken): 86
Bone Cancer: 94
Bone Pain: 86
Bone-Related Pain: 185
Boredom: 60
Brain Disorders: 86
Brain Tumor: 94
Breast Cancer: 94
Breastfeeding: 89
Broken Bones: 86

Bronchitis: 160
Brown Recluse Spider Bite: 151
Bruising: 90
Bunions: 129
Burns: 90
Bursitis: 92
Calcification Of Spine: 208
Cancer: 92
Candida Albicans (Intestinal): 131
Canker Sores: 101
Capsule: 68
Carbon Monoxide Poisoning: 101
Cardiovascular Conditions: 101
Carpal Tunnel Syndrome: 173
Carpet: 27
Cataracts And Glaucoma: 125
Cellulite: 103
Cervical Cancer: 95
Chapped, Dry, Or Cracked Skin: 201
Chemical Sensitivities: 16, 104
Chicken Pox (Herpes Zoster): 105
Chiggers (Mites): 151
Children's Headache: 140
Cholecystitis: 106
Cholera: 106
Chronic Pain: 185
Circulation Disorders: 107
Cleaning: 26
Clogged Pores: 202
Cold Packs: 22
Colds: 109
Cold Sores (Herpes Simplex
   Type 1): 108
Colitis, Ulcerative: 110
Colitis, Viral: 111
Colon Cancer: 96
Coma: 111
Compress: 67
Concentration: 60
Confusion: 60, 111

257

Congestive Cough: 110
Congestive Heart Failure: 112
Connective Tissue Trauma: 112
Constipation: 113
Convulsions: 114
Cooking: 28
Corns: 130
Cough: 211
Cramps and Charley Horses: 169
Cramps (Stomach): 117
Creating A Compress: 22
Crohn's Disease: 114
Cushing's Disease: 72
Cyst (Ganglion): 115
Dandruff: 137
Day-Dreaming: 60
Dental Pain and Infection Control: 182
Dental Visits: 182
Deodorant: 116
Deodorizing: 28
Depression: 61, 116
Despair: 61
Despondency: 61
Detoxification of Liver and Gall Bladder: 158
Diabetes (Blood Sugar Imbalance): 116
Diaper Rash: 202
Diarrhea: 118
Different Schools Of Application: 3
Diffusing: 24, 68
Digestion Problems: 117
Dilute 20-80: 67
Dilute 50-50: 67
Diptheria: 119
Direct: 68
Disappointment: 61
Discouragement: 61
Dishwashing Soap: 26
Disinfecting: 26
Diuretic (To Increase Urine Flow): 155
Diverticulosis/Diverticulitis: 119
Dizziness: 120
Dry Cough: 212
Dry, Cracked Nipples: 89
Dry Nose: 180
Dysentery: 121
Early History: 5
Ear Mites: 121

Ear Problems: 121
Eczema / Dermatitis: 202
Edema (Swelling): 122
Emotional Ear Chart: 56
Emotional Response: 59
Emotional Trauma: 123
Endocrine System: 123
Endometriosis: 165
Epilepsy: 124
Epstein-Barr Virus: 124
Excessive Bleeding: 166
Excessive Sexual Desire: 196
Eye Disorders: 125
Fainting: 126
Fatigue: 126
Fear: 61
Fertility: 127
Fever: 127
Fibrillation: 143
Fibroids: 128
Fibromyalgia: 128
Filters: 26
First-Aid Spray: 219
First-Degree Burns (Sunburn): 91
Flatulence (Gas): 129
Floors: 27
Food Allergies: 75
Food Poisoning: 129
Foot Problems: 129
Forgetfulness: 61
Freckles: 203
Frigidity: 196
Frustration: 61
Fungal Infections: 130
Fungal Skin Infection: 203
Gallbladder Infection: 134
Gallstones: 134
Gangrene: 134
Gargle: 67
Gas, Flatulence: 118
Gastritis: 135
Genital Warts: 197
Gingivitis & Periodontitis: 135, 182
Glaucoma: 135
Gonorrhea And Syphilis: 197
Gout: 136
Grief/Sorrow: 61
Guilt: 62
Hair And Scalp Problems: 136
Hair Loss: 138
Halitosis (Bad Breath): 138

Hardening Of The Arteries: 101
Hay Fever (Allergic Rhinitis): 75
Headaches: 139
Head Cold / Sinus Congestion: 110
Head Lice: 139
Hearing Impairment: 141
Heart: 142
Heart Attack (Myocardial Infarction): 143
Heartburn: 118
Heart Vita Flex: 142
Heavy Metals: 144
Hematoma: 145
Hemorrhages: 145
Hemorrhagic Strokes: 89
Hemorrhoids: 145
Hepatitis: 158
Herniated Disk / Disk Deterioration: 208
Herpes Simplex Type Ii: 196
Hiccups: 146
High Cholesterol: 102
Hives: 146
Hodgkin's Disease: 96
Hormone Imbalance: 166
Hot Tubs: 27
Huntington's Chorea: 177
Hyperactivity: 146
Hyperpnoea: 146
Hyperthyroid (Graves Disease): 214
Hypoglycemia: 147
Hypothyroid (Hashimoto's Disease): 214
Hysterectomy: 166
Impaired Concentration: 87
Impaired Memory: 87
Impotence: 147
Improve Lactation: 89
Indigestion: 119
Infection (Bacterial And Viral): 148
Infertility: 148
Inflammation: 149
Inflammation Due to Injury: 169
Influenza: 149
Ingestion: 68
Inhalation: 25, 68
Insect Bites: 150
Insecticide: 27
Insect Repellent: 151

Insomnia: 152
Insomnia From Bowel Toxicity: 152
Insomnia From Depression: 152
Insomnia From Thyroid Imbalance: 153
Irregular Periods: 166
Irritability: 62
Irritable Bowel Syndrome: 153
ISO: 11
Itching: 203
Jaundice: 153
Jealousy: 62
Joint Stiffness And Pain: 154
Juvenile Dwarfism: 154
Kidney Disorders: 154
Kidney Inflammation/Infection (Nephritis): 155
Kidney Stones: 156
Knee Cartilage Injury: 113
Lack of Libido: 195
Laryngitis: 212
Laundry: 26
Layering: 22
Liver Cancer: 97
Liver Disorders: 158
Liver Spots (Senile Lentigenes): 160
Loss of Smell: 181
Lumbago (Lower Back Pain): 208
Lung Cancer: 97
Lung Infections: 160
Lupus: 162
Lyme Disease: 162
Lymphatic Pump: 53
Lymphatic System: 163
Lymphoma (Cancer of Lymph Nodes): 98
Malaria: 164
Male Hormone Imbalance: 164
Massage: 22
Mastitis (Infected Breast): 89
M.C.T.: 163
Measles: 165
Melanoma (Skin Cancer): 99
Menstrual Conditions: 165
Menstrual Cramps: 167
Mental Fatigue: 88, 126
Metal Toxicity (Aluminum): 168
Migraines (Vascular-Type Headache): 140
Moles: 204

Mononucleosis: 124
Mood Swings: 62
Morning Sickness: 172
Motion Sickness: 172
Mouth Ulcers: 183
Mucus (Excess): 168
Multiple Sclerosis (Ms): 178
Mumps (Infectious Parotitis): 168
Muscle-Related Pain: 186
Muscles: 169
Muscle Weakness: 171
Muscular Dystrophy: 171
Nails (Brittle Or Weak): 171
Narcolepsy: 172
Nasopharyngitis: 198
Nausea: 172
Neat: 67
Neck Pain And Stiffness: 209
Nerve Disorders: 173
Nervous Fatigue: 175
Nervous System: 34
Nervous System (Autonomic): 176
Neuralgia: 174
Neuritis: 174
Neurological Diseases: 176
Neuropathy: 175
Night Sweats: 180
Nose: 180
Nosebleeds: 180
Obesity: 181
Obsessiveness: 62
Oral: 67
Oral Care (Teeth And Gums): 182
Oral Use: 29
Osteoarthritis: 79
Osteoporosis (Bone Deterioration): 184
Ovarian And Uterine Cysts: 184
Ovarian Cancer: 99
Pain: 185
Painting: 26
Pancreatitis: 186
Panic: 62
Parasites, Intestinal: 187
Parkinson's Disease: 179
Perforated Eardrum: 122
Perspiration (Excessive): 188
Petrochemicals: 64
Phlebitis: 103
Phlebitis - Thrombosis: 188
Physical Ear Chart: 57
Physical Fatigue: 126

Pleurisy: 188
Pneumonia: 161
Pointer Technique: 209
Poison Ivy: 204
Poison Oak: 204
Polio: 189
Polyps (Nasal): 181
Pregnancy: 189
Premature Graying: 137
Premenstrual Syndrome (PMS): 167
Prostate Cancer: 100
Prostate Problems: 190
Prostatitis: 191
Psoriasis: 204
Pyorrhea: 191
Radiation Damage: 191
Raindrop Technique: 35
Rectal: 67
Rectal Retention: 26
Resentment: 62
Restless Leg Syndrome: 192
Restlessness: 62
Retention: 67
Rheumatic Fever: 192
Rheumatoid Arthritis: 80
Rhinitis: 198
Rice Milk: 68
Ringworm And Skin Candida: 132
Rocky Mountain Spotted Fever: 162
Safe Use: 19
Sagging Skin: 204
Saunas: 27
Scabies: 192
Scar Tissue: 193
Schizophrenia: 193
Sciatica: 36, 210
Science and Application: 10
Scleroderma: 193
Scoliosis: 36, 194
Scurvy: 195
Second-Degree Burns (Blisters): 91
Seizures: 195
Sexual Dysfunction: 195
Sexually Transmitted Diseases: 196
Shingles: 105
Shock: 62, 197
Shower: 26
Sinus Congestion: 199
Sinus Headache: 141
Sinus Infections: 198

259

Sinusitis: 199
Skin Disorders: 200
Skin Ulcers: 205
Sleep Disorders: 206
Smoking Cessation: 206
Snake Bites: 206
Sore Feet: 130
Sore Muscles: 170
Sore Throat: 212
Spasms:: 113
Spina Bifida: 207
Spine Injuries and Pain: 207
Sprain: 210
Sprain/Torn Ligament: 113
Stimulate Pineal/Pituitary Gland: 88
Strep Throat: 212
Stress: 211
Stretch Marks: 205
Stroke: 88
Surface Cleansers: 26
Syrup: 68
Tachycardia: 143
Tampon: 67

Teeth Grinding: 183
Tension Headache: 141
Therapeutic-Grade: 9
Third-Degree Burns: 91
Throat Infections: 211
Thrombotic Strokes: 89
Thrush: 132
Thyroid Problems: 214
Tight, Spasmed or Torn Muscles: 170
Tinnitus (Ringing in the Ears): 142
To Improve Circulation: 107
Tongue: 67
Tonic-Stimulant: 144
Tonsillitis: 213
Toothache And Teething Pain: 183
Topical: 21, 67
To Stimulate Parasympathetic Nervous System: 176
To Stimulate Sympathetic Nervous System: 176
Toxemia: 215
Toxic Chemical Absorption: 105

Trauma (Emotional): 215
Trauma-Related Pain: 186
Tuberculosis: 215
Typhoid Fever: 217
Ulcers, Stomach: 119
Ureter Infection: 157
Urinary Tract/Bladder Infection: 217
Uterine Cancer: 100
Vaginal Retention: 26
Vaginal Yeast Infection: 133, 218
Vapor: 68
Varicose Veins (Spider Veins): 108, 218
Vascular Cleansing: 144
Vita Flex: 31, 67
Vita Flex Points: 32
Vitiligo: 205
Warm Packs: 22
Water Distillers: 26
Whooping Cough: 161
Wounds, Scrapes, or Cuts: 218
Wrinkled or Rough Skin: 205

Notes

Notes